Target Discovery and Validation

Methods and Principles in Medicinal Chemistry

Edited by R. Mannhold, H. Buschmann, J. Holenz

Previous Volumes of the Series

Swinney, D., Pollastri, M.

Neglected Tropical Diseases

Drug Discovery and Development

2019
ISBN: 978-3-527-34304-1
Vol.: 77

Bachhav, Y. (Ed.)

Innovative Dosage Forms

Design and Development at Early Stage

2019
ISBN: 978-3-527-34396-6
Vol.: 76

Gervasio, F. L., Spiwok, V. (Eds.)

Biomolecular Simulations in Structure-based Drug Discovery

2018
ISBN: 978-3-527-34265-5
Vol. 75

Sippl, W., Jung, M. (Eds.)

Epigenetic Drug Discovery

2018
ISBN: 978-3-527-34314-0
Vol. 74

Giordanetto, F. (Ed.)

Early Drug Development

2018
ISBN: 978-3-527-34149-8
Vol. 73

Handler, N., Buschmann, H. (Eds.)

Drug Selectivity

2017
ISBN: 978-3-527-33538-1
Vol. 72

Vaughan, T., Osbourn, J., Jalla, B. (Eds.)

Protein Therapeutics

2017
ISBN: 978-3-527-34086-6
Vol. 71

Ecker, G. F., Clausen, R. P., and Sitte, H. H. (Eds.)

Transporters as Drug Targets

2017
ISBN: 978-3-527-33384-4
Vol. 70

Martic-Kehl, M. I., Schubiger, P.A. (Eds.)

Animal Models for Human Cancer

Discovery and Development of Novel Therapeutics

2017
ISBN: 978-3-527-33997-6
Vol. 69

Holenz, Jörg (Ed.)

Lead Generation

Methods and Strategies

2016
ISBN: 978-3-527-33329-5

Target Discovery and Validation

Methods and Strategies for Drug Discovery

Edited by
Alleyn T. Plowright

WILEY-VCH

Series Editors

Prof. Dr. Raimund Mannhold
Rosenweg 7
40489 Düsseldorf
Germany

Dr. Helmut Buschmann
Aachen, Germany
Sperberweg 15
52076 Aachen
Germany

Dr. Jörg Holenz
GSK
R&D Neurosciences TAU
1250 S. Collegeville Road, PA
United States

Volume Editor

Alleyn T. Plowright
Sanofi-Aventis Deutschland GmbH
Integrated Drug Discovery Germany
Geb. H823
Industriepark Höchst
65926 Frankfurt am Main
Germany

Cover: iStock by Getty Images 497111243 / Thomas Vogel (jigsaw background) and Gunther Schulz (green arrow)

Library of Congress Card No.:
applied for

British Library Cataloguing-in-Publication Data
A catalogue record for this book is available from the British Library.

Bibliographic information published by the Deutsche Nationalbibliothek
The Deutsche Nationalbibliothek lists this publication in the Deutsche Nationalbibliografie; detailed bibliographic data are available on the Internet at <http://dnb.d-nb.de>.

Print ISBN: 978-3-527-34529-8
ePDF ISBN: 978-3-527-81825-9
ePub ISBN: 978-3-527-81826-6
oBook ISBN: 978-3-527-81824-2

Cover Design SCHULZ Grafik-Design, Fußgönheim, Germany
Typesetting SPi Global, Chennai, India
Printing and Binding Markono Print Media Pte Ltd, Singapore
Printed on acid-free paper

10 9 8 7 6 5 4 3 2 1

Contents

Preface

Target discovery and validation is perhaps the most critical discipline in the entire pharmaceutical research and development value chain. Where you start from is critically determining the success or failure of projects and selecting the "wrong" target, one that does not modify a disease in the desired way typically equates to late stage, expensive failures in clinical phase II (proof-of-concept) studies and beyond!

Although – over the recent decades – there has been significant progress in reducing the so-called "technical risks" associated with pharmaceutical projects through, e.g., improved understanding, prediction and measurement of drug-related DMPK (drug metabolism and pharmacokinetics), physicochemical properties, drug-likeness, toxicity or target engagement, and elicitation of downstream pharmacology (via biomarkers type 1 and 2), with many diseases we still lack a detailed understanding about the prospect of modulating a target or pathway to positively affect or even cure a disease in humans. A good example comes from recent failures in the Alzheimer's disease field, where modulating the "amyloid" cascade was long thought to be the holy grail in finding a medicine for this devastating disease, based on a thorough genetic understanding and validation of the relevance of this target. Although a plethora of clinical candidates (small molecules, antibodies, and vaccines) have been tested in recent years, each one of them has missed the primary end points in late-stage clinical trials and did not result in slower disease progression. How can we avoid late-stage clinical failures, improve Research and Development productivity, and speed up the delivery of truly innovative medicines and cures for patients in need? A lot of answers to these questions need to be asked while selecting the right target and pathway to work on while a new project is started.

As a consequence of the described failures, the field of target discovery and validation has undergone significant paradigm changes in the recent years, a few of them are listed here:

- **The importance of genetic validation of a target/pathway to increase its disease relevance**
  With the advent of measuring human DNA sequences fast, reliably and cost efficiently, and genotyping (the investigation of differences in the sequences)

broader patient populations and comparing them to healthy populations has been one of the key pillars for the identification of "genetically validated" targets in the hope to increase the odds for clinical success both by improving the degree of target validation and by better stratifying patients likely benefitting from a targeted therapy against this target/pathway. As one of the first genetically validated targets, mutations of the sodium channel subtype NaV1.7 have been found to provoke congenital insensitivity to pain in humans.

- **Disease understanding: from the "soup approach" to a detailed understanding of disease pathology**
  While only a few years ago drug discovery in many diseases relied heavily on general assumptions such as "increase or block protein A throughout the entire human system to improve a disease," today we increasingly believe that a successful therapy must be highly specific in tackling a specific target only at a certain compartment of the human body or even down to selectivity at the cellular level. Personalized medicines for a highly stratified patient population (often rare diseases) or even for an individual patient have delivered innovative medicines, while demonstrating high speed to market. A detailed understanding of the disease pathology and associated targets along with a deep understanding in which compartments and cells the drug needs to interfere is today believed to be a key for success.
- **The renaissance of phenotypic screening and advances in automation**
  With the desire to identify targets and pathways truly relevant in "authentic" disease conditions and prompted by late-stage clinical failures because of insufficient efficacy (as described above), one approach taken to frontload that risk was to employ phenotypic screens in highly relevant systems such as whole cells (native or induced pluripotent stem cells), as well as two- or three-dimensional organoids. A whole discipline coined chemical biology has been created around this concept, and a key step is to deconvolute the targets once a change in phenotype in the desired manner (e.g. decrease of survival in cancer cell lines) has been observed. Advances in automation as well as the advent of optogenetics have enabled a higher throughput screening capacity of those "high-content" assays, making them useful tools for target identification.
- **Target discovery and validation has become a truly multidisciplinary field strongly driven by medicinal chemists**
  Although target identification and validation has been traditionally a discipline dominated by biologists and pharmacologists, it is today truly a multidisciplinary team work, with the medicinal chemists being one of the key drivers in the team for identifying and validating novel targets that will work in clinical trials.

Alleyn Plowright and his team take on this important discipline both from the view of a medicinal chemist and from the view of the adjacent, critical disciplines. It is in our view a unique opportunity to learn from true experts in the field on not only the concepts and strategies but also to learn from the practical examples and case studies presented. The book is logically split into chemical-based approaches, biology-based approaches, and informatics-based approaches and provides deep, concise, and up-to-date answers to all questions the reader might have.

The editors would like to cordially thank Alleyn and the entire team of authors, as well as Frank Weinreich and the Wiley team for getting this project so quickly from concept to production, as we are hopeful that it will fill a large gap and be widely appreciated.

June 2019

Joerg Holenz, Boston
Helmut Buschmann, Aachen
Raimund Mannhold, Duesseldorf

A Personal Foreword

Diseases impacting human health are prevalent, and ones affected by lifestyle or age are on the rise throughout the world. Despite many drugs and treatments being available to patients, there is still massive unmet need, and those affected are waiting for new treatment options to improve their and their families' lives. As researchers pushing the boundaries of science, developing novel technologies, discovering the unknown, and creating new treatment options enables us to have a hugely positive impact on society and the lives of people.

Unfortunately discovering new medicines is fraught with difficulties and too infrequently successful. High rates of attrition in clinical trials and the associated high cost of developing a new medicine is a huge problem for drug discovery. Only 10% of molecules nominated as drug candidates that undergo initial phase I clinical trials are successful in transitioning through further phases of clinical development to complete regulatory approval and treat patients who are in need [1]. This unsatisfactory figure does not even include the projects that do not reach the drug candidate stage. If we could improve the drug discovery process and success rates, there is potential to have a massive impact on the lives of patients and society as a whole.

The major challenges and reasons for failure of clinical trials have been well documented with the most frequent reason being lack of efficacy or lack of differentiation of the development candidate over the current standard of care for the disease being treated [2, 3]. This is often due to inadequate target validation in the preclinical phases of drug discovery. On top of this, major bottlenecks we face are how to discover new biological targets and pathways relevant to human disease and the overall lack of validated targets in emerging areas of biology. However, science and technology are evolving at such a rapid pace that they are providing a wealth of opportunities for scientists across all fields of research and clinical medicine to contribute to the discovery of novel targets relevant to human disease. In addition, they are providing the necessary tools to more effectively validate these targets as well as understand the mechanisms of action of molecules in the early phases of drug discovery. Taking advantage of these tools will ensure that we focus our efforts and resources on those targets and mechanisms of action with the greatest probability of success to deliver drugs to the people who need them the most, the patients.

Drug discovery is truly a multidisciplinary endeavour. Scientists from different backgrounds and areas of science, informatics, and engineering need to come together, collaborate, and be curious how to utilize each other's diverse knowledge and capabilities to find the best solutions. Medicinal chemists have a key role to play in this along with chemical biologists, data scientists, chemo- and bioinformaticians, biologists, clinicians, and other disciplines. We need to continue to come together, join forces, and drive new ideas and innovation to translate novel science and discoveries into new medicines. Pharmaceutical companies, biotech companies, academia, and technology companies need to continue to forge collaborations and work together on solving critical questions to help us all drive forward. Good ideas can come from anywhere in the world, and working together will accelerate the discovery of novel validated targets that can be prosecuted with the armoury of therapeutic modalities we now have at our disposal. With the discovery of new modalities such as proteolysis targeting chimeras (PROTACs), clustered regularly interspaced short palindromic repeats (CRISPR)/Cas9 and diverse small to large molecule conjugates as well as new screening technologies to expand chemical space such as DNA-encoded libraries or cryo-electron microscopy (cryo-EM) and X-ray crystallography of membrane-bound proteins to understand the proteins and complexes we are aiming to modulate will enhance our ability to tackle challenging targets and understand mechanisms of action. All in all this provides many opportunities and makes it such an exciting time to work in the drug discovery arena.

This book is written by experts from academia and industry to highlight a range of techniques and approaches that are continuing to develop and provide utility and impact to help us all discover and validate novel biological targets. The aim of the book is not to be an exhaustive resource but rather to highlight diverse approaches and show the impact of new technologies on the discovery of new biological targets and in target validation studies and how these methods can support academic and drug discovery scientists in their target discovery and validation research. The book will describe both well-used and novel technologies and showcase recent examples where the methods have been applied. The chapters will be separated into chemistry-based approaches, biology-based approaches, and informatics-based approaches to highlight the range of techniques available and how multidisciplinary these studies are. Each of the approaches shown is complementary and has the ability to significantly impact target discovery and target validation, and a combination of approaches will most often be required to speed up and make this research more effective.

I would like to thank all of the authors for taking their time to share their knowledge and help us all increase our understanding of these important approaches and sharing tips on how we can apply them most effectively to increase our success with target discovery and validation.

Drug discovery is a challenging, innovation-driven, and large endeavour, and increasing our effectiveness in discovering and validating biological targets for human disease can increase our chances of success in delivering new medicines to patients to cure disease.

References

1 Hay, M., Thomas, D.W., Craighead, J.L. et al. (2014). Clinical development success rates for investigational drugs. *Nat. Biotechnol.* 32: 40–51.
2 Arrowsmith, J. (2011). Trial watch: phase III and submission failures: 2007–2010. *Nat. Rev. Drug Discovery* 10: 87.
3 Cook, D., Brown, D., Alexander, R. et al. (2014). Lessons learned from the fate of AstraZeneca's drug pipeline: a five-dimensional framework. *Nat. Rev. Drug Discovery* 13: 419–431.

Integrated Drug Discovery,
Sanofi-Aventis Deutschland GmbH,
Industriepark Höchst,
D-65926 Frankfurt am Main,
Germany

Alleyn T. Plowright

1

Chemical Strategies for Evaluating New Drug Targets

Adrian J. Carter[1], Raina Seupel[2], Paul E. Brennan[2], Michael Sundström[3], Andrea Introini[3], and Anke Mueller-Fahrnow[4]

[1] *Boehringer Ingelheim, Discovery Research Coordination, Binger Strasse 173, 55216 Ingelheim, Germany*
[2] *University of Oxford, Structural Genomics Consortium and Target Discovery Institute, Nuffield Department of Medicine, NDMRB, Roosevelt Drive, Oxford, OX3 7FZ, UK*
[3] *Karolinska Institutet, Structural Genomics Consortium, Karolinska Vägen 6, 17176, Sweden*
[4] *Bayer AG, Target Discovery, Muellerstrasse 178, 13342 Berlin, Germany*

1.1 Introduction

Discovering new drugs is difficult and expensive. Pharmaceutical companies typically spend at least $2.6 billion on average in research and development (R&D) for each drug before it reaches the market [1]. Interestingly, the high cost of R&D is not driven by the few programmes that succeed, but rather by the cost of pipeline projects that fail [2]. Only about 1 in 10 of drug candidates in phase I clinical trials actually makes it to become a new medicine [3, 4], and about half of the projects that fail in phase II clinical trials do so because of clinical efficacy [5, 6]. So why do so many drugs fail?

One answer is a lack of genetic evidence. An analysis of AstraZeneca's small molecule pipeline indicated that the success rate was over 70% for projects in phase II clinical trials with human genetic linkage of the target to the disease indication compared with 43% for projects without such a linkage [6]. Furthermore, another similar study concluded that selecting genetically supported targets can double the success rate in clinical development [7]. These observations have prompted some scientists to highlight the critical importance of the therapeutic hypothesis at the stage when a protein or gene is selected as a potential drug target [8]. However, it is often a long and difficult road between identifying a genetic link and understanding the underlying biological processes (see Chapter 6 for more details).

A major problem we are facing is that a large proportion of biomedical R&D focuses on only a small fraction of the genome despite the promised revolution in medicine following sequencing of the entire human genome [9]. Shortly after its announcement, scientists imagined that genome science would soon begin revealing the mysteries of hereditary factors in heart disease, cancer, diabetes, schizophrenia, and a host of other conditions and lead to new medicines [10]. Unfortunately, this has not happened. Indeed, more than 75% of protein research

Target Discovery and Validation: Methods and Strategies for Drug Discovery,
First Edition. Edited by Alleyn T. Plowright.

still focuses on the 10% of proteins that were known before the genome was mapped, even though many more have been genetically linked to disease [11]. A more recent analysis of drug targets highlights the continued dominance of a set of privileged target families across different disease areas, although there has also been a small growth of novel first-in-class mechanisms, particularly in oncology [12]. What can we do to help biomedical scientists worldwide to expand and prioritize the list of potential new drug targets?

One answer lies with high-quality chemical probes. We know that chemical tools can dramatically facilitate exploratory biomedical research. Let us take, for example, nuclear hormone receptors. When nuclear receptors were identified by sequence homology in the 1990s, all the family members were thought to have therapeutic potential. Scientists initially investigated those receptors that were found to have genetic links to disease or that had interesting knockout phenotypes. However, as time went on, research activity focused on a subset of eight of these receptors despite the fact that these eight were no more genetically interesting than the others. Indeed Edwards [11] postulated that the only connection among these eight receptors is that for each there exists a widely available, high-quality chemical probe that either enhances the receptor's activity or dampens it. In short, where high-quality tools are available, there is research activity; where there are no tools, there is none. What is a high-quality chemical probe and why are they so useful?

The Structural Genomics Consortium (SGC) (www.thesgc.org) is a large precompetitive public–private partnership between academia, private funders, and currently nine public pharmaceutical companies as well as patient advocacy and research organizations. The consortium has established a common set of principles for chemical probes, initially focused on epigenetic targets. A chemical probe is simply a small molecule that modulates the function of a protein in a specific and selective way. This allows a scientist to interrogate the biology and test hypotheses relating to the mechanism or role of the particular protein in a relevant cellular context [13]. The difference between specificity and selectivity is important to consider. Specificity is the capacity of a chemical probe to manifest only one kind of action. A chemical probe of perfect specificity of action might increase, or decrease, a specific function of a given cell type, but it would not do both, nor would it affect other receptors. In contrast, selectivity is the ability of a chemical probe to affect one cell population in preference to others, i.e. the ability of a chemical probe to affect one kind of cell, and produce effects, in doses lower than those required to affect other cells. This should not be confused with potency, i.e. the measure of the activity of a chemical probe, in terms of the concentration or amount required for producing a defined effect. Consequently, selectivity is actually a measure of the relative potency of a chemical probe in producing different effects.

The SGC has established a set of stringent criteria that a chemical tool compound must fulfil in order for its classification as a chemical probe (Figure 1.1). The compound must exhibit *in vitro* potency of less than 100 nmol/l for a single target or a small set (<5) of very similar targets and possess a minimum 30-fold selectivity relative to other sequence-related proteins of the same family. Furthermore, the probe must be profiled against a standard selection of other unrelated pharmacologically relevant targets and large protein families of relevance to drug discovery (specificity) and, finally, have demonstrated on-target effects in cells at less than 1 μmol/l (cellular activity) [13]. These criteria were developed jointly by academia and industry to help guide scientists to choose the best chemical probe for their needs because, unfortunately, there are numerous examples of less well-characterized tools that may generate misleading results. Although the chemical probe criteria could be stricter (e.g. 10 nmol/l potency, selectivity for a single target >100-fold, cellular activity <100 nmol/l), the chemical probe criteria outlined here are a pragmatic compromise between the cost of creating such a chemical probe and the potential value it brings to science.

Seven pharmaceutical companies have since worked together in a precompetitive collaboration to make available a large number of innovative, high-quality chemical probes from previous terminated pharmaceutical projects [14]. These probes have all been subject to a rigorous and independent scientific review by the SGC, are accompanied by comprehensive data packages, and include an appropriate structurally related yet inactive control compound. All of this is made available to the wide scientific community free of intellectual property restrictions via the portal https://opensciencprobes.sgc-frankfurt.de.

Regrettably, making a high-quality chemical probe entails a lot of effort especially for medicinal chemists. Indeed, the sort of efforts that are required to make such a tool are those that are only usually available for a full-fledged drug discovery project. How do we justify that level of investment if we do not know how important the target protein is *a priori*? Some scientists have likened it to a catch-22 situation. A scientist cannot justify the resources required for generating a chemical probe without knowing the importance of the target protein. On the other hand, the scientist cannot judge the importance of a protein without being able to interrogate its function with a chemical probe. But help is at hand. One way around this is to build chemogenomic sets of compounds for specific protein families known as chemogenomic libraries [15].

Chemogenomics was coined as a term to describe the use of target family-directed chemical libraries in target or cell-based assays as a means of accessing new areas of biology and accelerating drug discovery research based on the assumption that similar receptors bind similar ligands [16–18]. Such sets, although containing compounds that individually do not fulfil the stringent criteria of a chemical probe, nevertheless, can be used to interrogate multiple members of protein families to help prioritize the most therapeutically relevant ones that could then form the basis of a chemical probe project (Figure 1.1). A chemogenomic approach involves a systematic screening of a set of small molecules (chemogenomic library) with well-annotated pharmacology against target families of functionally related proteins such as G-protein-coupled receptors (GPCRs), kinases, and ion channels. Usually target families that are homologous at the protein level have similar properties. Consequently, compounds synthesized for the purpose of one family member will, with a high probability, be active against other members of the same family. This strategy allows an economical use of chemical and biological knowledge for more efficient drug discovery. A recent example is the public chemogenomic set, known as the comprehensive kinase chemogenomic set (KCGS) (Published Kinase

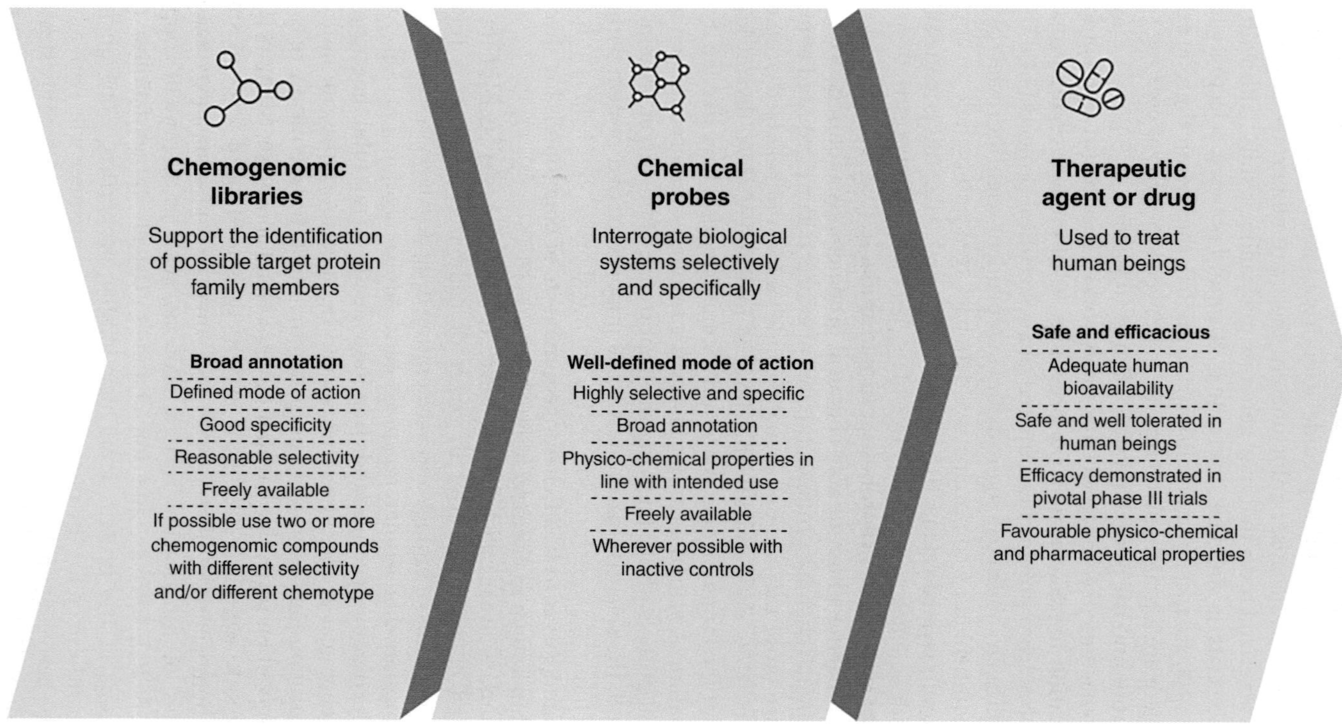

Figure 1.1 Chemogenomic tools support the identification of potential target proteins, and chemical probes help interrogate biological systems selectively and specifically with the goal of ultimately developing safe and efficacious medicines.

Inhibitor Set [PKIS]), that is being developed for the entire family of human protein kinases [19]. This is a large collaborative endeavour that will be made available as a public resource of both data and physical compound samples to support basic research to all scientists that agree to be trustees of the set. We believe that researchers will be able to use publicly available chemogenomic libraries and chemical probes to interrogate exciting areas of biology that genetic studies have helped to identify. We use the terms target evaluation and target prioritization as part of the target validation process. However, we appreciate that we can only truly validate a drug target after the clinical effects have been demonstrated in pivotal human phase III clinical trials. This chapter will outline the chemical strategies used to evaluate and prioritize such protein targets and provide examples that illustrate the successful application of these strategies.

1.2 Use Cases and Case Studies for Chemogenomic Compounds and Chemical Probes

The inappropriate use of chemical tools can have serious deleterious consequences for the interpretation of experimental results for several different reasons. Here are some examples:

- Insufficient selectivity might lead to the conclusion that a target is relevant for an observed effect, which, in reality, is caused by an uncharacterized off-target effect.
- Low permeability might lead to the conclusion that a compound does not modulate the activity of its target in a cellular setting when, in fact, it does not even reach the target.
- General cytotoxicity caused by an inappropriate tool compound might be confused with a specific effect on a cancer target.
- Limited solubility might lead to the conclusion that a compound is inactive because it has precipitated.

These reasons illustrate the importance of defining high-quality and well-characterized tool compounds. Limited reproducibility of published work [20, 21] might, in part, be caused by the use of compounds that are not suitable for the experiments in which they have been used. Other authors have published requirements for high-quality compounds that should be applied when carrying out biological experiments as described above [13, 14, 22–24].

Table 1.1 provides an overview of the data necessary to assess the suitability of tool compounds for different experiments. For work with a purified recombinant protein, e.g. for developing biochemical or biophysical assays, only a limited number of parameters need to be assessed. For all work in a cellular context or *in vivo,* we recommend a significantly more comprehensive dataset.

1.2.1 Chemogenomic Libraries

There are a number of available chemogenomic libraries available either commercially from chemical suppliers or via collaboration (Table 1.2). While

Table 1.1 Relevance of data for the use of chemical tools.

Data needed to assess suitability for intended use	Assay development (biochemical)	Assay development (cellular)	Target validation *in vitro*[a]	Target validation *in vivo*[a]	Drug	SGC criteria (epigenetic probes)
Biochemical potency	Yes	Yes	Yes	Yes	Yes	<100 nmol/l
Cellular potency		Yes	Yes	Yes	Yes	<1 μmol/l
Solubility	Yes	Yes	Yes	Yes	Yes	Yes
Selectivity	Yes	Yes	Yes	Yes	Yes	>30-fold within family
No Pan-assay interference compounds (PAINS)	Yes	Yes	Yes	Yes	Yes	Yes
Cellular permissibility		Yes	Yes	Yes	Yes	Yes
Metabolic stability		Yes	Yes	Yes	Yes	Yes
No general cytotoxicity		Yes	Yes	Yes	Yes	Yes
Adequate pharmacokinetic properties for *in vivo* studies				Yes	Yes	
Inactive control	Yes	Yes	Yes	Yes		Yes

Data needed for the corresponding applications are marked by 'yes'. No values are provided when the requirements will vary considerably between different targets/target families.
a) For intracellular targets.

most chemogenomic libraries contain compounds that are not potent enough or characterized sufficiently to be true chemical probes based on the definition above, they are still valuable in that they often have a broader coverage of target space (Table 1.2, Broad Libraries). Libraries that are composed of high-quality chemical probes cover far fewer targets and have fewer compounds due to the high cost associated with discovering and characterizing chemical probes (Table 1.2, Chemical Probe Libraries) because of the inherent capacity constraints of generating such high-quality probes.

1.2.2 Inactive Control

In addition to interaction with the intended target, chemicals can also cause uncharacterized off-target or cytotoxic effects. To exclude misinterpretation of the observed results and to confirm that the activity is indeed caused by the biochemical inhibition of the annotated, intended target, we strongly recommend using an inactive control compound. An inactive control compound is defined as a compound that is chemically similar to the chemogenomic compound, but is inactive at the annotated target. Inactivity is often rationally designed using

Table 1.2 Examples of libraries of chemogenomic tools and chemical probes.

Library	Number of compounds	Comments	Availability
Broad Libraries			
NCATS Pharmacologically Active Chemical Toolbox (NPACT)	>11 000	Collection from NCATS containing naturally occurring, nature-inspired, or synthetically created high-quality organism-agnostic and pharmacologically active compounds; diversity of physicochemical and pharmacological properties by a few best-in-class compounds with non-redundant chemotypes identified from the literature and worldwide patents https://ncats.nih.gov/preclinical/core/compound/npact	Available in collaboration with NCATS
NCATS Pharmaceutical Collection (NPC)	3 500	Collection from NCATS containing small molecular entities approved for clinical use by US, European Union, Japanese, and Canadian authorities; access to the collection through the Therapeutics for Rare and Neglected Diseases programme and the Toxicology in the 21st Century initiative https://ncats.nih.gov/expertise/preclinical/npc	Commercial and Collaborative
Sigma Library of Pharmacologically Active Compounds ($LOPAC^{1280}$)	1 280	Commercially available collection containing approved drugs and pharmaceutical compounds annotated with biological activities dominated by GPCR targets; in literature most widely used chemogenomic library https://www.sigmaaldrich.com/catalog/product/sigma/lo3300?lang=de&region=DE	Commercial
Prestwick Chemical Library	1 280	A collection of 1280 off-patent drugs with high chemical and pharmacological diversity, as well as known bioavailability and safety in humans http://www.prestwickchemical.com/libraries-screening-lib-pcl.html	Commercial
Published Kinase Inhibitor Set (PKIS) (GlaxoSmithKline)	367	Collection containing adenosine triphosphate (ATP)-competitive kinase inhibitors published by GSK for screening by external users; set represents >20 different chemotypes covering a total of 58 kinases https://www.ebi.ac.uk/chembl/	Collaborative and commercial

(*continued*)

Table 1.2 (Continued)

Library	Number of compounds	Comments	Availability
Published Kinase Inhibitor Set (PKIS2)	654	Collection containing small molecule inhibitors published by academia and industry collaborators; set represents 86 diverse chemotypes [19]	Collaborative
Chemical Probe Libraries			
SGC Chemical Probe Library	44	Probes developed by SGC with academic and industry collaborators; compounds are available from the website until they are commercially available; then order by suppliers (Sigma, Tocris, and Cayman) https://www.thesgc.org/chemical-probes	Commercially available
Chemical Probes Portal	189	Web-based resource with accessible recommendations about chemical probes based on expert input from its Scientific Advisory Board, supporting data and guidance are available [13] www.chemicalprobes.org	Information repository about high-quality probes
opnMe Portal	25	Chemical probes designed by Boehringer Ingelheim; access to the molecules to order (M2O), only for some exceptions for collaborative researcher (molecules for collaboration [M4C]); associated data and negative control compounds are available https://opnme.com	M2O are freely available, M4C collaborative
SGC Donated Probes	54	Chemical probes developed by pharmaceutical companies (Takeda, Merck, Bayer, Boehringer Ingelheim, AbbVie, Pfizer, Janssen); all probes and negative controls are available from the website by the SGC; *in vitro* and *in vivo* data with recommendations on their use [14] www.sgc-ffm.uni-frankfurt.de	Commercially available

knowledge of the target's preferred pharmacophore and inactive compounds are often taken from stereo- or regio-isomers to maximize chemical similarity.

1.2.3 Use of Biological Target Panels and Profiling

The value of a tool compound depends on different factors:

- Fit to the agreed criteria in line with its intended use as described above.
- Accessibility (cost, time, and effort needed to obtain compound).

- Versatility of use (e.g. physicochemical properties enabling use over a broad concentration range, over a long period of time).
- Extent of annotation.

To phrase it differently, the value of every chemical probe or chemogenomic compound can be increased significantly by in-depth profiling with large assay panels as this will increase the confidence that the effects observed with compound treatment are specific and reproducible.

We recognize that selectivity needs to be closely monitored for large target families with conserved binding sites such as GPCRs or kinases. The most pragmatic way to assess the selectivity profile of a tool compound is to measure the effect on target family members with the highest sequence identity, the highest predicted similarity of the binding pocket (e.g. for kinases assessed via Kinase SARfari [www.ebi.ac.uk/chembl/sarfari/kinasesarfari]) and the expected relevance of the biological effect.

Innovative technologies such as Kinobeads are very useful to explore selectivity in a cellular setting (for details see Chapter 4). In addition, service providers such as Eurofins (www.eurofins.com) have established large assay panels for several relevant target families, e.g. roughly 500 different biochemical and cell-based kinase assays to cover the majority of all kinases. Efforts like the kinase chemogenomic library and other broad profiling [25] are of high value as they provide the scientific community not only with a unique library of kinase inhibitors but also with the associated data from the profiling in the Eurofins panel. Many published kinase inhibitors still lack selectivity data, and we would like to stress that such compounds should not really be used as tools for target evaluation.

Off-target effects are, however, not restricted to targets from the same target family. Previous work has recently shown that several inhibitors developed to target specific kinases also potently inhibit diverse bromodomains (BRD) [26]. When testing 628 kinase inhibitors on BRD-containing protein 4 (BRD4), 9 compounds were identified with a strong effect on BRD4. Examples include BI-2536, a clinical-phase polo-like kinase 1 (PLK1) inhibitor, and TG-101348, a clinical-phase Janus kinase 2 – Fms related tyrosine kinase 3 (JAK2-FLT3) inhibitor, which both have nanomolar activity on BRD4. This was unexpected as the primary sequences of BRD4 and the kinases are not related. While activity on more than one target might even be beneficial for a drug, it is clearly not desirable for a tool compound used for evaluating new targets. Here we want to understand if the effect induced by a tool compound is caused via the target it has been optimized and characterized for or by an unknown off-target effect. Experience shows that many drugs still exhibit effects on different target proteins. It is not at all unusual to identify hits in a high-throughput screen that originate from another project, either from the same target family or from unrelated targets.

To understand potential issues with specificity and selectivity, tool compounds should be profiled as broadly as possible. The donated chemical probes released by the SGC are a good example for broad annotation: after acceptance, all donated probes are profiled in target specific assays, in relevant selectivity panels, in a panel of over 500 kinases as well as in over 100 ion channels, GPCRs, and proteases [14]. In this example, activity data related to more than 600 different targets are measured and made available. Nevertheless, these data relate mostly to well-known targets. To cover also underexplored targets, there is an urgent need to develop assays such as the thermal shift assay that are applicable to a broad range of targets with limited effort for specific assay development [27, 28].

Data supporting the selection of tool compounds for evaluating new drug targets are not always easy to find. Vendors usually provide some data and links to literature for the compounds they sell, but this is often limited to a few selected off-targets. Well established databases like ChEMBL are a very valuable source for activity data. In addition, new platforms like Probe Miner [29] and the Chemical Probes Portal [13] have recently been launched to help find information on tool compounds. Both platforms are user friendly and a valuable source of information when searching for the best tool compound for target validation.

1.3 Development of Chemical Probes

1.3.1 From BIX01294 to EPZ035544: Development and Improvement of G9a/GLP Inhibitors

The discovery of **EPZ035544** is an example of how a chemical probe was used to uncover a new biological link between epigenetic targets and haemoglobin expression and stimulate drug discovery for sickle cell anaemia.

The two closely related protein lysine methyltransferases (PKMTs) G9a (KMT1C/EHMT2) and G9a-like protein (GLP/KMT1D/EHMT1) are *S*-adenosyl methionine (SAM)-dependent enzymes responsible for the mono- and di-methylation of histone H3 lysine 9 (H3K9me1/H3K9me2) [30–33]. Dysregulation and overexpression of this post-translational epigenetic modification has been reported to be associated with a variety of human diseases, especially cancers [34, 35], including lung cancer [36–38], leukaemia [39–41], prostate carcinoma [39, 41, 42], breast carcinoma [43, 44], and hepatocellular carcinoma [45–47]. Over the past years, a number of selective G9a/GLP inhibitors have been used for the investigation of the cellular role of these PKMTs and developed as potential therapeutic drugs [35, 48].

The first selective and potent G9a/GLP inhibitor was discovered via high-throughput screening by Boehringer Ingelheim using a chemical library of 125 000 preselected compounds [49]. The only selective inhibition of G9a/GLP histone H3 lysine-9 di-methylation (H3K9me2) was observed for the diazepine-quinazoline-amine derivative **BIX01294** that competes with the peptide substrate and not with the methylation cofactor SAM (Figure 1.2). Although multiple studies of **BIX01294** have shown a successful application in cellular reprogramming [50, 51] and reactivation of latent HIV-1 [52], the use of the compound was limited due to the high cellular toxicity at concentrations (>4 μM) near the on-target cellular potency.

Further structure-based exploration of the **BIX01294** quinazoline scaffold [53, 54] led to the first potent, selective, and cell-active chemical probe **UNC0638** along with its inactive control **UNC0737** [55]. Additional optimization of

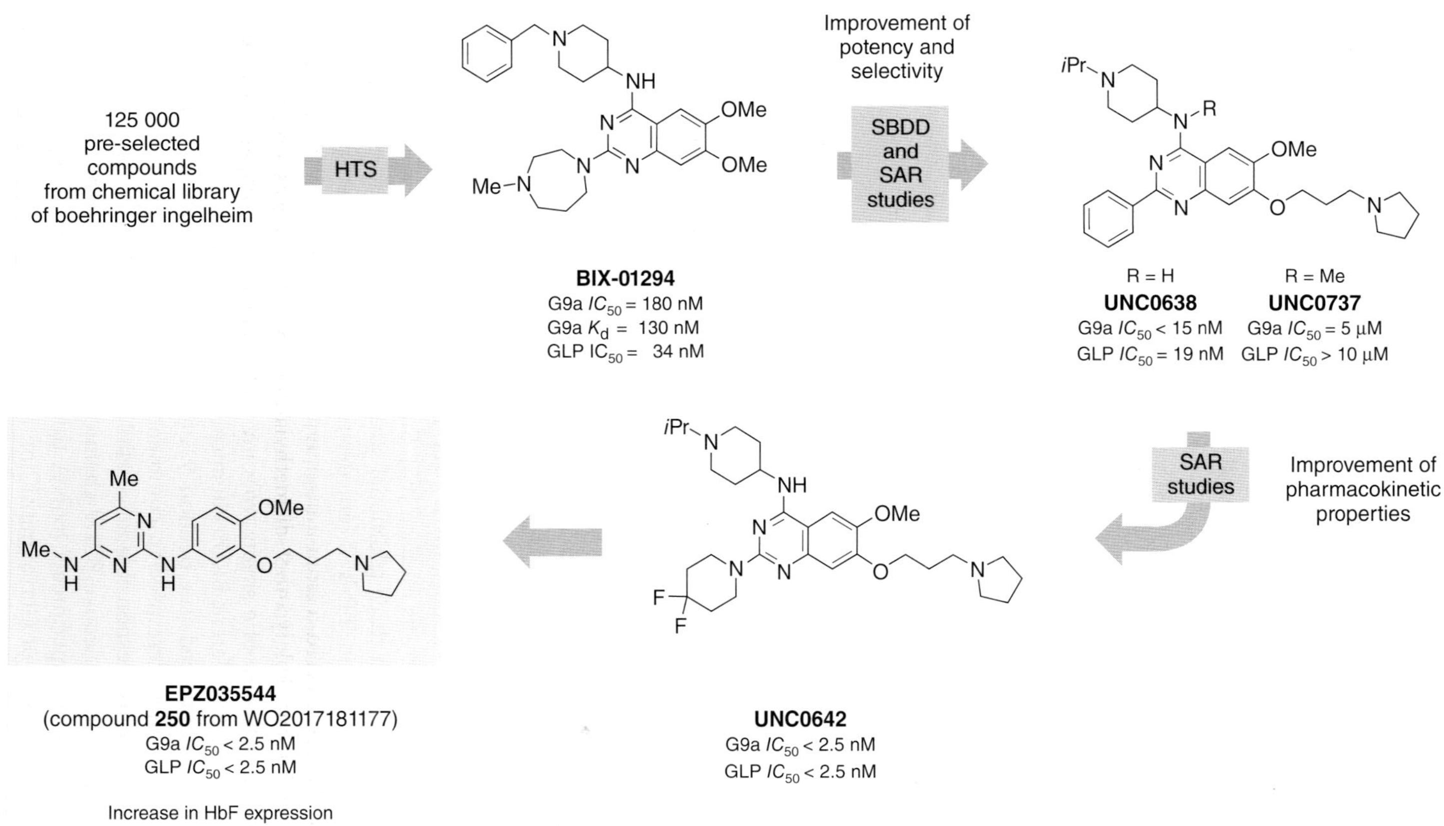

Figure 1.2 Development of G9a/GLP inhibitors. HTS, high-throughput screening.

pharmacokinetic properties produced **UNC0642**, a G9a/GLP chemical probe also suitable for *in vivo* use.

Although initially used in cancer studies, more recent work [56, 57] showed that **UNC0642** induced the expression of human foetal haemoglobin (HbF) in adult erythroid cells, despite its usual silencing after birth. Since the discovery of 5-azacytidine in 1982 [58], the reactivation of HbF synthesis has been widely explored for the treatment of blood disorders such as sickle cell anaemia and β-thalassaemia. Inspired by the results from **UNC0642**, the researchers at Epizyme developed additional G9a/GLP inhibitors as therapeutic agents to treat haemoglobin deficiency disorders [59]. Among the structures of a number of G9a/GLP inhibitors from an Epizyme patent application [60], **EPZ035544** (compound **205**), which shares some structural features to the previously disclosed chemical probes **UNC0638** and **UNC0642**, was identified as a potential candidate for the treatment of haemoglobin deficiencies such as sickle cell anaemia. The discovery of **UNC0642** and **EPZ035544** is an excellent example of using high-quality small molecule chemical probes to decipher new biology with the potential for great clinical benefit.

1.3.2 Development of BRD9 Inhibitors

The family of BRD are 'readers' of lysine acetylation (Kac) of proteins [61–64]. By reading histone acetylation, BRDs regulate gene transcription by serving as transcription factors themselves, thereby reorganizing the physical structure of chromatin (ATAD2) or recruiting transcription factors (BRD4) and chromatin remodellers (BRD7, BRD9). A dysfunction of BRD-containing proteins has been linked to diverse diseases such as cancer and inflammation.

For this reason, during the last decade, a number of single target and subfamily selective BRD chemical probes have been discovered [62–64]. All eight BRDs of the bromo- and extra-terminal (BET) subfamily were initially targeted, but chemical probes for most of the remaining BRD family have been described and allow near family-wide exploration of BRD effects on transcription and derived phenotypes. With the development of **LP99** from a fragment hit through structure-based drug design (SBDD), the first selective and potent BRD9 and BRD7 chemical probe was released [65]. Since the introduction of **LP99** by the SGC, there have been three additional structurally unrelated BRD9 and BRD7 inhibitors: I-BRD9 and **TP-472** [66] derived from BRD-focused libraries and **BI-9564** [67] also derived from a fragment hit (Figure 1.3). All of these BRD9 inhibitors are available to the scientific community to investigate the BRD9 biology, either by use of a single probe or a combination of several inhibitors. The availability of different BRD9 chemical probe chemotypes allows on-target effects to be confirmed (see Section 9.3 for further information on how cell biology techniques were used in combination to provide evidence that BRD9 target modulation is responsible for a cellular response).

I-BRD9, the first selective BRD9 chemical probe, has utility both in cellular assays and *in vivo* experiments [66]. A thienopyridone was identified as a hit by a cross-screening of GlaxoSmithKline (GSK) internal compounds to identify inhibitors of the BRD9 bromodomain. X-ray crystallography of analogues in

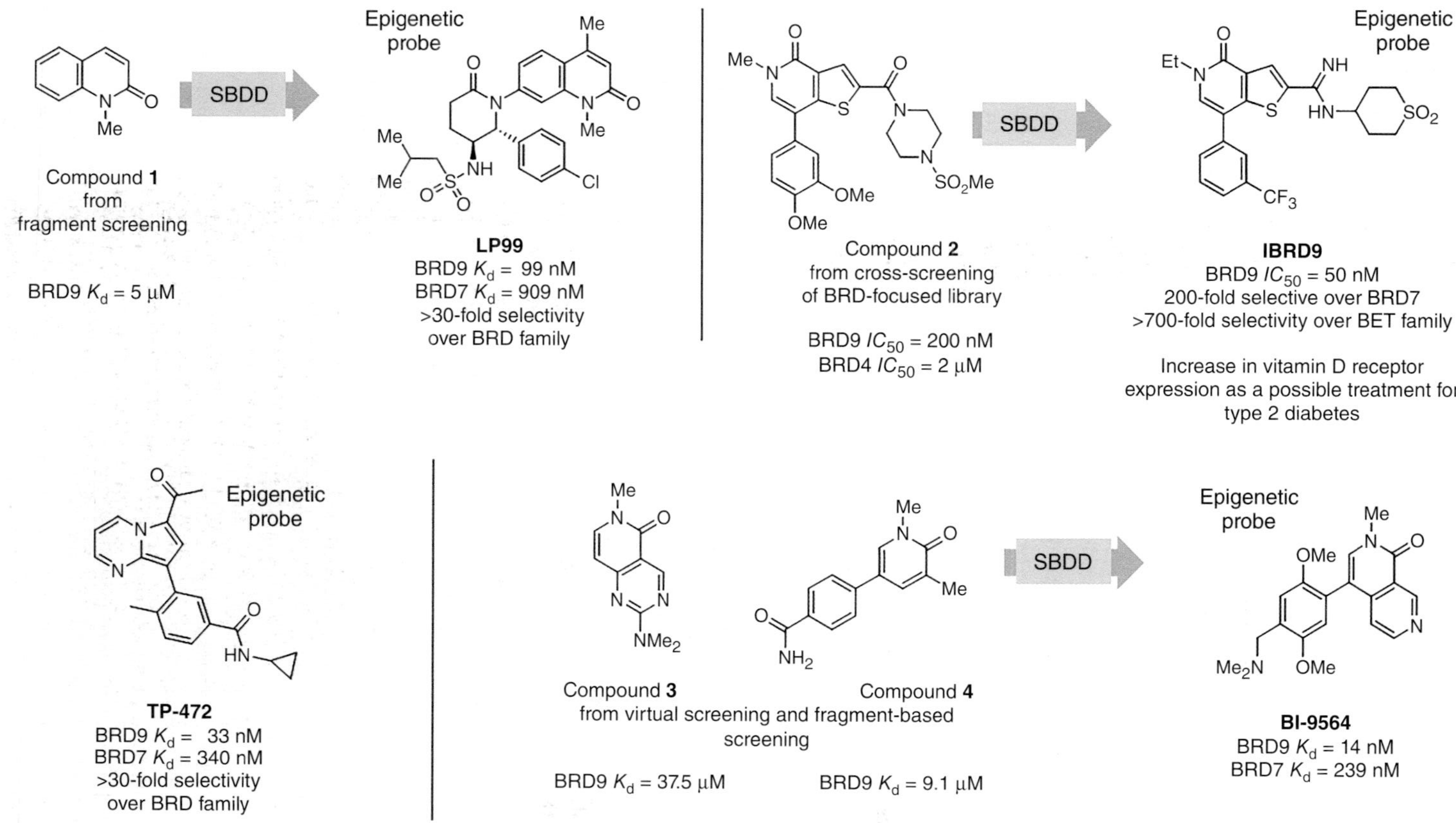

Figure 1.3 Development of BRD9 inhibitors with structure-based drug design (SBDD).

complex with BRD9 and BRD4 provided structural insight into substrate binding and selectivity for BRD9 over BRD4. Further optimization of the thienopyridone scaffold resulted in the synthesis of compounds with improved potency and selectivity for BRD9 culminating in the discovery of **I-BRD9** as a BRD9 chemical probe with nanomolar potency and a selectivity of greater than 700-fold over the BET family and greater than 200-fold over the highly homologous BRD7.

Besides the role of BRD9 in several cancer diseases, recent studies uncovered the utility of **I-BRD9** for treatment of progression of type 2 diabetes [68], which is caused by the dysfunction of pancreatic β-cells [69]. Previously, vitamin D receptors (VDRs) were identified as an important modulator of inflammation and pancreatic β-cell survival. Surprisingly, the use of **I-BRD9** [66] together with vitamin D [70] triggered an activation of VDRs and resulted in an enhanced survival of pancreatic β-cells and glucose homeostasis. Due to the restoration of pancreatic β-cell function by epigenetic regulation of VDR transcriptional response, BRD9 inhibitors consequently constitute a potential target for novel therapeutic approaches for the treatment of type 2 diabetes. The use of **I-BRD9** to link BRD9 to VDR expression and provide a new small molecule target for type 2 diabetes is another example of the utility of chemical probes in target discovery.

1.4 Compound-Based Target Evaluation with Patient-Derived Cells

Ideally, we need a cascade of assays from simple biochemical or physical tests all the way through to disease-relevant systems in order to discover new medicines (see Figure 1.4). In recent years, there has been an increased awareness of the limitations of conventional model systems (e.g. immortalized cell lines, rodent models). As a consequence, the interest to source and build translational assays and test systems using cells and tissue derived from patients has increased significantly in both industry and academia, since such systems hold the promise to recapitulate the disease state more accurately (also see Chapter 7 for more details) [71–73].

1.4.1 Compound-Based Target Evaluation

Translational medical research is to a large extent dependent upon high-quality antibody and chemical-based modulators of protein function for discovery and confirmation of target–disease associations. This can be carried out either as hypothesis-driven or as unbiased approaches. In hypothesis-driven studies, underlying data from genetic studies provide initial evidence for a specific protein target that is subsequently confirmed by the use of a functional antibody or chemical compound. An example of the unbiased and target agnostic approach is phenotypic cell-based screens with biomarker read-outs. Such screens will provide hit compounds in the absence of an initially identified target. Both approaches have their merits and drawbacks, but are complementary and can also be combined, as outlined below [74].

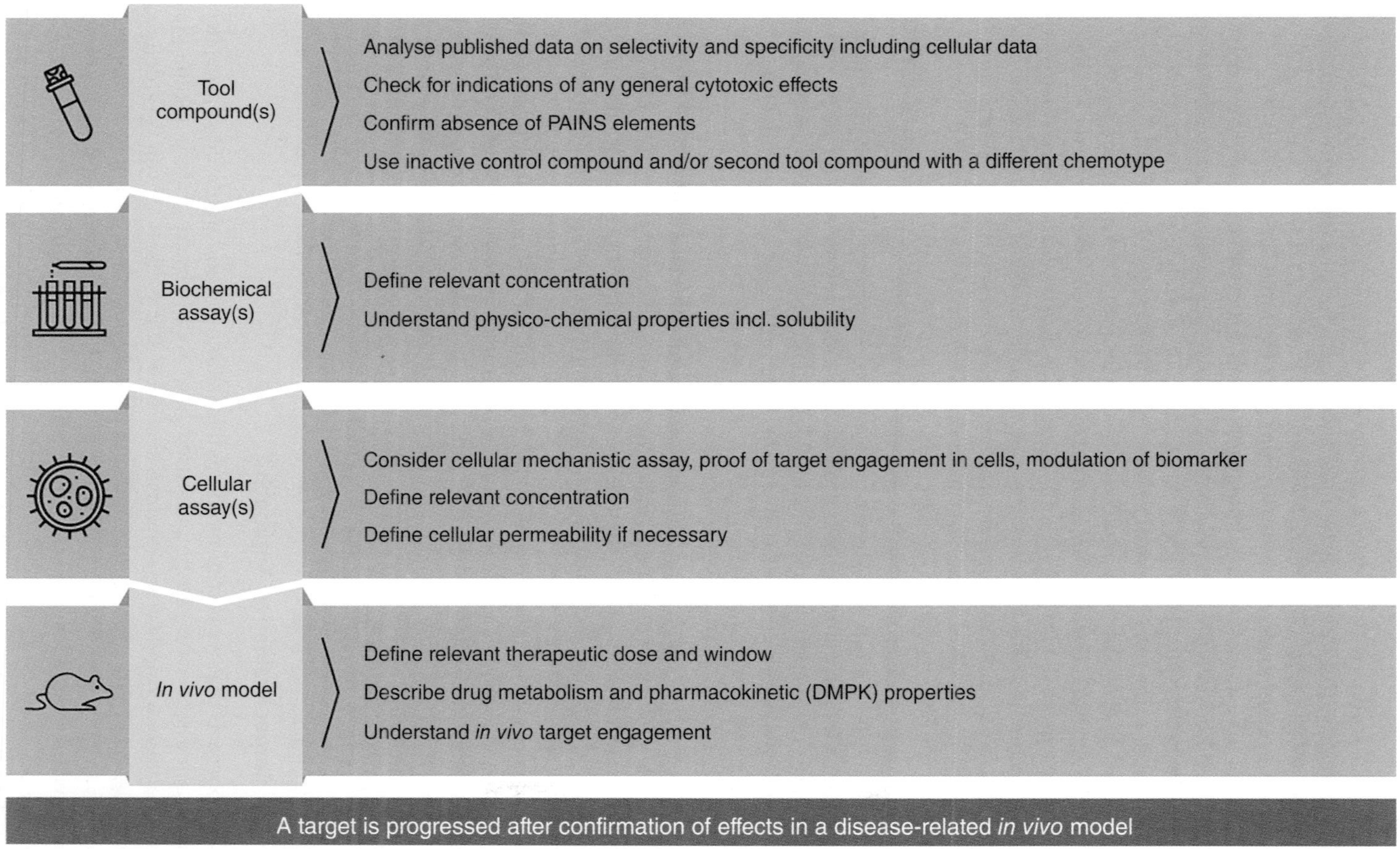

Figure 1.4 Workflow for target validation using tools compounds. Best practices are indicated for the individual steps.

1.4.2 Patient-Derived Cell Assays

Preclinical studies with conventional models of disease often fail to translate into clinical reality. This holds true for most therapeutic areas, ranging from infectious diseases to oncology [75, 76]. In addition, the path from discovery to clinical trials and ultimate market approval is long. For example, a recent analysis of the history of first-in-class kinase inhibitors revealed that often more than a decade transpired between the first published conclusive target–disease association and the initiation of clinical studies [77]. This delay occurred despite the fact that clinical success rates for kinase inhibitors and other targeted therapies are higher compared to classical small molecule medicines [78, 79]. One of the reasons for this is likely that multiple sources of data from different research groups need to, over time, provide converging and supporting disease-link evidence before the pharmaceutical or biotech industry became convinced of embarking on costly drug discovery and development programmes. However, there are also examples where the use of disease models based on patient cells has provided the necessary and supporting validation data. For example, therapeutic antibodies against tumour necrosis factor alpha for rheumatoid arthritis was developed with significant support from data using synovial cell samples from patients, enabled by the development and optimization of new more advanced cell culture conditions [80]. Thus, applying specific and high-quality probes as small molecules or antibodies to patient-derived test systems holds an enormous potential for target discovery and interrogation.

However, clinical samples are not always easily obtainable. The procurement involves direct collaboration with hospitals and clinicians and ethical approval of sample collection and analytical procedures and most importantly requires the consent of the patients themselves. Usually samples are of limited size or volume, remain in a near-native state for a short time, and often do not constitute the foundation for the generation of a renewable resource such as stem cells and organoids. The inherent variability between donors and patients, especially if combined with a relatively low number of samples available, results in observed trends rather than rigid statistical significance of effect. Hence, regular access to samples from multiple patients, along with stringent clinical as well as experimental inclusion and exclusion criteria, is required to allow sufficient amounts of data to be generated and analysed in a meaningful way.

1.4.3 Target Evaluation Approach

The approach that we recommend combines targeted and unbiased approaches: (i) targeted since the compounds used have well-defined protein specificities and if a disease modifying response is observed, it is likely driven by a defined modulation of that protein function, and (ii) unbiased since we apply all chemical probes to all assays, thereby allowing potential new discoveries in the absence of previously established disease-link evidence. Importantly, the same chemical probes are used in all assays from all disease areas, thereby allowing with time direct comparative studies (data integration and analysis) across all diseases studied.

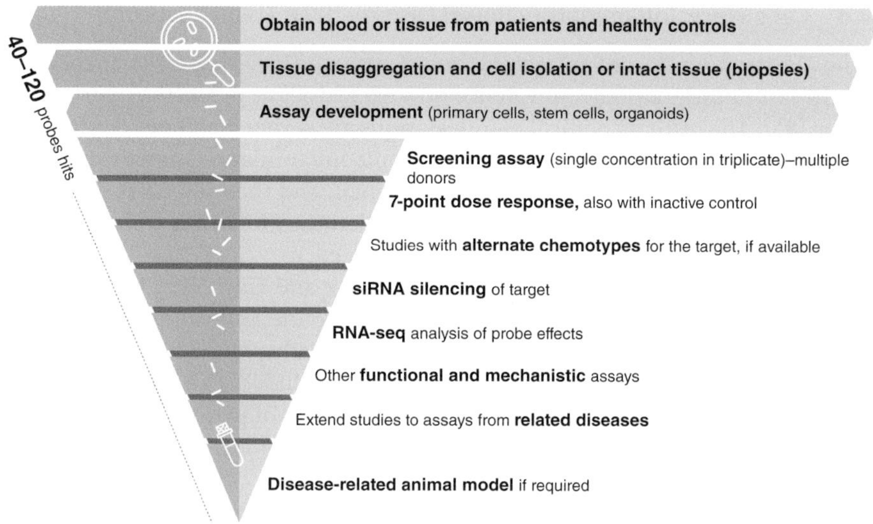

Figure 1.5 A generalized overview of the target validation process carried out at the SGC Tissue Platforms, from obtaining patient samples to functional studies. Source: Adapted from original by Fiona McCann, University of Oxford.

The general experimental approach at the platforms is as follows (Figure 1.5):

1. The initial assay is run at one single compound concentration, in triplicate. Depending on the compound properties, this normally ranges from 0.1 to 1 μmol/l concentration (proven non-toxic concentration). Typically, we include the SGC's chemical probes and compounds within the pharma donated probes collection [23, 24], as well as other compounds from academic and industrial collaborators. For compounds providing a positive response (hit compounds), the experimental steps 2–5 are usually carried out. Data from each step needs to be supportive and conclusive for it to pass on further in the validation cascade.
2. A dose–response curve is generated, typically with seven concentrations (0.1–10 μmol/l). The hit compound is used alongside an inactive control compound (using the aforementioned definition). The hit compound needs to exhibit reproducible dose–response effects, whereas the inactive control should not affect the assay read-outs.
3. If available, a compound with an alternate chemical or chiral structure and specificity profile, but hitting the same primary target, is used. If similar data are generated, this strengthens the case significantly.
4. Moreover, if the chemical probe screen identifies a promising target–disease association, an orthogonal genetic method is applied. Typically, siRNA is used for this purpose, as it is fast and relatively straightforward and, in our experience, mimics compound effects well in the patient-derived test systems.
5. Finally, and depending on the exact purpose of the study, other assays and technologies are applied. These can include gene expression profiling as a consequence of compound treatment, proteomics, and other functional or mechanistic studies, as well as collaborative studies in other related disease areas.

1.4.4 Case Story: Inflammatory Bowel Disease (IBD) Tissue Platform

In the Western world, inflammatory bowel disease (IBD) has been increasing over the last decade, and the prevalence now exceeds 0.3% in North America and Europe [81]. The primary clinical manifestations are severe diarrhoea, abdominal pain, and weight loss resulting from gut chronic inflammation, in particular the colon. Treatment options are few and suboptimal, and the molecular drivers of the disease are poorly understood. Thus, the identification of new intervention points for improved IBD therapies is greatly needed.

The IBD Tissue Platform at Karolinska Institutet and University Hospital was initiated in mid-2017. The aim of the study is to define and validate new intervention points for future therapies. The study is initially planned for three years, during which up to 300 consenting patients can be included. Patients will provide samples of blood and colon biopsies for the generation of patient-based assays.

To date, two assay formats have been generated, one directly on biopsies of colon mucosa, which are maintained under specific culture conditions for 24 hours, and thereafter spontaneous cytokine release is measured. Biopsies retain their inflammatory phenotype during culture, and a clear distinction is observed between non-inflamed and inflamed tissue. The biopsies also respond as expected to drugs in clinical use, such as prednisolone (Figure 1.6).

Since a limited number of biopsies per patient can be obtained and used to study only very few prototype drugs, we also needed to develop blood-based screening assays. Here, the first is a whole blood assay in which we induce inflammation by stimulating nucleotide-binding oligomerization domain-containing protein 2 (NOD2) signalling with muramyl dipeptide (MDP), and thereafter cytokine release is measured. Around 70 open-source chemical probes have been tested to date, reconfirming the effect of previously published kinase inhibitors (such as mitogen-activated protein kinase (MAPK) and receptor-interacting serine/threonine-protein kinase 2 (RIPK2) inhibitors), but also implicating other novel targets; verification studies are currently underway. The study also includes the generation of novel screening platforms based on colon organoids as well as a deep *-omics* patient characterization study of approximately 60

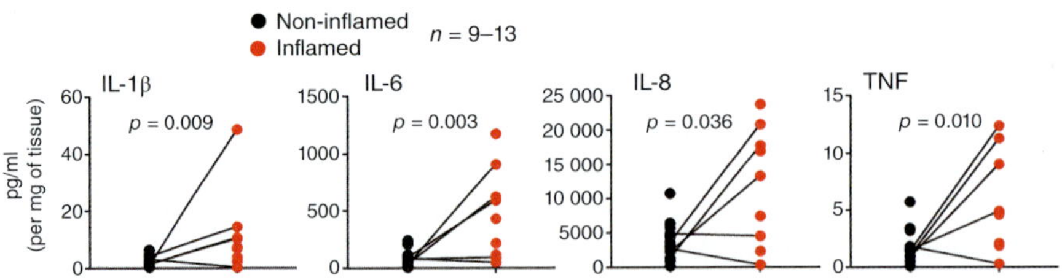

Figure 1.6 Preliminary results (Mann–Whitney test) on spontaneous pro-inflammatory cytokine release in colon tissue culture supernatant, comparing inflamed (red) and non-inflamed (black) mucosa from 17 IBD patients with heterogeneous inflammation and medication profiles. Donor-matched inflamed and non-inflamed tissues were available for five patients (connecting lines). IL, interleukin; TNF, tumour necrosis factor.

patients, including whole genome sequencing (blood and colon mucosa) and gene expression profiling studies.

In conclusion, patient-derived cell and tissue assays can be a powerful tool and complement in preclinical research as described above. However, the establishment of such test systems is complex and resource intense as compared to conventional disease-related models with animals. Hence, it is of utmost importance that the research tools and reagents used, such as chemical probes, are of the highest quality to ensure high-quality assay read-outs and best use of precious patient samples.

1.5 Summary and Outlook

The evaluation of potential new drug targets can be performed in a variety of different ways. Genetic approaches such as gene editing [82] are routinely used to study the function of a target of interest by suppressing its expression (see Chapter 9 for more details). As genetic methods usually remove or suppress the entire protein, they cannot easily reveal the function of an individual domain. Furthermore, the effects are not reversible, which limits their value as a stand-alone method of prioritizing a target for small molecule drug discovery. In contrast, we can use chemical probes and chemogenomic compounds to interrogate any particular function of a targeted protein or protein domain in a dose- and time-dependent manner, and such chemical tools should be used whenever possible to complement other approaches for evaluating and prioritizing new potential targets.

In-depth understanding of the potential and limits of each tool compound is needed to correctly interpret the results. Indeed, there are several examples where tools of poor quality and compounds being used incorrectly have generated misleading results [13]. Nevertheless, user-friendly tools are available to support scientists' search for an appropriate tool compound for target evaluation. Even with the very broad annotation, we must expect effects from uncharacterized off-targets and therefore highly recommend using several tool compounds with different chemotypes whenever possible, as well as applying orthogonal approaches to strengthen the validation case.

The different steps in the path towards evaluating a new target using chemicals tools are depicted in Figure 1.4 along with best practices that we suggest for the individual steps. Biochemical and cellular assays performed with carefully selected tools compounds provide valuable information on the relevance of a novel drug target, but we wish to stress that a target is only fully validated after successful pivotal phase III clinical studies in humans. The number of open-access chemical probes and chemogenomic compounds has significantly increased over the last few years, supported by both academia and pharma companies, such as the recent donated probes initiative [14]. Still, there is an urgent need to identify high-quality chemical tools for a large area of the underexplored druggable genome, as well as de-orphanize new druggable target families. A concerted worldwide effort is needed to fill this gap.

References

1 DiMasi, J.A., Grabowski, H.G., and Hansen, R.W. (2016). Innovation in the pharmaceutical industry: new estimates of R&D costs. *J. Health Econ.* 47: 20–33.
2 Paul, S.M., Mytelka, D.S., Dunwiddie, C.T. et al. (2010). How to improve R&D productivity: the pharmaceutical industry's grand challenge. *Nat. Rev. Drug Discovery* 9 (3): 203–214.
3 Hay, M., Thomas, D.W., Craighead, J.L. et al. (2014). Clinical development success rates for investigational drugs. *Nat. Biotechnol.* 32: 40–51.
4 Smietana, K., Siatkowski, M., and Moller, M. (2016). Trends in clinical success rates. *Nat. Rev. Drug Discovery* 15 (6): 379–380.
5 Arrowsmith, J. (2011). Trial watch: phase III and submission failures: 2007–2010. *Nat. Rev. Drug Discovery* 10 (2): 87.
6 Cook, D., Brown, D., Alexander, R. et al. (2014). Lessons learned from the fate of AstraZeneca's drug pipeline: a five-dimensional framework. *Nat. Rev. Drug Discovery* 13 (6): 419–431.
7 Nelson, M.R., Tipney, H., Painter, J.L. et al. (2015). The support of human genetic evidence for approved drug indications. *Nat. Genet.* 47 (8): 856–860.
8 Plenge, R.M., Scolnick, E.M., and Altshuler, D. (2013). Validating therapeutic targets through human genetics. *Nat. Rev. Drug Discovery* 12: 581–594.
9 Oprea, T.I., Bologa, C.G., Brunak, S. et al. (2018). Unexplored therapeutic opportunities in the human genome. *Nat. Rev. Drug Discovery* 17: 317–332.
10 Collins, F.S., Morgan, M., and Patrinos, A. (2003). The human genome project: lessons from large-scale biology. *Science* 300 (5617): 286–290.
11 Edwards, A. (2011). Too many roads not taken. *Nature* 470: 163–165.
12 Santos, R., Ursu, O., Gaulton, A. et al. (2017). A comprehensive map of molecular drug targets. *Nat. Rev. Drug Discovery* 16 (1): 19–34.
13 Arrowsmith, C.H., Audia, J.E., Austin, C. et al. (2015). The promise and peril of chemical probes. *Nat. Chem. Biol.* 11 (8): 536–541.
14 Müller, S., Ackloo, S., Arrowsmith, C.H. et al. (2018). Donated chemical probes for open science. *eLife* 7: e34311.
15 Jones, L.H. and Bunnage, M.E. (2017). Applications of chemogenomic library screening in drug discovery. *Nat. Rev. Drug Discovery* 16: 285–296.
16 Caron, P.R., Mullican, M.D., Mashal, R.D. et al. (2001). Chemogenomic approaches to drug discovery. *Curr. Opin. Chem. Biol.* 5 (4): 464–470.
17 Bredel, M. and Jacoby, E. (2004). Chemogenomics: an emerging strategy for rapid target and drug discovery. *Nat. Rev. Genet.* 5: 262–275.
18 Klabunde, T. (2007). Chemogenomic approaches to drug discovery: similar receptors bind similar ligands. *Br. J. Pharmacol.* 152 (1): 5–7.
19 Drewry, D.H., Wells, C.I., Andrews, D.M. et al. (2017). Progress towards a public chemogenomic set for protein kinases and a call for contributions. *PLoS One* 12 (8): e0181585 https://doi.org/10.1371/journal.pone.0181585. https://www.ebi.ac.uk/chembl/.

20 Prinz, F., Schlange, T., and Asadullah, K. (2011). Believe it or not: how much can we rely on published data on potential drug targets? *Nat. Rev. Drug Discovery* 10: 712–713.

21 Begley, C.G. and Ellis, L.M. (2012). Raise standards for preclinical cancer research. *Nature* 483: 531–533.

22 Bunnage, M.E., Chekler, E.L., and Jones, L.H. (2013). Target validation using chemical probes. *Nat. Chem. Biol.* 9 (4): 195–199.

23 Blagg, J. and Workman, P. (2017). Choose and use your chemical probe wisely to explore cancer biology. *Cancer Cell* 32 (1): 9–25.

24 Frye, S.V. (2010). The art of the chemical probe. *Nat. Chem. Biol.* 6 (3): 159–161.

25 Jacoby, E., Tresadern, G., Bembenek, S. et al. (2015). Extending kinome coverage by analysis of kinase inhibitor broad profiling data. *Drug Discovery Today* 20 (6): 652–658.

26 Ciceri, P., Müller, S., O'Mahony, A. et al. (2014). Dual kinase-bromodomain inhibitors for rationally designed polypharmacology. *Nat. Chem. Biol.* 10: 305–312.

27 Niesen, F.H., Berglund, H., and Vedadi, M. (2007). The use of differential scanning fluorimetry to detect ligand interactions that promote protein stability. *Nat. Protoc.* 2: 2212–2221.

28 Molina, D.M. and Nordlund, P. (2016). The cellular thermal shift assay: a novel biophysical assay for in situ drug target engagement and mechanistic biomarker studies. *Annu. Rev. Pharmacol. Toxicol.* 56 (1): 141–161.

29 Antolin, A.A., Tym, J.E., Komianou, A. et al. (2018). Objective, quantitative, data-driven assessment of chemical probes. *Cell Chem. Biol.* 25 (2): 194–205.e5.

30 Shinkai, Y. and Tachibana, M. (2011). H3K9 methyltransferase G9a and the related molecule GLP. *Genes Dev.* 25 (8): 781–788.

31 Tachibana, M., Ueda, J., Fukuda, M. et al. (2005). Histone methyltransferases G9a and GLP form heteromeric complexes and are both crucial for methylation of euchromatin at H3-K9. *Genes Dev.* 19 (7): 815–826.

32 Tachibana, M., Sugimoto, K., Fukushima, T., and Shinkai, Y. (2001). Set domain-containing protein, G9a, is a novel lysine-preferring mammalian histone methyltransferase with hyperactivity and specific selectivity to lysines 9 and 27 of histone H3. *J. Biol. Chem.* 276 (27): 25309–25317.

33 Tachibana, M., Sugimoto, K., Nozaki, M. et al. (2002). G9a histone methyltransferase plays a dominant role in euchromatic histone H3 lysine 9 methylation and is essential for early embryogenesis. *Genes Dev.* 16 (14): 1779–1791.

34 Casciello, F., Windloch, K., Gannon, F., and Lee, J.S. (2015). Functional role of G9a histone methyltransferase in cancer. *Front. Immunol.* 6: 487.

35 Liu, Q. and M-w, W. (2016). Histone lysine methyltransferases as anti-cancer targets for drug discovery. *Acta Pharmacol. Sin.* 37: 1273–1280.

36 Watanabe, H., Soejima, K., Yasuda, H. et al. (2008). Deregulation of histone lysine methyltransferases contributes to oncogenic transformation of human bronchoepithelial cells. *Cancer Cell Int.* 8 (1): 15.

37 Chen, Y., Liu, X., Li, Y. et al. (2018). Lung cancer therapy targeting histone methylation: opportunities and challenges. *Comput. Struct. Biotechnol. J.* 16: 211–223.

38 Chen, M.W., Hua, K.T., Kao, H.J. et al. (2010). H3K9 histone methyltransferase G9a promotes lung cancer invasion and metastasis by silencing the cell adhesion molecule Ep-CAM. *Cancer Res.* 70 (20): 7830–7840.

39 Huang, J., Dorsey, J., Chuikov, S. et al. (2010). G9a and Glp methylate lysine 373 in the tumor suppressor p53. *J. Biol. Chem.* 285 (13): 9636–9641.

40 Kondengaden, S.M., L-F, L., Huang, K. et al. (2016). Discovery of novel small molecule inhibitors of lysine methyltransferase G9a and their mechanism in leukemia cell lines. *Eur. J. Med. Chem.* 122: 382–393.

41 Jung, H., Chae, Y.-C., Kim, J.-Y. et al. (2017). Regulatory role of G9a and LSD1 in the transcription of olfactory receptors during leukaemia cell differentiation. *Sci. Rep.* 7: 46182.

42 Kondo, Y., Shen, L., Ahmed, S. et al. (2008). Downregulation of histone H3 lysine 9 methyltransferase G9a induces centrosome disruption and chromosome instability in cancer cells. *PLoS One* 3 (4): e2037.

43 Curry, E., Green, I., Chapman-Rothe, N. et al. (2015). Dual EZH2 and EHMT2 histone methyltransferase inhibition increases biological efficacy in breast cancer cells. *Clin. Epigenet.* 7 (1): 84.

44 Wang, Y.-f., Zhang, J., Su, Y. et al. (2017). G9a regulates breast cancer growth by modulating iron homeostasis through the repression of ferroxidase hephaestin. *Nat. Commun.* 8 (1): 274.

45 Kondo, Y., Shen, L., Suzuki, S. et al. (2007). Alterations of DNA methylation and histone modifications contribute to gene silencing in hepatocellular carcinomas. *Hepatol. Res.* 37 (11): 974–983.

46 Yokoyama, M., Chiba, T., Zen, Y. et al. (2017). Histone lysine methyltransferase G9a is a novel epigenetic target for the treatment of hepatocellular carcinoma. *Oncotarget* 8 (13): 21315–21326.

47 Wei, L., Chiu, D.K.-C., Tsang, F.H.-C. et al. (2017). Histone methyltransferase G9a promotes liver cancer development by epigenetic silencing of tumor suppressor gene RARRES3. *J. Hepatol.* 67 (4): 758–769.

48 Ye, T. and Hui, C. (2015). Synthesis of lysine methyltransferase inhibitors. *Front. Chem.* 3: 44.

49 Kubicek, S., O'Sullivan, R.J., August, E.M. et al. (2007). Reversal of H3K9me2 by a small-molecule inhibitor for the G9a histone methyltransferase. *Mol. Cell* 25 (3): 473–481.

50 Shi, Y., Tae Do, J., Desponts, C. et al. (2008). A combined chemical and genetic approach for the generation of induced pluripotent stem cells. *Cell Stem Cell* 2 (6): 525–528.

51 Shi, Y., Desponts, C., Do, J.T. et al. (2008). Induction of pluripotent stem cells from mouse embryonic fibroblasts by Oct4 and Klf4 with small-molecule compounds. *Cell Stem Cell* 3 (5): 568–574.

52 Imai, K., Togami, H., and Okamoto, T. (2010). Involvement of histone H3 lysine 9 (H3K9) methyltransferase G9a in the maintenance of HIV-1 latency and its reactivation by BIX01294. *J. Biol. Chem.* 285 (22): 16538–16545.

53 Liu, F., Chen, X., Allali-Hassani, A. et al. (2010). Protein lysine methyltransferase G9a inhibitors: design, synthesis, and structure activity relationships of 2,4-diamino-7-aminoalkoxy-quinazolines. *J. Med. Chem.* 53 (15): 5844–5857.

54 Liu, F., Chen, X., Allali-Hassani, A. et al. (2009). Discovery of a 2,4-diamino-7-aminoalkoxyquinazoline as a potent and selective inhibitor of histone lysine methyltransferase G9a. *J. Med. Chem.* 52 (24): 7950–7953.

55 Liu, F., Barsyte-Lovejoy, D., Li, F. et al. (2013). Discovery of an in vivo chemical probe of the lysine methyltransferases G9a and GLP. *J. Med. Chem.* 56 (21): 8931–8942.

56 Krivega, I., Byrnes, C., de Vasconcellos, J.F. et al. (2015). Inhibition of G9a methyltransferase stimulates fetal hemoglobin production by facilitating LCR/γ-globin looping. *Blood* 126 (5): 665–672.

57 Renneville, A., Van Galen, P., Canver, M.C. et al. (2015). EHMT1 and EHMT2 inhibition induces fetal hemoglobin expression. *Blood* 126 (16): 1930–1939.

58 DeSimone, J., Heller, P., Hall, L., and Zwiers, D. (1982). 5-Azacytidine stimulates fetal hemoglobin synthesis in anemic baboons. *Proc. Natl. Acad. Sci. U.S.A.* 79 (14): 4428–4431.

59 Chan-Penebre, E., Gibaja, V., Campbell, J. et al. (2017). Reawakening of human fetal hemoglobin and an epigenetic path to the clinic for sickle cell disease and beta-thalassemia: identification of an orally-available, potent, and selective euchromatic histone lysine methyltransferase 1 and 2 (EHMT1/2) inhibitor. *Blood* 130 (Suppl 1): 537.

60 Campbell, J.E., Duncan, K.W., Foley, M.A., et al. (2017). Amine-substituted aryl or heteroaryl compounds as EHMT1 and EHMT2 inhibitors. WO2017181177, filed 15 April 2016.

61 Filippakopoulos, P. and Knapp, S. (2014). Targeting bromodomains: epigenetic readers of lysine acetylation. *Nat. Rev. Drug Discovery* 13: 337–356.

62 Fujisawa, T. and Filippakopoulos, P. (2017). Functions of bromodomain-containing proteins and their roles in homeostasis and cancer. *Nat. Rev. Mol. Cell Biol.* 18: 246–262.

63 Ferri, E., Petosa, C., and McKenna, C.E. (2016). Bromodomains: structure, function and pharmacology of inhibition. *Biochem. Pharmacol.* 106: 1–18.

64 Meslamani, J., Smith, S.G., Sanchez, R., and Zhou, M.-M. (2016). Structural features and inhibitors of bromodomains. *Drug Discovery Today* 19: 3–15.

65 Clark, P.G.K., Vieira, L.C.C., Tallant, C. et al. (2015). LP99: discovery and synthesis of the first selective BRD7/9 bromodomain inhibitor. *Angew. Chem. Int. Ed.* 54 (21): 6217–6221.

66 Theodoulou, N.H., Bamborough, P., Bannister, A.J. et al. (2016). Discovery of I-BRD9, a selective cell active chemical probe for bromodomain containing protein 9 inhibition. *J. Med. Chem.* 59 (4): 1425–1439.

67 Martin, L.J., Koegl, M., Bader, G. et al. (2016). Structure-based design of an in vivo active selective BRD9 inhibitor. *J. Med. Chem.* 59 (10): 4462–4475.

68 Olokoba, A.B., Obateru, O.A., and Olokoba, L.B. (2012). Type 2 diabetes mellitus: a review of current trends. *Oman Med. J.* 27 (4): 269–273.

69 Wei, Z., Yoshihara, E., He, N. et al. (2018). Vitamin D switches BAF complexes to protect β cells. *Cell* 173 (5): 1135–49.e15.

70 Takiishi, T., Gysemans, C., Bouillon, R., and Mathieu, C. (2012). Vitamin D and diabetes. *Rheum. Dis. Clin.* 38 (1): 179–206.
71 Edwards, A.M., Arrowsmith, C.H., Bountra, C. et al. (2015). Preclinical target validation using patient-derived cells. *Nat. Rev. Drug Discovery* 14 (3): 149–150.
72 Han, C., Chaineau, M., Chen, C.X.-Q. et al. (2018). Open science meets stem cells: a new drug discovery approach for neurodegenerative disorders. *Front. Neurosci.* 12: 47.
73 Drost, J. and Clevers, H. (2018). Organoids in cancer research. *Nat. Rev. Cancer* 18 (7): 407–418.
74 Moffat, J.G., Vincent, F., Lee, J.A. et al. (2017). Opportunities and challenges in phenotypic drug discovery: an industry perspective. *Nat. Rev. Drug Discovery* 16 (8): 531–543.
75 McGonigle, P. and Ruggeri, B. (2014). Animal models of human disease: challenges in enabling translation. *Biochem. Pharmacol.* 87 (1): 162–171.
76 Seok, J., Warren, H.S., Cuenca, A.G. et al. (2013). Genomic responses in mouse models poorly mimic human inflammatory diseases. *Proc. Natl. Acad. Sci. U.S.A.* 110 (9): 3507–3512.
77 Knapp, S. and Sundström, M. (2014). Recently targeted kinases and their inhibitors—the path to clinical trials. *Curr. Opin. Pharmacol.* 17: 58–63.
78 Walker, I. and Newell, H. (2009). Do molecularly targeted agents in oncology have reduced attrition rates? *Nat. Rev. Drug Discovery* 8 (1): 15–16.
79 Toniatti, C., Jones, P., Graham, H. et al. (2014). Oncology drug discovery: planning a turnaround. *Cancer Discovery* 4 (4): 397–404.
80 Brennan, F.M., Chantry, D., Jackson, A. et al. (1989). Inhibitory effect of TNF alpha antibodies on synovial cell interleukin-1 production in rheumatoid arthritis. *Lancet* 2 (8657): 244–247.
81 Ng, S.C., Shi, H.Y., Hamidi, N. et al. (2018). Worldwide incidence and prevalence of inflammatory bowel disease in the 21st century: a systematic review of population-based studies. *Lancet* 390 (10114): 2769–2778.
82 Mali, P., Yang, L., Esvelt, K.M. et al. (2013). RNA-guided human genome engineering via Cas9. *Science (New York, NY)* 339 (6121): 823–826.

2

Affinity-Based Chemoproteomics for Target Identification

Annika Jenmalm Jensen[1] *and Ivan Cornella Taracido*[2]

[1] *Karolinska Institutet, Chemical Biology Consortium Sweden, Science for Life Laboratory, Department of Medical Biochemistry and Biophysics, Tomtebodavägen 23a, Solna 171 65, Sweden*
[2] *Cedilla Therapeutics, Inc., 38 Sidney Street, Cambridge, MA 02139, USA*

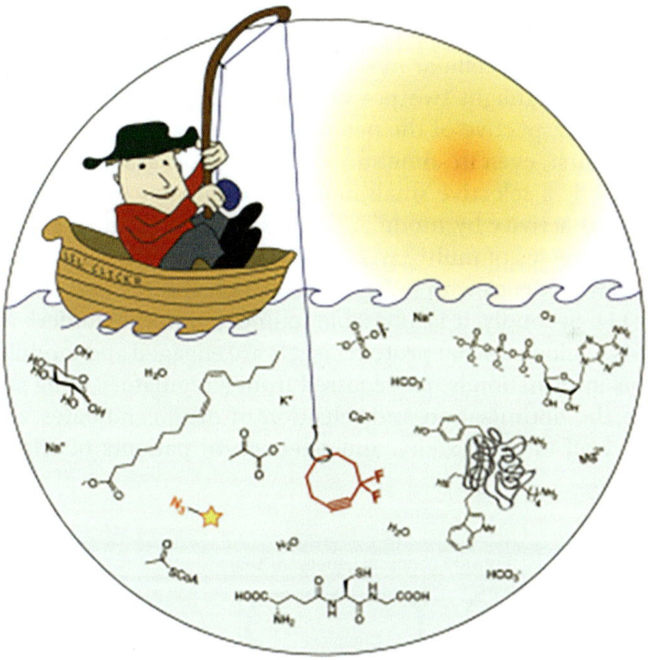

2.1 Introduction

Phenotypic screening (PS) is experiencing a comeback in academic and industrial drug discovery [1–5]. Three main factors can be attributed to its renaissance: the advancement of cell culture techniques, miniaturization, and computational technologies that enable the use of primary human cells, organoids, or tissues in

Target Discovery and Validation: Methods and Strategies for Drug Discovery,
First Edition. Edited by Alleyn T. Plowright.

complex assays with multiplexed read-outs (see Chapter 7 for more details) [6–8]; the limited diversity of safe, validated drug targets in drug discovery portfolios; and the statistically modest discovery and validation achievements attributable to the dominance of target-based approaches in the last decades.

Cell-based PS can be prosecuted with genetic perturbagens, such as collections of targeted short hairpin ribonucleic acids (shRNAs) or deoxyribonucleic acid (DNA) gene-editing clustered regularly interspaced short palindromic repeats (CRISPR) reagents (see Chapter 9 for more details) or small molecules (SMs). Arguably, the value proposition for SM PS in disease-relevant cell-based assays, followed by mechanism of action (MoA) deconvolution, resides in the opportunity to identify cell-active SMs that provide a springboard towards novel biological targets with strong disease relevance and 'first-in-class' therapeutics. Herein we will not add arguments to the debate on whether a reductionist 'one drug–one target–one disease' paradigm may or may not still be the best path to drug discovery or whether it should be overhauled with genetically informed phenotypic approaches [1, 2, 6]. We commend successful target-based drug discovery (TDD) leading to approved drugs and advocate for investing in both avenues when possible. When selecting only one, we ponder on the understanding of disease genetics and biology, the wealth or lack thereof of validated protein targets, and the availability and scalability of cellular models of disease. Notwithstanding the choice, it is important to highlight two powerful incentives for investing in SM MoA deconvolution, irrespective of the penchant for one or another discovery tactic (Figure 2.1). At first, even in some successful TDD programmes, what originally was thought to be a selective small molecule drug later turned out to exert its pharmacological activity by modulation of several protein targets [10]. Moreover, clinical successes of multi-targeted kinase inhibitors demonstrate that it is possible to identify drugs with polypharmacological MoA and optimal selectivity profiles [11]. Secondly, it is advisable to understand the underlying MoA for bioactive SMs, including what protein targets are engaged and modulated *in vivo*. Although this information is not required from a regulatory filing standpoint, it will facilitate the optimization and selection of drug candidates, evaluation of selectivity and off-target toxicity, and selection of patients to effectively test a drug candidate.

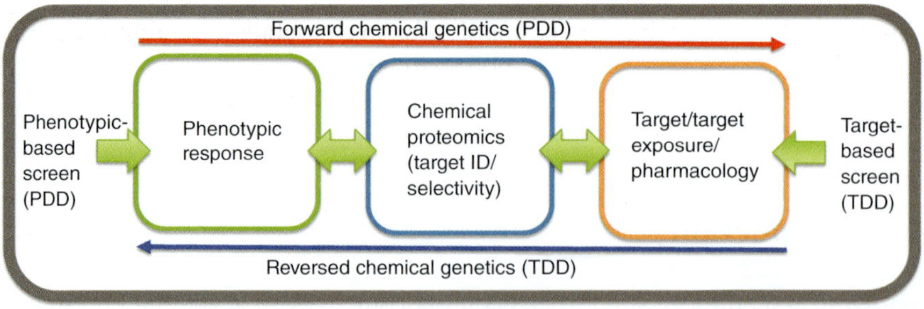

Figure 2.1 The role of chemical proteomics in forward chemical genetics (PDD) and reversed chemical genetics (TDD). Source: Jenmalm Jensen et al. 2015 [9]. Modified with permission of Future Science.

However, MoA deconvolution remains a major challenge despite the growing number of chemical biology approaches to target identification. Through recent developments and availability of several new experimental techniques, MoA elucidation is now more feasible, and the number of successful examples steadily grows. However, a generic methodology that can be successfully applied in the majority of cases has not yet been established. There is a need to combine different methods to generate and prioritize plausible hypotheses and, like solving a puzzle, step by step pin down the protein target(s) and the molecular MoA. It is tempting to select a single tactic for scientific or financial reasons, but we remind the reader that even for time-tested, straightforward MoA deconvolution methods, such as developing resistant mutant bacterial strains to identify the molecular target of antibacterial SMs emerging from whole organism phenotypic screens, each individual technique has limitations. In the case of antibacterials, resistance due to reliance on mutations of a cellular binding partner may lead to altered permeability, transport, or up-regulation of a compensatory pathway, which complicates the analysis of the MoA of a compound [12]. Not to mention that, arguably, MoAs that can be discovered by raising resistance to a particular gene product may not be the best to provide long-term benefits to patients and society, compared with those druggable targets for which pathogenic bacteria cannot defeat through resistance.

Several useful complementary methodologies for SM target identification exist, of which some are covered in this book. Irrespective of the cell type or indication, it has become mainstream to leverage high-throughput screening (HTS) historical data for SM libraries, by means of in-depth computational methods to create 'biological signatures' and classify hit MoAs (see Chapter 11 for more details) [13, 14]. Comparing a SM biological signature to sets of MoA-annotated SMs to infer MoA can also be prospectively achieved during post-HTS triaging by leveraging different read-outs such as imaging, for example, the 'cell painting' methodology developed by scientists at the Broad Institute [15, 16], gene fingerprints and molecular phenotyping approaches, such as the pathway reporter gene signature developed at Novartis [17], Roche's reporter gene method [18], transcriptomic signatures, like the '1000 gene transcription signature' L1000 panel developed by the US National Institutes of Health/Broad Institute Library of Integrated Network-based Cellular Signatures (LINCS) [16] (see Chapter 11 for more details), or recently developed functional genomic technologies [19] (see Chapters 6, 8 and 9 for more details). In addition to the aforementioned tactics, arguably one of the most validated MoA deconvolution approaches is chemical proteomics, or chemoproteomics, generally defined as the collection of biochemical and analytical techniques that address MoA elucidation through the design and use of non-covalent and covalent SM bait probes to interrogate the cell- or tissue-specific proteome and enrich a relevant protein or collection of proteins (Figure 2.2). This method has been utilized in a broad range of studies to identify ligand binding partners and has recently even been expanded to pull down specific species of RNA [20]. Chemoproteomic experimental read-outs are usually based on protein detection with specific antibodies following polyacrylamide gel electrophoresis (PAGE) separation and western blotting (WB) or coupled with quantitative high-resolution mass

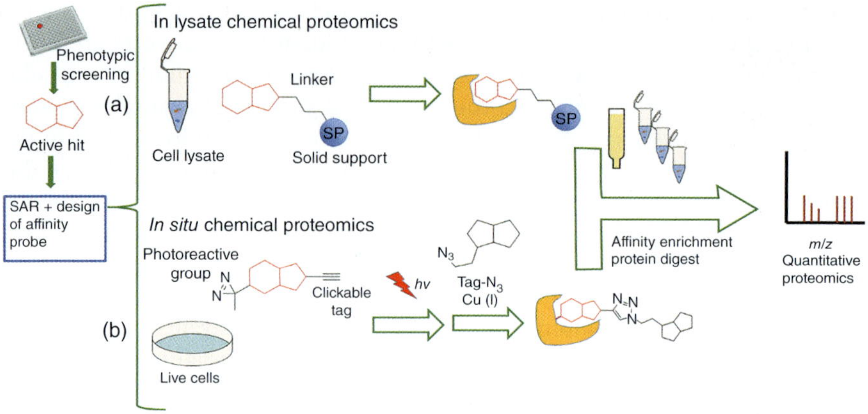

Figure 2.2 Different affinity-based chemical proteomic methods: (a) classical 'in-lysate' affinity-based chemoproteomic 'pulldown', where cell lysates are incubated with non-covalent SM affinity 'baits' to enrich non-covalent binding partners, and (b) *'in situ'* affinity-based chemoproteomics, where live cells are incubated and labelled with photoreactive covalent SM probes.

spectrometry (HRMS) as a more generally exhaustive protein detection and analysis method.

Among chemoproteomic workflows, methods differ in two main aspects: (i) the design and physico-chemical features of the SM enrichment bait and (ii) the proteome fraction accessible. Activity-based proteome profiling (ABPP) chemoproteomics leverage reactive SM biomimicry of enzyme substrates to functionally interrogate protein enzyme classes such as hydrolases [21], yet it cannot interrogate MoA in an unbiased proteome-wide cellular setting (see Chapter 3 for more details). Thermal proteome profiling (TPP) chemoproteomics leverages the possibility to observe a shift in protein stability against thermal denaturation upon temperature increases by SM binding, with *bona fide* SM–protein interactions characterized by a measurable shift in thermal stability, but certain proteins do not undergo a measurable change in precipitation rate (see Chapter 5 for more details) [22]. Herein, we will focus on current methods within affinity-based chemical proteomics: (a) classical 'in-lysate' affinity-based chemoproteomics (also known as 'pulldown'), where cell lysates are incubated with resin bound SM 'baits' to enrich non-covalent binding partners, and (b) '*in situ*' affinity-based chemoproteomics, where live cells are incubated and labelled with photoreactive covalent SM probes (Figure 2.2). Many reviews have covered the general principles of these two approaches [23–26]; thus we do not aim to give the reader a complete coverage but rather provide an overview of the various steps of these workflows, illustrating with well-validated examples the main aspects and challenges related to the design of the affinity probe, the general experimental workflow and its limitations for the readers to be able to robustly recapitulate these workflows in their own laboratories.

2.2 Small Molecule Phenotypic Mechanism of Action Elucidation

In the past decades, SM TDD has been the dominant approach in the pharmaceutical industry, but in recent years there has been a regained interest in phenotypic drug discovery (PDD) approaches [27]. This transition has been enabled by access to human tissues and human-derived induced pluripotent stem cells (iPSCs) to design complex phenotypic screens with the aim to improve translatability in clinical settings (see Chapter 7 for more details). Well-designed PS campaigns are utilized to identify innovative novel targets but can also generate chemical starting points for further optimization. The translatability of phenotypic cellular assays varies with the type of disease and indication i.e. for infectious diseases, where the end-point phenotype is selective death of infected mammalian cells while sparing non-infected cell pools, translatability and probability of success are high, whereas in other diseases, areas such as neoplasia, metabolism, immunobiology, and neuroscience are notoriously more difficult due to large cellular heterogeneity in genotypes, germlines, and the often time-dependent and subtle phenotypic effects.

Vincent et al. proposed a set of guiding principles for PDD and emphasize three key factors (rule of 3) of the phenotypic assay to consider carefully: the assay system, stimulus, and read-out [7]. In order to increase the probability of clinical translation of compounds and mechanisms identified by PS, assays should strive to replicate the disease of interest in terms of the assay system and stimulus while ideally using a miniaturized version of the clinical end point as the assay read-out.

A variety of approaches are reported for the choice of screening libraries for phenotypic-based screening largely depending on the overall project goal. If the primary objective is to identify novel physiology for known targets and/or explore possibilities for drug repurposing, annotated chemogenomic libraries are commonly used. Several recent articles describe the characterization and applications of such chemogenomic libraries with particular regard to understanding the specificity of the MoA and the curation of nominal target identity (see Chapter 1 for more details) [28]. The Chemical Probes Portal acts as a valuable public repository of such information.

If the identification of novel targets is the goal, diverse collections of novel compounds should be screened, and even though annotated compounds can be reported as selective from selectivity panel screening, they may well hit other targets than those already known. In an analysis by Santos et al., they estimate that molecular targets of known drugs and existing tool compounds constitute only 3% and 6% of the human proteome, although, as they also indicate, this only reflects what has been identified to date [29]. Natural products and their derivatives have lately received a lot of interest to be used in PS campaigns, and they occupy an orthogonal chemical space to the majority of synthetic compounds.

Fragment-based libraries are normally not a natural choice for PDD. However, in a recent paper from the Cravatt laboratory, they demonstrated that low-molecular-mass (~250 Da) fragment-like libraries can yield selective functionally active hits. The important factor in making this fragment-based PS useful, in spite of the reduced binding specificity with low molecular weight (MW) fragments, was that each compound was functionalized with a photoreactive crosslinking moiety and an affinity tag, enabling any functional hits to be rapidly profiled for promiscuity of binding and target identity (see Section 4.4.4 for details of this example) [30]. A similar approach was described in a recent paper from Nomura and coworkers using cysteine-targeted covalent ligand screening [31].

Taken together it is widely recognized that PS provides a useful addition to target-based approaches in drug discovery. Moffat et al. have recently given their industry perspective of opportunities and challenges with PDD [5]. They conclude that rather than being viewed as opposing alternatives, PDD and TDD should be seen as complementary approaches that can together increase the odds of discovering and developing drugs with novel efficacious molecular MoA. The unique promise of PDD is its ability to exploit a disease phenotype and discover novel treatments for diseases for which the root cause is unknown, complex, or multifactorial and for which scientific understanding is insufficient to provide valid molecular targets. However, they stress that PDD should not be regarded simply as an alternative screening technology or as an easy fix to the challenges of clinical attrition rates or R&D productivity. Finally, the authors highlight that determination in determining the molecular MoA, even in a simple cell system, is at the heart of any successful PDD approach and that the identification of the molecular targets of compounds from PDD screens remains a key bottleneck and requires significant resources.

2.3 Quantitative High-Resolution Mass Spectrometry as a Protein Detection Read-Out

Affinity chromatography coupled to the recent technology developments in mass spectrometry (MS) and bioinformatics has provided the most sensitive and unbiased methods for target identification. Quantitative HRMS analytics can be efficiently applied to the identification and quantitation of protein–SM interactions [32–34]. In the context of target identification, typically HRMS proteomic workflows follow a shotgun, or so-called bottom-up, proteomic approach where proteins are digested by trypsin into their sequence peptides to facilitate their separation by high-performance liquid chromatography (HPLC). They are subsequently identified and quantified by consecutive injections into a mass spectrometer and investigated using an ion trap mass analyser followed by dedicated software applications that will reconstitute and identify *in silico* the protein from peptides unique to its sequence. To achieve quantitative information at the peptide level and allow comparison with control experiments, two different quantitative techniques are traditionally used, so-called label-free peptide quantitation or label-based peptide quantitation (see review in quantitative proteomics [34]). The latter can be broadly divided into metabolic and chemical labelling of the trypsin-digested peptides (Figure 2.3).

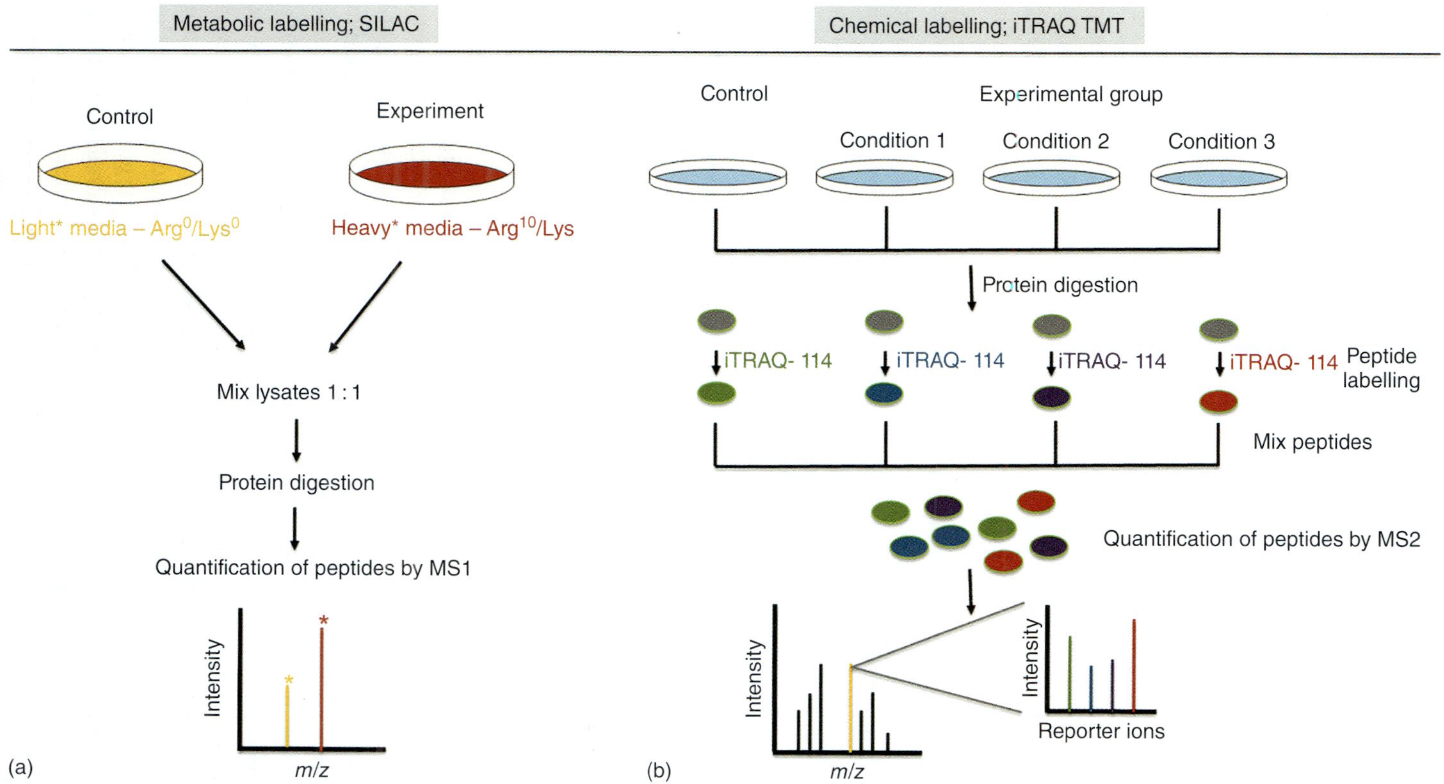

Figure 2.3 Quantitative approaches for chemical proteomic experiments. (a) Stable isotope labelling by amino acids in cell culture (SILAC): cells are cultured with medium containing heavy or light isotope labelled amino acids; cells are treated differently (e.g. probe or vehicle control/untreated) and lysed, and samples combined for all downstream analysis. (b) Chemical labelling approaches (iTRAQ, TMT) in which samples are isotope labelled separately and combined before mass spectrometry.

In metabolic labelling, isotope labelled amino acids are added to the cell culture media and, upon uptake, incorporated into newly synthesized proteins. The use of stable isotope labelling by amino acids in cell culture (SILAC) [35] has been successfully used in chemoproteomic experiments where an unmodified SM is incubated in live cells prior to cell lysis and the resulting protein mixture is affinity enriched with an SM-derived affinity bait to provide unbiased identification of multiple direct as well as indirect targets (Figure 2.3a) [36]. Metabolic labelling has the advantage of allowing sample pooling early in the process, eliminating quantification errors due to sample handling. A disadvantage is that it limits the workflow, as well as the biological sample types, due to requirements of extensive culturing of cells prior to the experiment.

Chemical isotopic labelling offers an alternative to SILAC that adds isotopic tags through an amide bond formation between an *N*-hydroxysuccinimide (NHS) modified reagent and the lysine residues and *N*-termini of peptides generated after cell lysing and post-protein tryptic digestion. Isobaric tags for relative and absolute quantitation (iTRAQ) (Figure 2.3b), coupled with free soluble competitor for elution as a control, has been used to profile kinases enriched by affinity purification with non-selective kinase-binding SMs. Similar chemical labelling reagents are mass differential tags for relative and absolute quantitation (mTRAQ), providing quantitation on precursor ion level, tandem mass tags (TMTs) and stable isotope dimethyl labelling. These chemical labelling strategies are more versatile regarding the type and amounts of biosamples that can be labelled, significantly increasing single experiment multiplexing, as many isotopic tagging reagents are commercially available. Initially these methods were more prone to variation and less accuracy, but MS instrumentation with more sophisticated ion trap analysers has overcome most of these limitations. Cost aside, the fact that labelling requires a chemical reaction and occurs later in the proteomic workflow must be considered when planning experiments since it adds additional steps to the workflow.

Recently, label-free quantitation approaches have gained interest as a suitable alternative because they allow for a more simplistic experimental set-up avoiding expensive and time-consuming labelling protocols. However, labelling-facilitated workflows are often needed in MS-based proteomics due to the high complexity of samples requiring multiple fractionation steps, as well as the possibility to perform inter-experiment comparisons with appropriate references to the relative abundance, and signal intensity, of the identified peptides. Label-free quantitation methods can be used efficiently in affinity chemoproteomic experiments, due to 'simplification by enrichment' of analysed proteome samples. There is no restriction for the number of samples that are to be compared, and it is easier to adapt the experimental design. Disadvantages of label-free quantitation are the dependency on very stable HPLC separation and spray conditions and the requirement of larger amounts of biosamples due to the need for technical replicates. Furthermore, if the enriched sample is complex with hundreds of proteins, several of these can be missed due to the only one-dimensional fraction by liquid chromatography–mass spectrometry (LC-MS) or due to the low peptide coverage in such an experiment. Label-free quantitation has been used extensively in shotgun proteomics, and several examples are reported in the literature for its use in combination with ABPP or affinity-based chemoproteomics.

Once the HRMS experimental workflow is completed, computational proteomic analytical methods allow for the comparison of acquired spectra against databases of theoretical spectra obtained from *in silico* protein digestion utilizing open-access or proprietary software packages such as Mascot (developed by Perkins et al.) [37] or Andromeda [38], part of the freeware MaxQuant package. State-of-the-art HRMS instruments now achieve analytical depths of close to 10 000 protein identifications per biosample, with raw data file sizes on the order of several gigabytes (GB). That is, the raw data file from a TMT multiplexed with 11 distinct peptide labelling reagents, followed by HPLC peptide separation and injections over a 24 hour MS experimental run, will easily surpass 10 GB of size.

2.4 In-Lysate Affinity-Based Chemical Proteomics

Classical affinity-based chemical proteomics, in which binding partners are enriched from cells or tissue ('pulldown') lysates, has been used for target identification for many years and is still evolving in line with the continuous technical advancement of experimental procedures, MS instrumentation, and computational methods [33, 36, 39].

A typical pulldown workflow consists of the following steps:

(1) Preparation of the SM-derived affinity probe with a suitable linker and a chemical moiety that, as a handle, allows its attachment to a solid support ('bead') at an optimal controlled concentration and packing density.
(2) Preparation of cell or tissue lysate by reagent-based (e.g. usually detergents) methods or physical methods such as mechanical disruption, liquid homogenization, high frequency sound waves, freeze/thaw cycles, or manual grinding.
(3) Incubation of the affinity probe-bearing beads with a cell or tissue lysate results in non-covalent SM–protein interactions.
(4) Gentle washing of the beads to remove non-specific stochastically bound proteins.
(5) Strong wash to elute bead-bound proteins followed by trypsin digestion to peptides or on-bead trypsin digestion to recover peptides.
(6) Finally the resulting enriched peptides are separated by HPLC and identified and quantified by MS using the aforementioned software packages.

A vehicle control (often dimethyl sulfoxide [DMSO]) is processed in parallel to provide a benchmark list of proteins that bind non-specifically to the beads. Hits are therefore identified as those proteins enriched over background. A detailed useful protocol has recently been published by Huber and Superti-Furga [40]. Some of the important steps that need to be carefully considered are outlined below. In a modification of the above described workflow, in (1) the chemical handle attached to the SM contains a, usually shorter, linker with a terminal reactive group such as an alkyne or azide moiety amenable to 'click' chemistry. The resulting SM affinity bait is more structurally similar to the 'parent' SM bioactive molecule, which will hopefully retain cell permeability (e.g. otherwise impeded by the presence of the bead). This modification of the protocol allows for a change in the order of steps (2–4) and, importantly, the SM–proteome incubation to occur in live cells with preserved organelle integrity and proteome subcellular localization, followed by lysis and ligation to immobilize the enriched proteins to the bead.

2.4.1 Design of the Affinity Probe

The SM-derived affinity bait of interest is chemically modified installing a linker or spacer and a terminal functional group (i.e. primary or secondary aliphatic amine) that allows the immobilization of the affinity bait by reacting it with a solid support matrix reagent (i.e. NHS-activated agarose). It is imperative that such chemical modification of the 'parent' SM to incorporate a linker or handle is performed in a position that does not alter its phenotypic activity. For this critical aspect of the affinity probe design, sufficient knowledge of the SM structure–activity relationship (SAR) is required.

A variety of linkers have been explored and all share an issue with unspecific target binding to the linker. However, the use of appropriate controls can reduce this effect, and unspecific binding to the compound of interest is still a larger problem. In general, a hydrophilic linker with a linear length of 5–10 atoms is sufficient and beneficial to extend the ligand away from the solid support matrix. Among them, a polyethylene glycol (PEG) linker is one of the most commonly used [41].

Alternative functional groups to aliphatic amines can be used (e.g. alcohols, thiols, carboxylic acids) for immobilization onto a solid matrix, e.g. crosslinked beaded forms of agarose such as Sepharose™ or Affi-Gel 102. In addition, modification of the SM with a chemical tag such as biotin, followed by the use of streptavidin for affinity enrichment, or an alkyne to apply 'click' chemistry can be used for immobilization of the molecule and subsequent enrichment. Several successful examples of using affinity probes including the choice of matrix, the parent compounds, controls, and quantitative MS detection method are shown in Table 2.1.

As highlighted above, it is important to build confidence that the immobilized affinity probe has the same phenotypic activity as the parent compound. This is normally performed by synthesizing a capped precursor affinity probe (with the same functional group being formed when reacted with solid matrix) and test for its activity in the relevant phenotypic assay. An appropriate linker position needs to be defined based on previous SAR information or can be determined based on medicinal chemistry SAR studies on the hit molecule. Alternatively, the attachment of the solid support can be positioned on two or more sites on the molecule, hoping that at least one would result in retained binding capacity. A drawback of not using the parent compound for the pulldown experiment is that the modified affinity probe will most likely have a different binding pattern. However, the immobilized affinity probe, due to its higher MW and more complex structure,

Table 2.1 Examples of bioactive affinity probe precursor structure and matrix of choice in comparison with the parent compound structure.

	A	B	C	D
	Bioactive affinity probe precursor + choice of matrix	**Parent compound (SM)**	**Choice of controls and proteomic method**	**References**
1	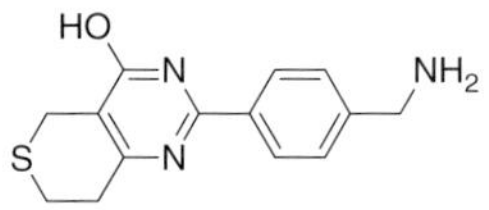 + NHS-activated Sepharose™	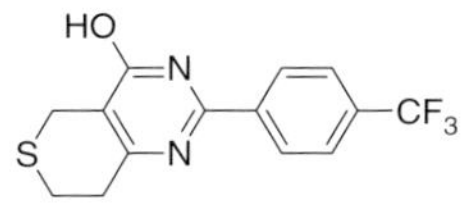	Competition SM + inactive analogue Chemical labelling (iTRAQ)	[42]
2	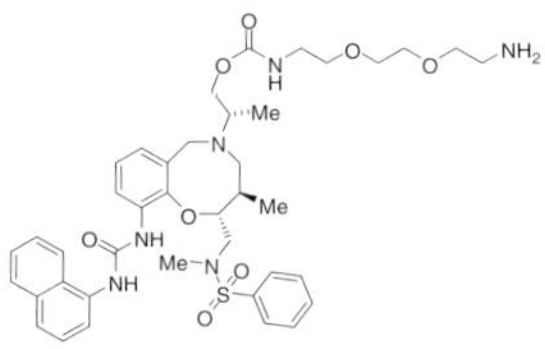 + Affi-Gel 102	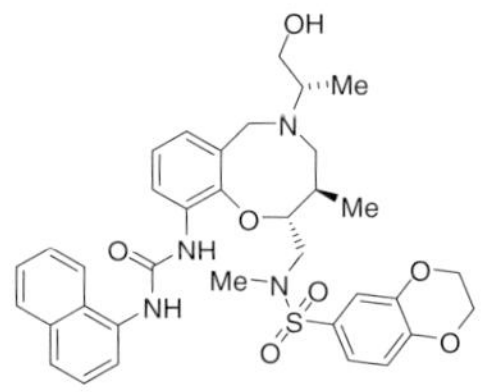	Competition with SM SILAC	[43]
3	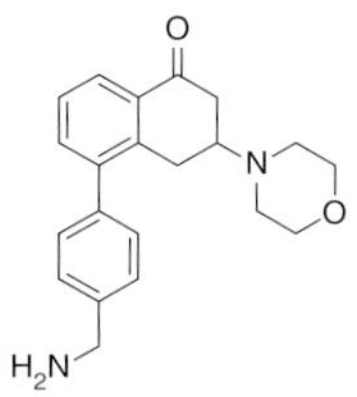 + NHS-activated Sepharose™	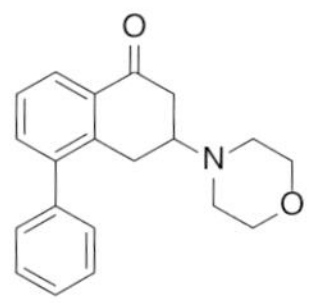	Comparison with inactive analogue TMT labelling	[44]
4	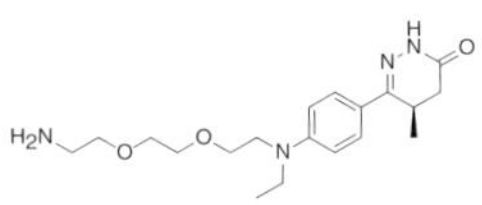 + Affi-Gel 102	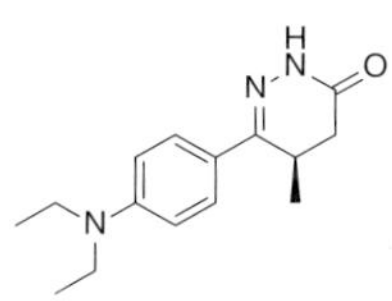	DMSO; competition with SM + inactive analogue iTRAQ	[45]
5	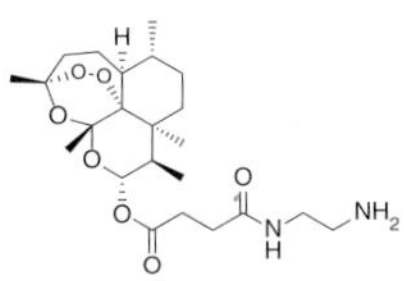 + NHS-activated Sepharose™	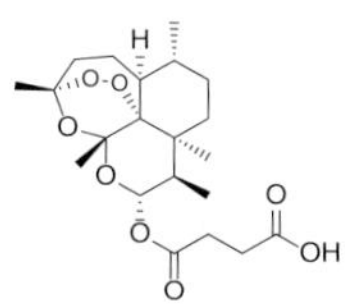		[46]
6	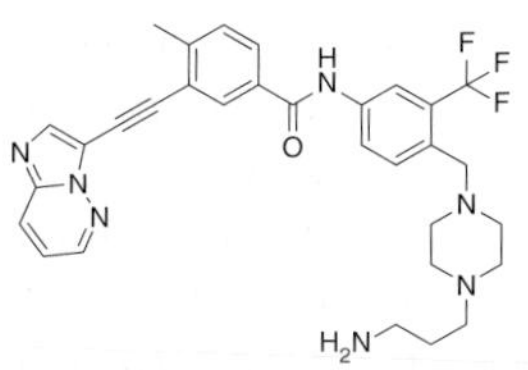 + NHS-activated Sepharose™	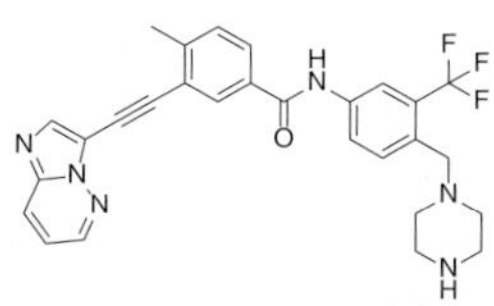	Competition with SM Gel-free one-dimensional LC-MS	[47]

(*continued*)

Table 2.1 (Continued)

	A	B	C	D
	Bioactive affinity probe precursor + choice of matrix	**Parent compound (SM)**	**Choice of controls and proteomic method**	**References**
7	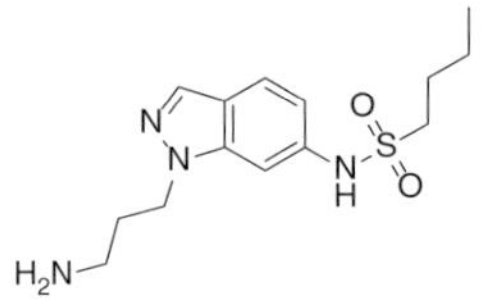 + NHS-activated Sepharose™	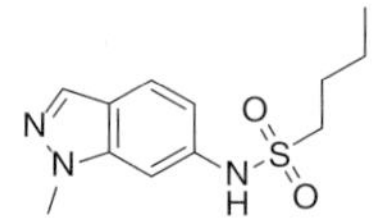	Competition with SM and inactive analogue In-gel quantitative (HRMS); TMT isobaric tags	[48]
8	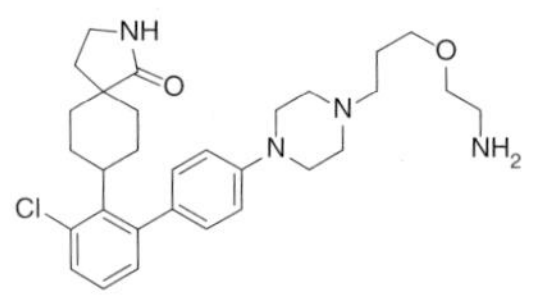 + NHS-activated Sepharose™	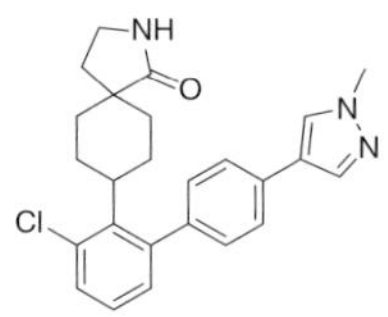	Competition with SM, potent analogue, and inactive analogue	[49]

In column C the choice of controls and the quantitative proteomic method used are stated.

will presumably bind to fewer 'non-specific' targets, thus resulting in a shorter list of potential targets that needs to be confirmed after pulldown.

2.4.2 General Experimental Pulldown Workflow

Considering the fact that cells are packed with several thousands of different proteins that have different biophysical properties and abundances and that the small molecule does not only bind to a single protein but to many proteins non-specifically, it is a challenge to identify the true specific targets from the non-specific background. In addition and as mentioned above, proteins are also enriched through non-specific binding to the linker or bead. Moreover, affinity probes can enrich not only their direct binding targets but also protein complexes associated with those targets, which on the other hand could give useful information about the MoA.

To avoid undesired protein steric hindrance effects and reduce non-specific binding events, special attention must be paid to the loading density of the SM affinity bait on the surface of the solid support matrix in the affinity bead-preparation step. It is never advisable to reach loading capacity as often stated, but rather leave a significant ratio of unreacted bead functional moieties. A bead too 'packed' with SM baits will decrease the amount and diversity of proteins enriched, while a bead too sparsely functionalized with the SM bait runs the risk of affinity enriching a suboptimal amount of protein to survive subsequent washing steps, digestion and MS analysis. Typical ranges of bead loading, measured as micromoles (μM) of affinity bait per millilitre (ml) of settled beads slurry, are 1–4 μM/ml.

Typically, the excess of functional groups present on the solid support need to be 'capped' through a chemical reaction to make them inert and provide a hydrophilic surface with low background binding. In the case of NHS-activated agarose, the excess of NHS moieties are usually reacted with ethanolamine. Upon amide bond formation, the result is a surface with hydroxy groups. When all of the experiments are performed against this background, it becomes more straightforward to identify and minimize unspecific binding events.

In the washing step that follows contacting the affinity bead with the protein lysate, it is difficult to balance specificity and sensitivity. Too gentle washes result in high levels of non-specific proteins being co-eluted with the target, while stringent washes can lead to severe target loss particularly of low abundant or weakly binding partners. Typically for non-covalent affinity enrichment pulldowns, it is advisable to err on the side of gentleness and apply informatics filters to identify (i) co-enriched proteins that are known to interact with each other and (ii) flag 'frequent' unspecific binders that, irrespective of the SM bait, tend to be enriched against the solid support background. Short-lived weak interactions will be lost even with gentle washes, but other protein interactions can be preserved and offer additional insights into the experiment.

A solution to capture weak interactors and interacting complexes is to use crosslinking as part of the pulldown protocol. Another solution is to use affinity probes that covalently link to the proteins (see Section 2.5) although this methodology also has its challenges. A crucial strategy to circumvent the problem is to use carefully designed control experiments coupled with quantitative proteomics. A classical control includes repeating the experiment with an inactive analogue and removing hits enriched by the inactive probe matrix. Alternatively, competition experiments can be used in which free compound is added to either the live cell or the lysate before incubation with the affinity probe, and specifically bound proteins are identified as those with reduced binding in the presence of free compound compared with a vehicle control. Often a combination of control experiments is performed to build evidence of true binding targets.

These strategies were successfully applied by Dale et al. in a study where they identified the targets for compound **1**, which was developed from a micromolar hit in a cell-based phenotypic screen of the Wnt pathway [49, 50]. Knowledge of the SAR gave information about a suitable linker position, and compound **2** was synthesized as a precursor affinity probe. Compound **3**, a closely related potent analogue, and compound **4**, an inactive analogue, were also used in the experimental set-up (Figure 2.4).

Through the careful choice of control experiments, the authors could conclude that **1** was a selective inhibitor for the human mediator complex-associated protein kinases CDK8 and CDK19 with >100-fold selectivity over 291 other kinases. The experimental set-up was as follows: LS174T cells were SILAC encoded (light, medium, or heavy) (Figure 2.5). Cell lysates were incubated with control beads or beads coupled to **2** in the presence of 3 nM to 30 μM of

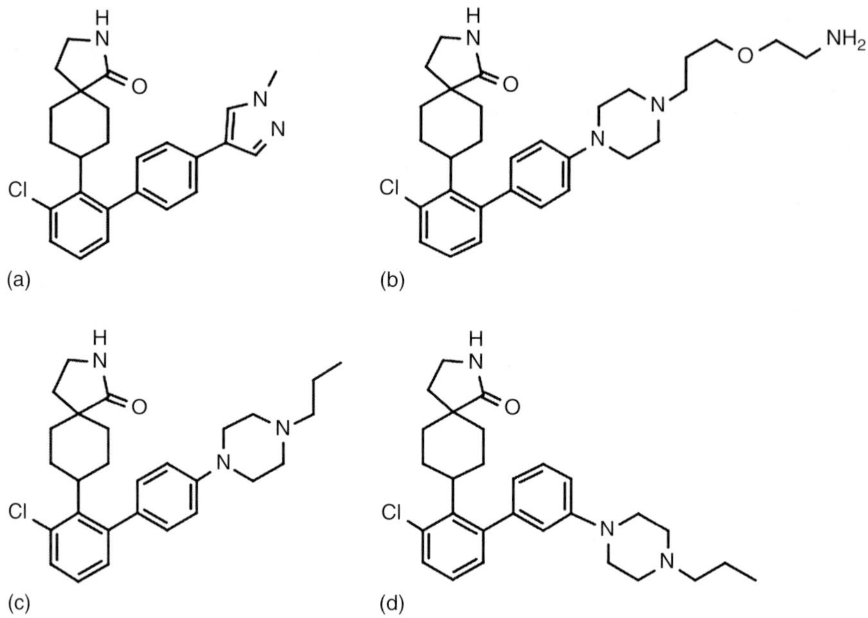

Figure 2.4 Compounds used in chemoproteomic experiment: (a) parent **SM 1** (0.005 μM), (b) precursor affinity probe **2** (0.006 μM), (c) potent close analogue **3** (0.007 μM), and (d) inactive analogue **4** (>5 μM). Source: Dale et al. 2015 [49]. Reproduced with permission of Springer Nature.

1, **3**, or inactive control **4** (Figure 2.4b). After washing, proteins that remained bound were eluted, separated by Sodium Dodecyl Sulphate PolyAcrylamide Gel Electrophoresis (SDS-PAGE), trypsinized, and analysed by LC-MS/MS. In total 53 proteins bound to compound **2** conjugated beads and were displaced by compound **1**. These proteins were ranked according to binding affinity, of which CDK8 and CDK19 exhibited the highest affinities (K_d values = 36 and 102 nM, respectively).

2.4.3 Limitations

In-lysate affinity-based chemical proteomics has been widely and, in many cases, successfully applied for SM target identification and selectivity assessment but as already indicated suffers from several limitations: weak or low abundant true protein binders are sometimes missed (false negatives), and non-specific interactions with high abundant proteins may give rise to false positives if not properly tracked with 'frequent hitter' filters. At the cellular level, lysing affects protein interactions, disruption of subcellular localization of pools of proteins, and loss of 'insoluble' fractions such as multipass transmembrane proteins (i.e. G-protein coupled receptors [GPCRs], ion channels, etc.). On the SM front, limitations usually occur on the modification to the probe to append a linker

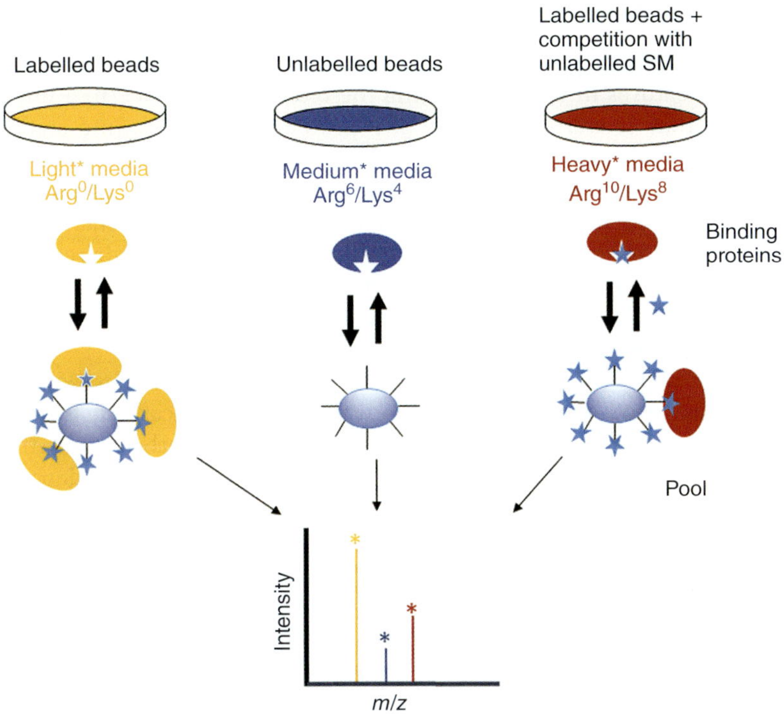

Figure 2.5 SILAC-encoded (light, medium, or heavy) experimental set-up with controls of unlabelled bait and competition with the unlabelled small molecule used in Ref. [49]. Source: Dale et al. 2015 [49]. Reproduced with permission of Springer Nature.

since its installation may alter at least a subset of the native proteome binding to the SM. In addition, in some cases, the chemistry to attach the SM to the solid support may be incompatible with the SAR. For example, in the example of utilizing NHS-activated agarose, if the bioactive SM pharmacophore presents primary or secondary amines required for bioactivity, these would prevent bioorthogonal amide coupling with the N-terminus of the linker, and other chemistries must be tolerated.

A solution that addresses part of these issues is to use cell-permeable photoreactive affinity probes derived from the bioactive investigational SM that, upon mild light-mediated activation, covalently attach to native proteins *in situ*.

2.5 In-Cell Light-Activated Affinity-Based Chemoproteomics

In situ affinity-based chemoproteomics are performed in live cells and use photoreactive affinity ligation (PAL) probes that, upon light-mediated activation at certain wavelengths, covalently react with proteins.

2.5.1 Design of the Reactive Photoaffinity Probe (PAL Probe)

The photoreactive affinity probes typically comprise the following elements: (i) the structural features in the SM exerting the biological activity; (ii) a photoreactive group that converts reversible SM–protein interactions into stable covalent adducts upon irradiation with UV light; and (iii) an alkyne moiety, serving as a sterically minimized reporter allowing conjugation to azide tags by copper-catalysed azide–alkyne cycloaddition (CuAAC) (or 'click') chemistry. The photoreactive group and the alkyne can either be added via a single reagent such as with Yao's minimalist linkers that incorporate both the photoreactive moiety and the 'clickable' reporter [51] or attached to different suitable sites on the parent compound based on known SAR information.

The most commonly used photoreactive groups are benzophenones, azides, and aryl or alkyl diazirines that undergo a diradical, nitrene, and carbene formation upon UV irradiation, respectively (Table 2.2). They all have their strengths and limitations [52–55], and the matter of choice seems highly context dependent. However, there has been a recent focus in alkyl diazirines, probably influenced by improvements in synthetic methodology, access to convenient building blocks, their small size, and the relatively undamaging wavelengths required for their activation, and this is in spite of their disadvantage in forming rearrangement side reactions upon irradiation. Another favourable photoreactive group is the trifluoromethyl phenyl diazirine due to the fact that a significant proportion of drug-like compounds contain phenyl rings and incorporation into a bioactive motif is often possible [53].

Similar to affinity probes described in Section 2.4.1, there is a need to confirm that the photoreactive affinity probe has the same or similar biological activity as the parent compound in live cells. The advantage here is that the probe itself can be tested in the relevant assay compared to evaluating a linker-bearing precursor compound. Table 2.3 highlights several examples of photoaffinity probes and the parent compound. Also disclosed is the choice of controls and quantitative proteomic approach.

2.5.2 General Experimental Workflow

A decade ago MacKinnon and Taunton described a general protocol for diazirine photocrosslinking and click chemistry that can be adapted to a variety of systems and photoaffinity probe designs [62]. At a high level, the experimental workflow consists of the following steps: (i) Cells are incubated with photoreactive affinity probes to allow the probes to associate with their targets. The time and condition for probe incubation should reflect the conditions of the biological assays being used to detect the phenotypic response of the SM. In terms of concentrations of the probe, typically these will be incubated at high concentrations (IC_{90}) to ensure high target occupancy. (ii) Samples are then irradiated with a specific wavelength of light to activate the photoreactive group and covalently crosslink with proximate proteins. (iii) Cells are lysed to expose the PAL probe–protein

Table 2.2 Commonly used photoreactive groups and their reaction under UV light.

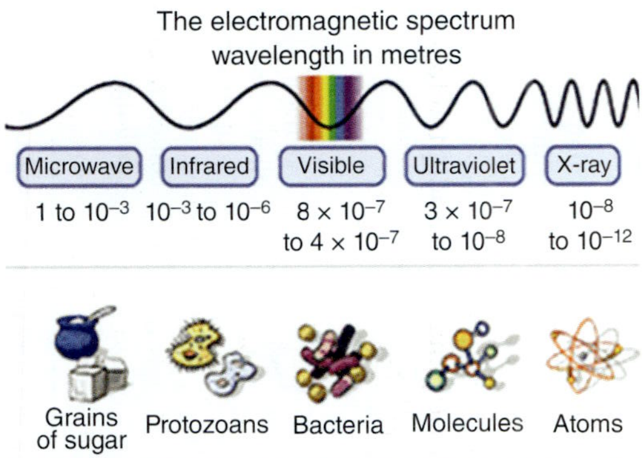	**Aryl azides** 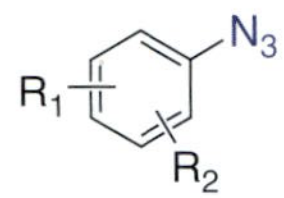	**Benzophenone** Color Fig 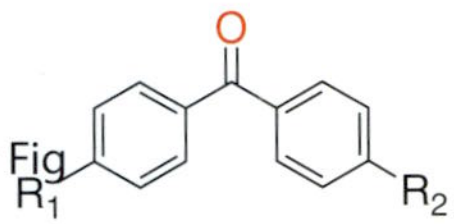	**Diazirines** 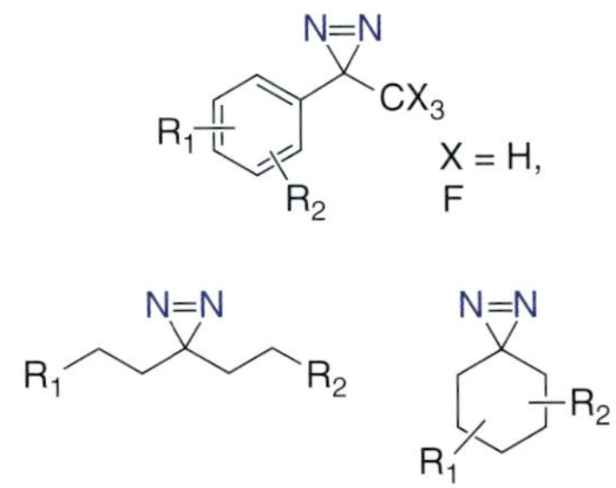
$h\nu$ (nM)	254	360	360
Reactive species	Nitrene	C–O bi-radical	Carbene
Bond	Irreversible	Reversible	Irreversible
Live cell compatibility	Toxic	Biocompatible	Biocompatible
Size	++	–	+++
Synthetic versatility	+	–	+++

Table 2.3 Examples of photoaffinity probes in comparison with the parent small molecule (SM).

	A Bioactive affinity probe	B Parent compound (SM)	C Controls and quantitative proteomic method	D References
1	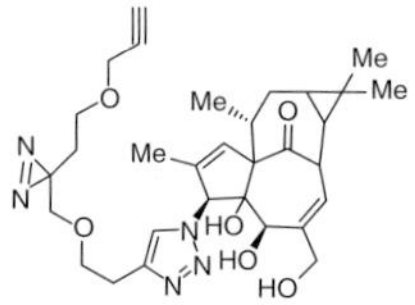	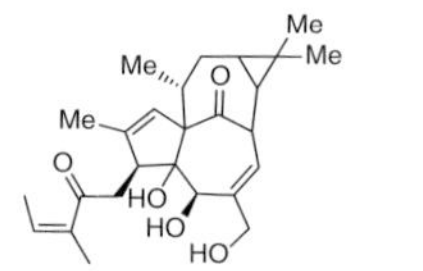	No UV or competition with SM SILAC	[56]
2	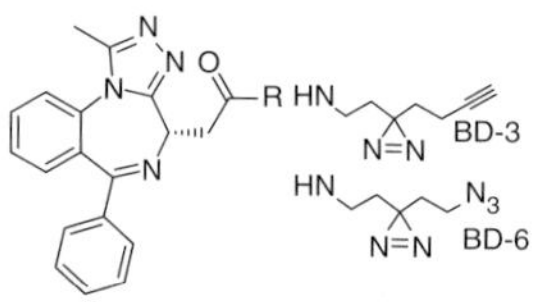	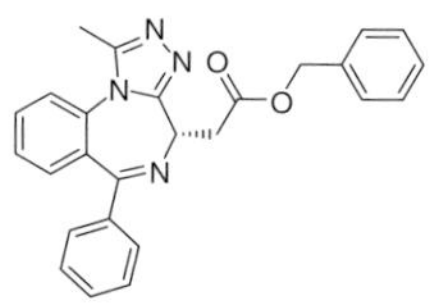	No UV or competition with SM SILAC	[52]
3	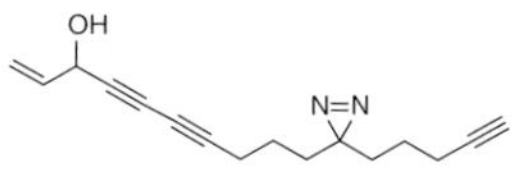	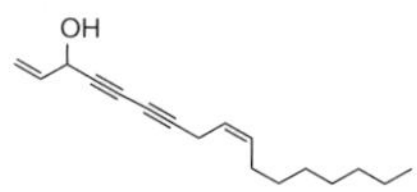	DMSO control SILAC	[57]
4	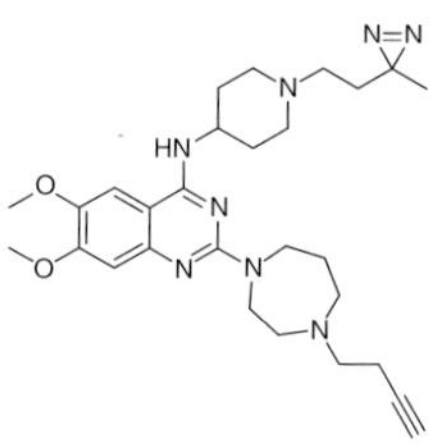	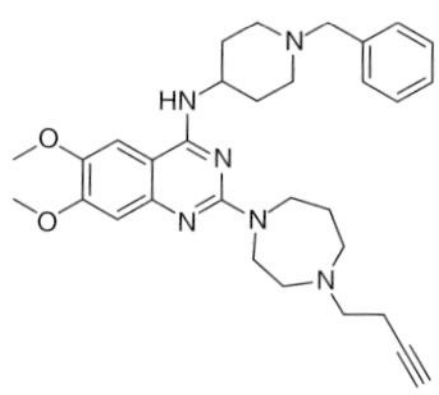	DMSO control Label-free	[58]
5	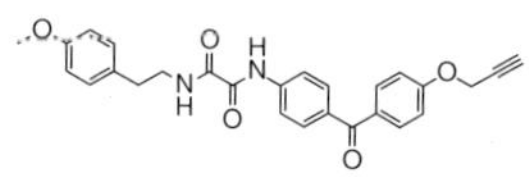	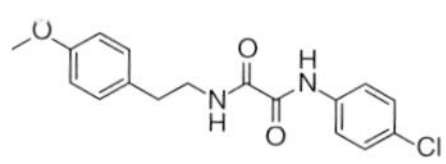	Competition with SM Label-free	[59]
6	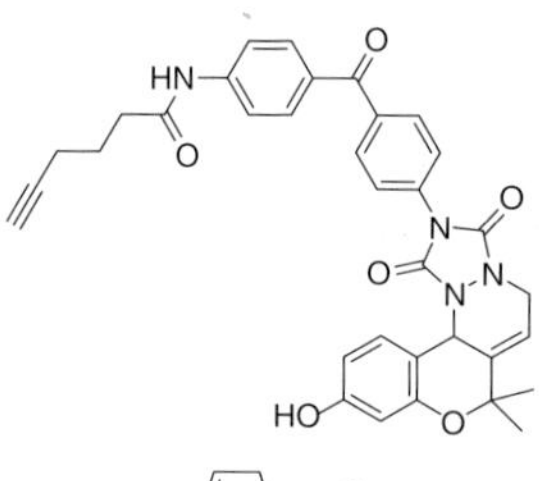	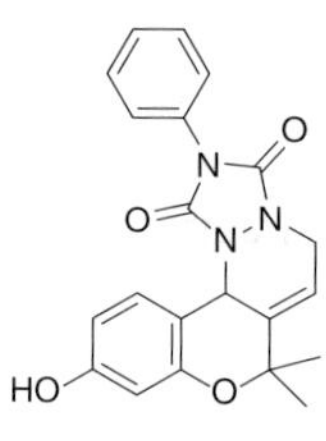	Competition with SM Label-free	[60]
7	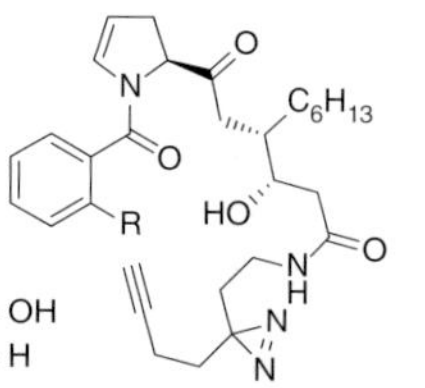 (a) R = OH (b) R = H	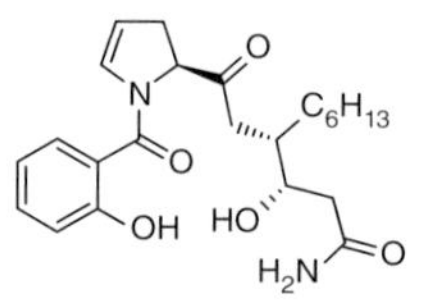	Inactive analogue photoaffinity probe Competition with SM Dimethyl-isotope labelling	[61]

Also enclosed are controls used and the quantitative proteomic method.

conjugates that will undergo click chemistry conjugation with the reporter tag moiety for affinity enrichment. (iv) Labelled and tagged SM–protein covalent adducts are separated from the rest of the proteome by affinity purification using the reporter/affinity tag. (v) Affinity-enriched proteins undergo digestion to produce peptide fragments. (vi) The peptide fragments are sequenced using MS to determine the identity of the isolated proteins.

2.5.3 Limitations

It is often the case that the observed activity of the parent unmodified SM probe is greater than the corresponding photoaffinity probe analogue, usually measured by phenotypic potency. One can speculate that such bioactivity disparity could be extrapolated to differences in binding affinity towards protein binders and the potency shift due to interference of the photolabile moiety on the SM–protein interactions. Intuitively, it is ideal to aim for the position of the photoreactive functional group to be optimized for productive modification of the protein backbone, but this is not always feasible due to lack of binding information. Even in cases where the SM–protein interactions are known or can be modelled (for example, with photocrosslinking experiments aimed to map SM–protein binding sites), such optimization is not always possible without altering the pharmacophore properties and thus binding. Paradoxically, positioning of the PAL moiety in a region of the SM that allows retention of bioactivity, such as a solvent-facing region of the protein–SM interaction, on the other hand, poses a risk of minimal reaction with the target protein (unproductive quenching) or the enhancement of non-specific crosslinking of bystander or high abundant 'sticky' proteins. In this second scenario, off-target labelling is usually exacerbated particularly when the probe is incubated at concentrations much higher than those needed to maximize target occupancy. To distinguish between background and specific labelling, several control experiments can be applied. Sometimes it is useful to perform a competition experiment incubating cells with increasing concentration of the parent unlabelled SM, co-incubating a constant concentration of the PAL probe, to outcompete the PAL probe from the target prior to photo-irradiation. In addition, Sieber and coworkers recently suggested the use of a minimalist photoreactive probe without the binding moiety to identify photocrosslinker-specific off-targets [63].

2.6 Target Validation and Mode of Action

Once a list of potential protein hits has been identified, the challenging follow-up task is to validate which ones are true binders that link SM modulation to the phenotypic response. Typically, the corroboration of chemoproteomic observations is a two-step process that involves validating binding and phenotype recapitulation via orthogonal methods (see also Chapter 8). There are several ways to approach this challenge, and the choice often depends on pre-existing knowledge as well as the biological context. As we briefly discussed in Section 2.2 of this chapter, in some cases, such as for infectious disease phenotypes, the cellular models are well characterized, and genetic tools allow the validation to be streamlined, for example, relying on growing resistant mutant strains for the proteins identified during MoA elucidation; when the mutation cancels the effect of the bioactive SM, one can confidently state that the interaction of the SM with the wild-type protein was the driver for the cellular phenotype.

More generally, common ways to confirm SM–protein binding involve the use of recombinant proteins and biophysical technologies such as isothermal titration calorimetry (ITC), surface plasmon resonance (SPR), and differential scanning fluorimetry (DSF) [64] or the use of a cell-based thermal shift assay (CETSA) (see Chapter 5 for more details) enabled with an antibody against the target protein. Subsequently, the most common approach to demonstrate that target binding is involved in the pathway causing the phenotypic response is to use genome editing (e.g. CRISPR/Cas9) or RNA interference applied to the differentially enriched proteins and evaluate whether cellular knockouts (or knockdowns) phenocopy the effect of the parent compound (see Chapter 9 for more details). To firmly demonstrate that a phenotypic response is due to target binding, several representatives from the chemical series with different potencies in the cell assay can be evaluated to see if there is a correlation with in cell target engagement. An interesting recent approach utilized the CETSA method for target engagement with imaging as a read-out in adherent cells [65]. A simultaneous monitoring of downstream relevant events or biomarkers to the phenotypic response would enable a direct measure of target engagement coupled to phenotypic effect.

In the earlier described work of Dale et al., the authors initially identified 53 potential target proteins binding to the affinity matrix **2** (Figure 2.4) [49]. Of these, CDK8 and CDK19 exhibited by far the highest affinities in a displacement assay (K_d = 36 and 102 nM, respectively) together with additional subunits of the overall CDK mediator complex. Competition with potent analogue **3** also identified CDK8 and CD19 as high-affinity specific binding proteins. In contrast, the structurally similar but inactive analogue **4** failed to compete with CDK8 and CDK19 or any of the subunits of the mediator complex. Moreover, both **1** and **3** interacted with an additional three unrelated protein complexes, but since the inactive analogue **4** also interacted with the same three proteins in the same potency range, it was regarded unlikely that these contributed to the cellular activity. Altogether this shows that intelligent use of control experiments using both active and inactive close analogues in competition could in this case single out few potential targets to be validated. Confirmation of the binding was performed using SPR experiments and finally through co-crystallization studies. The involvement of CDK8 and CDK19 in the phenotypic cell activity (Wnt signalling) was confirmed by among other experiments comparing the induced transcriptional signature of compound **1** with the transcriptional signature obtained from gene silencing of CDK8 and CDK19. Finally, *in vivo* activity of **1** in Wnt-dependent tumours could be demonstrated.

2.7 Concluding Remarks

Elucidation of the MoA and cellular targets of candidate compounds is essential for chemical biology research and drug discovery and development. Although the growing trend towards unbiased PS strategies in live cells and organisms has the potential to identify new aspects of biology, the target-naïve character of these screens results in what is commonly known as 'black-box pharmacology' and will require follow-up methods for elucidating the MoA. The deconvolution of the MoA of SMs remains a major challenge, and no one method can exquisitely reveal all types of drug efficacy targets, and combinations are often required to be successful. As described, useful methodologies can be grouped into (i) affinity-based methods, identifying physical interactors of 'targets' (both label-free methods and methods requiring SM modified affinity probes); (ii) cellular profiling methods, which use SM-induced biological signatures (morphological, transcriptional, and protein profiling); (iii) knowledge-based approaches, using reference collections of compounds with known targets and MoA; and (iv) genetic approaches, identifying genes relevant for the compound-induced phenotype that does not only inform about binding targets but also other components involved in the MoA.

This chapter has focused on affinity enrichment-based methods using modified SMs as a bait to identify the direct physical interactors. Although label-free methods are preferred because they do not require time- and resource-intensive modification of the original compound, affinity purification-based methods have their advantages: the affinity enrichment considerably decreases the complexity of proteome analysis, and the modified SM, with a similar level of cellular potency, is likely to have fewer off-targets due to its more complex structure, resulting in a shorter list of potential targets to validate.

Important success factors for affinity-based chemoproteomics include careful optimization of cellular potency (ideally nanomolar activity) including thorough understanding of SAR and with minimal loss of potency for the modified affinity reagent. In addition, the use of negative control SMs and repetition of experiments in 'insensitive' cell lines of biosamples where the SM does not show a phenotype are informative. Note, however, that the protein of interest may still be expressed, perhaps in different cellular compartments or forming different protein complexes, which may confuse the interpretation. Moreover, the importance of developing bioinformatics tools for pathway analysis, flagging false positives, and inter-experiment comparisons (e.g. comparing in-lysate versus PAL or comparing different cell lines) is emphasized.

Finally it is for a good reason that a multitude of approaches to target deconvolution and MoA exist and are actively being developed. As already stressed, no one method can exquisitely reveal all types of efficacy targets or pinpoint the exact MoA. Future developments and trends covering methods for PDD and target deconvolution will be exciting and necessary to follow, and importantly, the continuous addition of new compound–target relationships should be integrated into core knowledge-based tools and used to feed back into the PDD machinery. This will support the future identification of new targets and help enable target validation studies.

References

1 Swinney, D.C. and Anthony, J. (2011). How were new medicines discovered? *Nat. Rev. Drug Discovery* 10 (7): 507–519.

2 Moffat, J.G., Rudolph, J., and Bailey, D. (2014). Phenotypic screening in cancer drug discovery – past, present and future. *Nat. Rev. Drug Discovery* 13 (8): 588–602.

3 Haasen, D., Schopfer, U., Antczak, C. et al. (2017). How phenotypic screening influenced drug discovery: lessons from five years of practice. *ASSAY Drug Dev. Technol.* 15 (6): 239–246.

4 Eder, J., Sedrani, R., and Wiesmann, C. (2014). The discovery of first-in-class drugs: origins and evolution. *Nat. Rev. Drug Discovery* 13 (8): 577–587.

5 Moffat, J.G., Vincent, F., Lee, J.A. et al. (2017). Opportunities and challenges in phenotypic drug discovery: an industry perspective. *Nat. Rev. Drug Discovery* 16 (8): 531–543.

6 Lee, J.A. and Berg, E.L. (2013). Neoclassic drug discovery: the case for lead generation using phenotypic and functional approaches. *J. Biomol. Screening* 18 (10): 1143–1155.

7 Vincent, F., Loria, P., Pregel, M. et al. (2015). Developing predictive assays: the phenotypic screening "rule of 3". *Sci. Transl. Med.* 7 (293): 293ps15.

8 Horvath, P., Aulner, N., Bickle, M. et al. (2016). Screening out irrelevant cell-based models of disease. *Nat. Rev. Drug Discovery* 15 (11): 751–769.

9 Jenmalm Jensen, A., Martinez Molina, D., and Lundbäck, T. (2015). CETSA: a target engagement assay with potential to transform drug discovery. *Future Med. Chem.* 7 (8): 975–978.

10 Imming, P., Sinning, C., and Meyer, A. (2006). Drugs, their targets and the nature and number of drug targets. *Nat. Rev. Drug Discovery* 5 (10): 821–834.

11 Apsel, B., Blair, J.A., Gonzalez, B.Z. et al. (2008). Targeted polypharmacology: discovery of dual inhibitors of tyrosine and phosphoinositide kinases. *Nat. Chem. Biol.* 4 (11): 691–699.

12 Lakemeyer, M., Zhao, W., Mandl, F.A. et al. (2018). Thinking outside the box – novel antibacterials to tackle the resistance crisis. *Angew. Chem. Int. Ed.* 57: 14440–14475.

13 Delves, B.J., Miguel-Blanco, C., Matthews, H. et al. (2018). A high throughput screen for next-generation leads targeting malaria parasite transmission. *Nat. Commun.* 9: 3805.

14 Gamo, F., Sanz, L.M., Vidal, J. et al. (2010). Thousands of chemical starting points for antimalarial lead identification. *Nature* 465 (7296): 305–310.

15 Wawer, M.J., Li, K., Gustafsdottir, S.M. et al. (2014). Toward performance-diverse small-molecule libraries for cell-based phenotypic screening using multiplexed high-dimensional profiling. *Proc. Natl. Acad. Sci. U.S.A.* 111 (30): 10911–10916.

16 Subramanian, A., Narayan, R., Corsello, S.M. et al. (2017). A next generation connectivity map: L1000 platform and the first 1,000,000 profiles. *Cell* 171 (6): 1437–1452.

17 King, F.J., Selinger, D.W., Mapa, F.A. et al. (2009). Pathway reporter assays reveal small molecule mechanisms of action. *J. Assoc. Lab. Autom.* 14 (6): 374–382.

18 Zhang, J.D., Küng, E., Boess, F. et al. (2015). Pathway reporter genes define molecular phenotypes of human cells. *BMC Genomics* 16: 342.

19 Nijman, S.M. (2015). Functional genomics to uncover drug mechanism of action. *Nat. Chem. Biol.* 11 (12): 942–948.

20 Velagapudi, S.P., Cameron, M.D., Haga, C.L. et al. (2016). Design of a small molecule against an oncogenic noncoding RNA. *Proc. Natl. Acad. Sci. U.S.A.* 113 (21): 5898–5903.

21 Liu, Y., Patricelli, M.P., and Cravatt, B.F. (1999). Activity-based protein profiling: the serine hydrolases. *Proc. Natl. Acad. Sci. U.S.A.* 96 (26): 14694–14699.

22 Schűrmann, M., Janning, P., Ziegler, S., and Waldmann, H. (2016). Small-molecule target engagement in cells. *Cell Chem. Biol.* 23 (4): 435–441.

23 Moellering, R.E. and Cravatt, B.F. (2012). How chemoproteomics can enable drug discovery and development. *Chem. Biol.* 19 (1): 11–22.

24 Schirle, M., Bantscheff, M., and Kuster, B. (2012). Mass spectrometry-based proteomics in preclinical drug discovery. *Chem. Biol.* 19 (1): 72–84.

25 Schenone, M., Dančík, V., Wagner, B.K., and Clemons, P.A. (2013). Target identification and mechanism of action in chemical biology and drug discovery. *Nat. Chem. Biol.* 9 (4): 232–240.

26 Wright, M.H. and Sieber, S.A. (2016). Chemical proteomics approaches for identifying the cellular targets of natural products. *Nat. Prod. Rep.* 33 (5): 681–708.

27 Plowright, A.T. and Drowley, L. (2017). Phenotypic screening. In: *Platform Technologies in Drug Discovery and Development*, Annual Reviews in Medicinal Chemistry, vol. 50 (ed. R.A. Goodnow Jr.,), 263–299. Cambridge, MA: Academic Press.

28 Jones, L.H. and Bunnage, M.E. (2017). Applications of chemogenomic library screening in drug discovery. *Nat. Rev. Drug Discovery* 16 (4): 285–296.

29 Santos, R., Ursu, O., Gaulton, A. et al. (2016). A comprehensive map of molecular drug targets. *Nat. Rev. Drug Discovery* 16 (1): 19–34.

30 Parker, C.G., Galmozzi, A., Wang, Y. et al. (2017). Ligand and target discovery by fragment-based screening in human cells. *Cell* 168 (3): 527–541.

31 Counihan, J.L., Wiggenhorn, A.L., Anderson, K.E., and Nomura, D.K. (2018). Chemoproteomics-enabled covalent ligand screening reveals ALDH3A1 as a lung cancer therapy target. *ACS Chem. Biol.* 13 (8): 1970–1977.

32 Ong, S.E. and Mann, M. (2005). Mass spectrometry–based proteomics turns quantitative. *Nat. Chem. Biol.* 1 (5): 252–262.

33 Rix, U. and Superti-Furga, G. (2009). Target profiling of small molecules by chemical proteomics. *Nat. Chem. Biol.* 5 (9): 616–624.

34 Domon, B. and Aebersold, R. (2010). Options and considerations when selecting a quantitative proteomics strategy. *Nat. Biotechnol.* 28 (7): 710–721.

35 Ong, S., Blagoev, B., Kratchmarova, I. et al. (2002). Stable isotope labeling by amino acids in cell culture, SILAC, as a simple and accurate approach to expression proteomics. *Mol. Cell. Proteomics* 1 (5): 376–386.

36 Ong, S.-E., Schenone, M., Margolin, A.A. et al. (2009). Identifying the proteins to which small-molecule probes and drugs bind in cells. *Proc. Natl. Acad. Sci. U.S.A.* 106 (12): 4617–4622.

37 Perkins, D.N., Pappin, D.J., Creasy, D.M., and Cottrell, J.S. (1999). Probability-based protein identification by searching sequence databases using mass spectrometry data. *Electrophoresis* 20 (18): 3551–3567.

38 Cox, J., Neuhauser, N., Michalski, A. et al. (2011). Andromeda: a peptide search engine integrated into the MaxQuant environment. *J. Proteome Res.* 10 (4): 1794–1805.

39 Ziegler, S., Pries, V., Hedberg, C., and Waldmann, H. (2013). Target identification for small bioactive molecules: finding the needle in the haystack. *Angew. Chem. Int. Ed.* 52 (10): 2744–2792.

40 Huber, K.V.M. and Superti-Furga, G. (2016). Profiling of small molecules by chemical proteomics. In: *Proteomics in Systems Biology*, Methods in Molecular Biology, vol. 1394 (ed. J. Reinders), 211–218. New York, NY: Humana Press.

41 Sato, S., Kwon, Y., Kamisuki, S. et al. (2007). Polyproline-rod approach to isolating protein targets of bioactive small molecules: isolation of a new target of indomethacin. *J. Am. Chem. Soc.* 129 (4): 873–880.

42 Huang, S.M.A., Mishina, Y.M., Liu, S. et al. (2009). Tankyrase inhibition stabilizes axin and antagonizes Wnt signalling. *Nature* 461 (7264): 614–620.

43 Chou, D.H., Vetere, A., Choudhary, A. et al. (2015). Kinase-independent small-molecule inhibition of JAK-STAT signaling. *J. Am. Chem. Soc.* 137 (24): 7929–7934.

44 Dittmann, A., Werner, T., Chung, C.W. et al. (2014). The commonly used PI3-kinase probe LY294002 is an inhibitor of BET bromodomains. *ACS Chem. Biol.* 9 (2): 495–502.

45 De Waal, L., Lewis, T.A., Rees, M.G. et al. (2015). Identification of cancer-cytotoxic modulators of PDE3A by predictive chemogenomics. *Nat. Chem. Biol.* 12 (2): 102–108.

46 Li, J., Casteels, T., Frogne, T. et al. (2017). Artemisinins target $GABA_A$ receptor signaling and impair α cell identity. *Cell* 168 (1–2): 86–100.

47 Fauster, A., Rebsamen, M., Huber, K.V.M. et al. (2015). A cellular screen identifies ponatinib and pazopanib as inhibitors of necroptosis. *Cell Death Dis.* 6 (5): e1767.

48 Abrahams, K.A., Chung, C.W., Ghidelli-Disse, S. et al. (2016). Identification of KasA as the cellular target of an anti-tubercular scaffold. *Nat. Commun.* 7: 12581.

49 Dale, T., Clarke, P.A., Esdar, C. et al. (2015). A selective chemical probe for exploring the role of CDK8 and CDK19 in human disease. *Nat. Chem. Biol.* 11 (12): 973–980.

50 Mallinger, A., Crumpler, S., Pichowicz, M. et al. (2015). Discovery of potent, orally bioavailable, small-molecule inhibitors of WNT signaling from a cell-based pathway screen. *J. Med. Chem.* 58 (4): 1717–1735.

51 Li, Z., Wang, D., Li, L. et al. (2014). "Minimalist" cyclopropene-containing photo-cross-linkers suitable for live-cell imaging and affinity-based protein labeling. *J. Am. Chem. Soc.* 136 (28): 9990–9998.

52 Pan, S., Jang, S.-Y., Wang, D. et al. (2017). A suite of "minimalist" photo-crosslinkers for live-cell imaging and chemical proteomics: case study with BRD4 inhibitors. *Angew. Chem. Int. Ed.* 56 (39): 11816–11821.

53 Hill, J.R. and Robertson, A.A.B. (2018). Fishing for drug targets: a focus on diazirine photoaffinity probe synthesis. *J. Med. Chem.* 61 (16): 6945–6963.

54 Peng, Z. and Chang, C. (2015). Recent developments and applications of clickable photoprobes in medicinal chemistry and chemical biology. *Future Med. Chem.* 7 (16): 2143–2171.

55 Smith, E. and Collins, I. (2015). Photoaffinity labeling in target- and binding-site identification. *Future Med. Chem.* 7 (2): 159–183.

56 Parker, C.G., Kuttru, C.A., Galmozzi, A. et al. (2017). Chemical proteomics identifies SLC25A20 as a functional target of the ingenol class of actinic keratosis drugs. *ACS Cent. Sci.* 3 (12): 1276–1285.

57 Heydenreuter, W., Kunold, E., and Sieber, S.A. (2015). Alkynol natural products target ALDH2 in cancer cells by irreversible binding to the active site. *Chem. Commun.* 51 (87): 15784–15787.

58 Lubin, A.S., Rueda-Zubiaurre, A., Matthews, H. et al. (2018). Development of a photo-cross-linkable diaminoquinazoline inhibitor for target identification in *Plasmodium falciparum*. *ACS Infect. Dis.* 4 (4): 523–530.

59 Theodoropoulos, P.C., Gonzales, S.S., Winterton, S.E. et al. (2016). Discovery of tumor-specific irreversible inhibitors of stearoyl CoA desaturase. *Nat. Chem. Biol.* 12 (4): 218–225.

60 Lee, S., Nam, Y., Koo, J.Y. et al. (2014). A small molecule binding HMGB1 and HMGB2 inhibits microglia-mediated neuroinflammation. *Nat. Chem. Biol.* 10 (12): 1055–1060.

61 Keohane, C.E., Steele, A.D., Fetzer, C. et al. (2018). Promysalin elicits species-selective inhibition of *Pseudomonas aeruginosa* by targeting succinate dehydrogenase. *J. Am. Chem. Soc.* 140 (5): 1774–1782.

62 Mackinnon, A.L. and Taunton, J. (2009). Target identification by diazirine photo-cross-linking and click chemistry. *Curr. Protoc. Chem. Biol.* 1 (415): 55–73.

63 Kleiner, P., Heydenreuter, W., Stahl, M. et al. (2017). A whole proteome inventory of background photocrosslinker binding. *Angew. Chem. Int. Ed.* 56 (5): 1396–1401.

64 Renaud, J., Chung, C., Danielson, U.H. et al. (2016). Biophysics in drug discovery. *Nat. Rev. Drug Discovery* 15 (10): 679–698.

65 Axelsson, H., Almqvist, H., Otrocka, M. et al. (2018). In situ target engagement studies in adherent cells. *ACS Chem. Biol.* 13 (4): 942–950.

3

Activity-Based Protein Profiling

Nattawadee Panyain, Cassandra R. Kennedy, Ryan T. Howard, and Edward W. Tate

Imperial College London, Department of Chemistry, Molecular Sciences Research Hub, White City Campus, 80 Wood Lane, London, W12 0BZ, UK

3.1 Introduction

The drug discovery pipeline can be limited by a large investment of time and money as well as the human and technological resources necessary to drive the process. Small molecule drug discovery is often underpinned by *in vitro* screening of the interaction between the target, which could be DNA, RNA, or protein, and potential ligands [1]. From this screening, compounds that exhibit high affinity and selectivity for the target are optimized and hit series taken forward for further validation using biochemical and cell-based assays. Although these assays can provide basic information such as binding affinity and selectivity of the molecule, knowledge of a compound's complete interaction profile inside a living biological system is still absent. Understanding these interactions can validate the molecule's mechanism of action and is especially important in cases where the molecule was identified via phenotypic screening, meaning the likely biomolecular target is not yet known. Furthermore, uncovering any off-target interactions could be crucial in preventing costly late-stage failure of the molecules [2]. To help address this limitation, proteomic analysis has become a powerful tool to interrogate the proteome of biological systems of interest.

Proteomics is the study of the full complement of proteins in a sample, including, but not limited to, their identification and quantification. The development of key proteomic tools has benefitted drug discovery and medical research. One of these key tools is liquid chromatography–mass spectrometry (LC-MS) [3, 4] coupled to chemical probes that enable the accurate assessment of changes in protein levels and activity in endogenous cells or tissues. Expressed protein level does not necessarily correlate with protein activity due to protein post-translational modifications (PTMs) and protein–protein interactions. To assess the activity profile of proteins, a method called activity-based protein profiling (ABPP) has been widely established to directly identify and characterize the catalytic activity in complex native systems [4–6]. This ABPP approach has been pioneered and developed by several groups including Cravatt, Boygo, and Tate [4, 5, 7–10].

Target Discovery and Validation: Methods and Strategies for Drug Discovery,
First Edition. Edited by Alleyn T. Plowright.

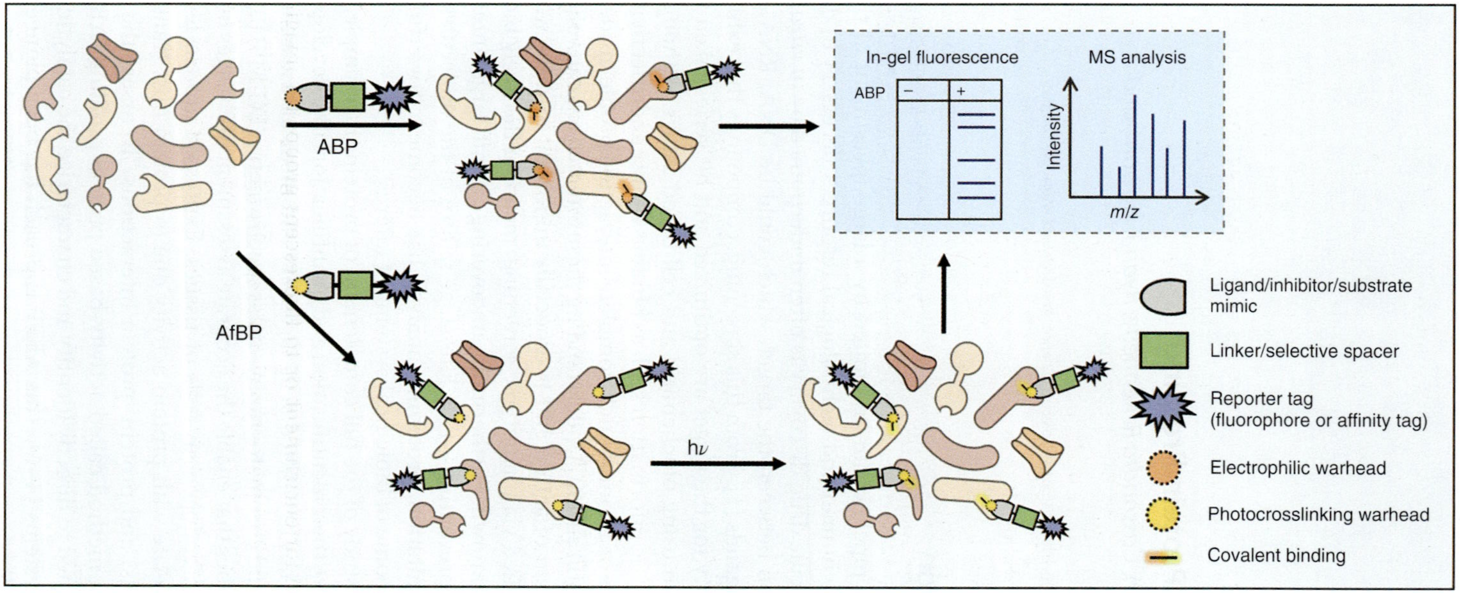

Figure 3.1 Activity-based probes (ABPs) versus affinity-based probes (AfBPs). ABPs covalently bind to the active site of target proteins, whereas AfBPs bind to the active site before covalent conjugation is achieved through a photocrosslinking warhead. Both ABPs and AfBPs contain the following key components: warhead moieties, linker groups, and reporter tags.

ABPP uses small molecule probes, termed activity-based probes (ABPs), which are designed from irreversible inhibitors or suicide substrates of the target. ABPs covalently bind to the catalytically active site of the target protein through the functional reactivity of the enzyme (Figure 3.1) [11]. By attaching a suitable reporter, with fluorescent and/or biotin affinity tags, to the ABP, the probe–protein complexes are further analysed by gel-based and LC-MS approaches. In addition to profiling the activity of target proteins and enzymes [4, 7, 12], ABPs have been used for the characterization of protein functions in disease states, the discovery and development of enzyme inhibitors [8, 13–15], target identification (ID) for ligands [16–18], and the study of enzyme activity and localization in living organisms [19, 20].

Recently, affinity-based protein profiling (AfBPP) has been widely developed for target ID and quantification of both non-covalent and reversible inhibitors and drugs [5, 21]. Unlike ABPs, affinity-based probes (AfBPs) are designed from *reversible* inhibitors and contain an additional chemical moiety that adds a photoreactive group. After non-covalent engagement of the target protein(s), this group can be converted to a hyper-reactive intermediate, such as a carbene or a radical species, by photo-irradiation. This species then facilitates covalent linkage of the probe to the protein, as shown in Figure 3.1 [22]. Both ABPP and AfBPP can be used during drug discovery and development in order to identify and validate the on- and off-target proteins of a compound prior to clinical trials [16, 17].

3.2 Activity-Based Probe (ABP) and Affinity-Based Probe (AfBP) Design

The crucial element of the ABPP or AfBPP approach is the design of the probe. Several key properties such as target selectivity, biological compatibility, membrane permeability, and solubility are required. The design of ABPs and AfBPs is generally based on known and effective covalent irreversible or reversible inhibitors, respectively.

Generally, the A(f)BP consists of three essential components: a warhead moiety, a linker group, and a reporter tag (Figure 3.2). The warhead is a reactive component that can react with the active site (ABP) or ligand binding site (AfBP) of the target protein, binding irreversibly and covalently. The reporter tag allows for direct detection and isolation of the probe-bound proteins, for example, by conjugation to biotin for enrichment or to fluorescent groups for imaging. The linker component connects the warhead and the reporter tag, providing enough space between the two moieties to maintain the selectivity and reactivity of the warhead and reducing steric congestion. All three components should ideally be bioorthogonal, causing minimal disruption to complex biological systems.

3.2.1 Warheads (Reactive Groups)

The warhead is the most important part of the ABP or AfBP, ensuring the selective modification of one or more protein active site(s). Warheads have been developed

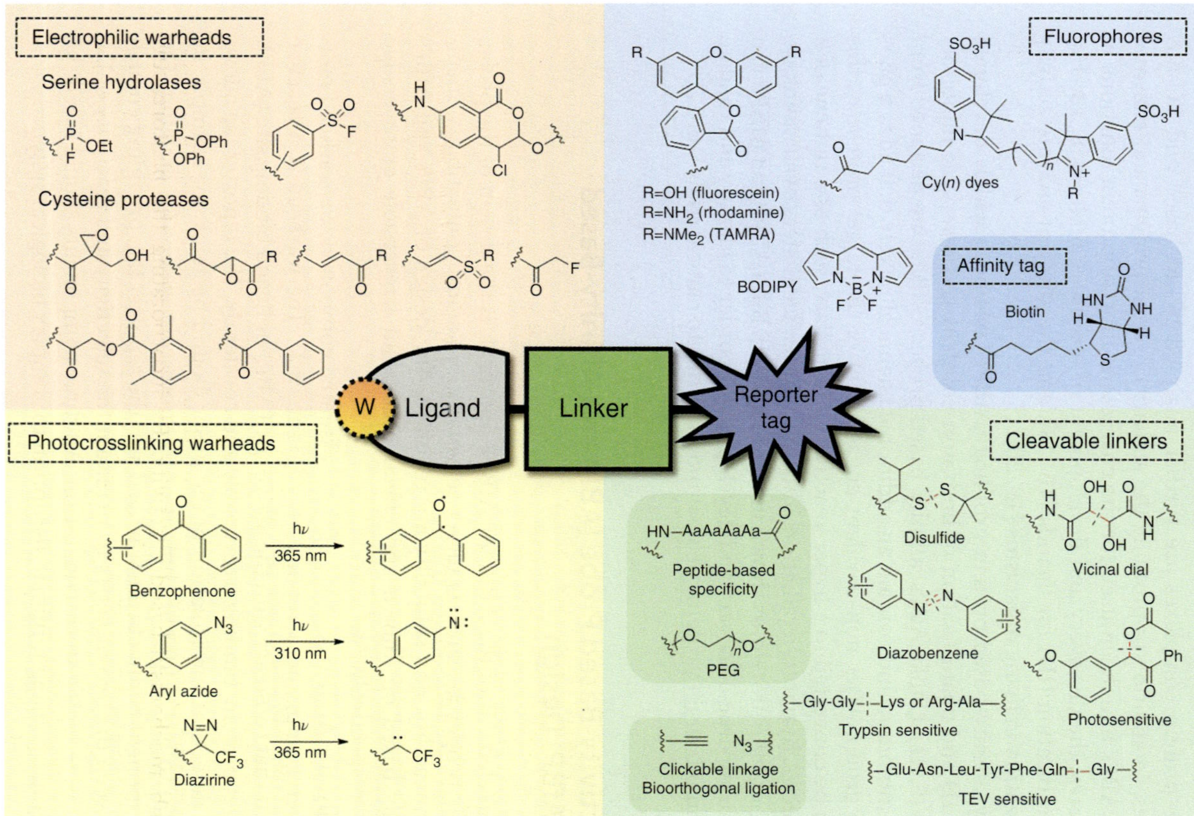

Figure 3.2 Essential components of activity-based probes (ABPs) including a reactive warhead, a linker, and a reporter tag with some representative examples. The reactive warhead irreversibly and covalently binds with the target proteins. The warhead (W) is classified as either an electrophilic (orange) or a photocrosslinking (yellow) warhead depending on whether the inhibitor works via a covalent or non-covalent mechanism, respectively. The linker (green) can be used as a specificity element, e.g. a peptide recognition sequence, or as a cleavable element for selectively cleaving the probe from the protein or peptide. The reporter tag allows for visualization using a fluorophore and/or purification using an affinity handle (e.g. biotin). Some probes eliminate the reporter group entirely, separating protein labelling and reporter conjugation into two steps by incorporating a 'clickable' linkage in place of a linker and reporter tag. The reporter group can then be incorporated by a downstream bioorthogonal ligation step (as discussed in Section 3.2.4) to mitigate reductions in cell

based on non-covalent or covalent inhibitors and can be divided into two groups: electrophilic warheads for ABPs and photocrosslinkers for AfBPs.

3.2.1.1 Electrophilic Warheads

Canonical examples are ABP warheads for cysteine, serine, and threonine hydrolases (e.g. proteases, lipases), which are generated from electrophilic traps based on their respective hydrolytic mechanisms, but there exists a very wide range of potential starting points for ABPs, including natively reactive natural products [23–25], several of which are discussed in Section 3.4. For cysteine, serine, and threonine hydrolases, the nucleophilic enzyme active site residues react with the electrophilic warhead, forming an irreversible covalent bond to the ABP. The wide variety of hydrolase-specific electrophilic warheads is shown in Figure 3.2, along with their specific target enzymes. A notable example is fluorophosphonate-biotin (FP-biotin), which was designed based on the diisopropyl fluorophosphate (DFP) inhibitor of serine hydrolases [26]. FP-biotin is widely used to profile the activity of serine hydrolase enzymes, of which more than 80 have been identified in both mouse and human proteomes [27–29], and this probe enabled numerous novel serine hydrolases to be identified [30]. Despite its success and widespread use, FP is not specific for serine proteases (e.g. over lipases), with diphenyl phosphonates [31–33] and isocoumarins [34–36] reacting more specifically with different classes of proteases.

Another key mechanistic enzyme class is cysteine proteases; here, ABPs exploit the specific arrangement of a cysteine residue as a nucleophile and a histidine residue to facilitate proton transfer in order to target the protease with an electrophilic warhead. Several warheads have been developed to react with the cysteine active site, including acyloxymethyl ketone [37], diazomethyl ketone [38], epoxide [39, 40], α-haloketones [41], α,β-unsaturated ketones [42], and vinyl sulfones [43, 44]. Cysteine proteases, for example, papain [39, 45–47], caspases [48], and deubiquitinating [43, 49–51] families, have been extensively studied using these probes, as they are involved in many diseases including cancer and parasitaemia.

3.2.1.2 Photocrosslinking Warheads

AfBPs are commonly used for studying reversible inhibitors, as these require a photocrosslinking warhead to form a covalent connection between probe and protein. AfBPs rely on target selectivity through binding affinity as opposed to through mechanism-based reactivity. By incorporating the photoreactive group onto the reversible inhibitor structure, a hyper-reactive intermediate can be formed upon UV irradiation, enabling a covalent bond to form between the probe and the proximal protein or enzyme. The labelling efficiency of this method mainly depends on the type of the photoreactive warhead used to generate the reactive species, as well as the similarity of probe structure to the parent inhibitor scaffold.

Commonly used photocrosslinking warheads [22, 52, 53] include aryl azides, benzophenones, and diazirines [54, 55], each of which generates a different reactive species under UV irradiation (Figure 3.2). The nitrene, diradical, and carbene reactive species can insert into proximal C—, O—, N—, or S—H bonds, forming a covalent link between the probe and whatever is in the local environment, e.g. a bound protein target. These warheads can be used in several solvents, including water, and in ambient light, making them useful tools for biological systems [56]. This technique has allowed chemical proteomic identification and activity profiling of the aspartic proteases [57] and metalloproteases [58–60], as well as protein–protein [22] and protein–lipid interactions [61]. Incorporating photocrosslinking warheads onto reversible small molecule inhibitors or drugs has become a powerful strategy for on-and off-target ID [62, 63].

3.2.2 Reporter Tags

Reporter tags allow for the detection and/or isolation of the target protein or enzyme–probe conjugate and should enable visualization, identification, quantification, or purification of probe–protein adducts. Some simple probes have the warhead attached via a linker to a fluorophore, such as TAMRA, fluorescein, rhodamine, BODIPY, and Cy dyes (Figure 3.2). These probes can be used for direct fluorescence visualization, separating the proteins using sodium dodecyl sulfate-polyacrylamide gel electrophoresis (SDS-PAGE) and identifying tagged proteins using in-gel fluorescence. They can also be used in conjunction with fluorescence microscopy for studying *in situ* (live cells) or *in vivo* protein localization. Alternatively, the attachment of an affinity tag, such as biotin, enables enrichment and purification of probe-labelled proteins from the background protein pool or lysate. The enriched proteins can be further identified and quantified by mass spectrometry (MS) techniques.

However, fluorescent dyes and affinity binding groups add significant steric bulk to probes and therefore might interrupt the biological uptake of the ABP or disrupt biological processes in *in situ* or *in vivo* systems. To address this issue, bioorthogonal ligation chemistry can be used, separating the probe–protein conjugation and reporter tagging into a two-step labelling process, which is discussed in Section 3.2.4.

3.2.3 Linkers

The linker is the central part of the probe that connects the reactive warhead to the reporter tag. It can be made from a variety of functionalities, and it can be used to change or optimize different properties of the probe such as solubility, uptake, specificity, and cleavability, playing a critical role in fine-tuning the behaviour of a reactive warhead.

To increase the selectivity of the probe, the linker can be tuned to favour binding to the target protein(s). An example of this is the use of peptide chains or amino acids, which are known to bind to a specific target, as a linker [64]. Alternatively, some deubiquitinating enzymes (DUBs) have been profiled using probes containing ubiquitin protein as the linker, as it helps to direct the probe to the desired class of enzymes [50, 51]. Alternatively, to increase the solubility of the probe linker, groups such as polyethylene glycol (PEG) can be added.

It can be useful to add a cleavable linker to the ABP to simplify the identification and quantification of labelled proteins through MS techniques. Labelled proteins are often enriched using biotin-streptavidin pulldown prior to MS, and harsh elution conditions are required to recover labelled proteins due to the high binding affinity between biotin and streptavidin ($K_d \sim 10^{-15}$ M). This can lead to high levels of background noise from endogenously biotinylated proteins and proteins bound non-specifically to the streptavidin or its solid support, which can produce false positive hits. One approach to avoid a high background signal involves using a cleavable linker within the ABP, removing the need for harsh elution of bound proteins off the streptavidin. Several cleavable linkers have recently been developed for chemical proteomic and ABPP applications, such as diazobenzenes [65, 66], disulfides [67], vicinal diols [68], and photosensitive [69], acid-sensitive [70], and enzymatically cleavable linkers [71, 72] as shown in Figure 3.2.

Two cleavage enzymes typically used in chemical proteomics are *tobacco etch virus* (TEV) and trypsin proteases. A TEV-cleavable probe developed by the Cravatt and Speers groups has been widely used in combination with a bioorthogonal handle and a biotin affinity tag, as well as isotopically labelled valine for MS-based protein quantification [71, 73]. However, trypsin is more commonly used for protein digestion in MS-based proteomics. Recently, the Tate group has developed a multifunctional capture reagent called AzRTB that contains biotin for enrichment, a TAMRA fluorophore for imaging purposes, and a trypsin cleavable linker, as well as an azide for bioorthogonal ligation to labelled proteins [72] (see Section 3.2.4). This capture reagent has been used in several applications including the identification of proteome-wide myristoylation and validation of *N*-myristoyl transferase (NMT) inhibitors in malaria parasites [74, 75].

3.2.4 Bioorthogonal Ligation Chemistry

In order to ensure efficient uptake of the ABP and mitigate disruption of the biological system *in situ* or *in vivo*, a two-step labelling process is applied to facilitate ABPP. The active molecules or inhibitors are first modified with a small reactive group designed to minimize the change in structure from the parent compounds and retain their activity and cell permeability. The reactive group is designed to be *bioorthogonal* (that is, the chemistry operates independently from and without interaction with a complex biological environment such as a cell) to minimize interference with/from the biological milieu. Once ABP treatment is complete, any labelled proteins now containing this reactive handle can be ligated to a reporter tag containing a complementary bioorthogonal group using the appropriate bioorthogonal reaction. This reporter tag contains chemical species such as fluorophores or affinity handles, allowing downstream biochemical manipulation (Table 3.1).

Bioorthogonal ligation reactions are those that are compatible with aqueous conditions, are highly selective, and have efficient covalent bond formation. Above all, they must be suitable for biological systems. There are four different key bioorthogonal ligation reactions that have been used in chemical proteomics (Table 3.1) [82, 87].

Table 3.1 Some common bioorthogonal reactions used in chemical proteomics. The most common orientation of tag and capture reagent is shown, with alkyne/strained alkene on the probe; however, these are in principle interchangeable (e.g. azide tag can be used on the probe, with an alkyne on the capture reagent).

Reactions	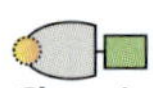 Chemical tag	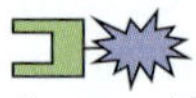 Capture/detection reagent	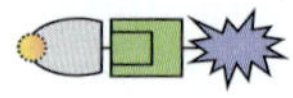 Product	References
Staudinger ligations		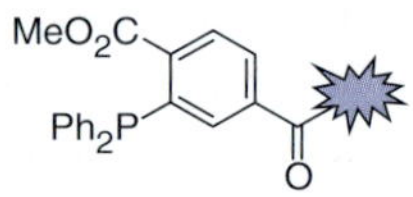	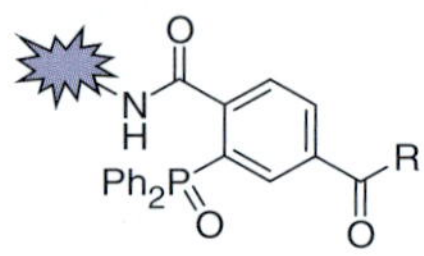	[76–78]
CuAAC	R—N_3 azide	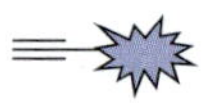	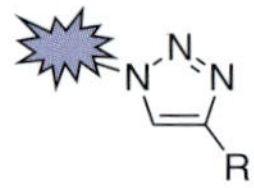	[17, 24, 79–81]
SPAAC		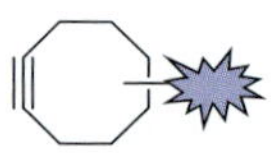	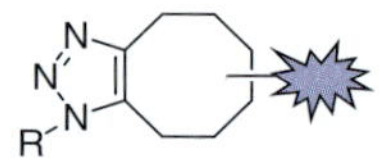	[82, 83]
Diels–Alder cycloadditions	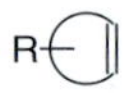 alkene, strained alkene	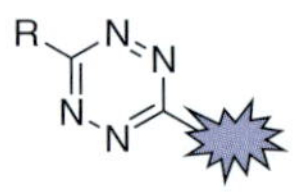	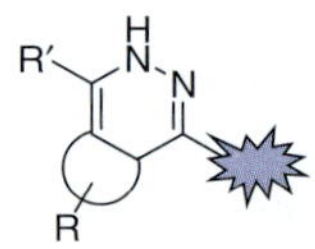	[84–86]

3.2.4.1 Staudinger Ligation

The Staudinger ligation was described by Hermann Staudinger in 1919 and developed for bioorthogonal ligation by Carolyn R. Bertozzi and is a reaction between an azide and a phosphine to form a stable amide [88]. The advantages of this method are the mild conditions required, with no additional reagents or organic solvents needed. This ligation method has been applied in several ABPP studies both *in situ* and *in vivo*, including cysteine cathepsin profiling in macrophages [77] and proteasome profiling [78]. Although this method does not require harsh reaction conditions and the reagents have relatively low toxicity, the phosphines are oxygen sensitive and have poor solubility in water, and the rate of ligation is relatively slow compared with other bioorthogonal ligation reactions [87].

3.2.4.2 Copper(I)-Catalysed Azide-Alkyne Cycloaddition (CuAAC)

Copper(I)-catalysed azide-alkyne cycloaddition (CuAAC), discovered by Rolf Huisgen and developed for bioorthogonal ligation by the Sharpless group, is a reaction between terminal alkynes and azides to form a 1,2,3-triazole [89, 90]. It has been extremely popular in chemical proteomics and materials science due to its outstanding characteristics, and it has become known as simply a 'click' reaction. CuAAC ligations can occur quickly under mild reaction conditions with no organic solvent, proceeding with a high product yield and high selectivity. The alkyne and azide functional groups are widely employed 'tags' as they are small, chemically inert, and easy to incorporate into a probe. Their small size and relative inertness make them excellent biological tags with minimal interference with the native environment of cells and are the most commonly used bioorthogonal ligation reactions in ABPP, first introduced in this context by the Cravatt group [80]. Alkyne handles are commonly used to characterize target proteins of small molecule inhibitors or drug molecules as the size, potency, and cell permeability of the parent compounds are largely retained. Several target protein identification studies have been performed on FDA-approved drugs using ABPP such as orlistat [91], aspirin [92], andrographolide [93], and ampicillin [94]. To do this, these drugs were modified with an alkyne tag, enabling subsequent bioorthogonal ligation to reporter molecules and identification of the exact target or the off-target proteins. Importantly this information can be used to obtain more details about the cause of drug side effects and the mode of action of these biologically active molecules. Despite all the advantages of CuAAC reactions, due to the toxicity of copper, it is not possible to perform this reaction *in situ* or *in vivo*, so probe–protein labelling and capture reagent coupling must be performed in two steps. Furthermore, the azide and alkyne tags are not entirely orthogonal, with azides undergoing slow background redox chemistry with thiols and alkynes susceptible to metabolic oxidation, e.g. by cytochrome P450 enzymes [95].

3.2.4.3 Strain-Promoted Azide-Alkyne Cycloaddition (SPAAC)

The strain-promoted azide-alkyne cycloaddition (SPAAC) or copper-free azide–alkyne cycloaddition developed by the Bertozzi group avoids the potential toxicity from the copper catalyst. SPAAC forms a triazole by the reaction between an azide and a strained alkyne, such as cyclooctyne [96, 97]. The release of strain provides a thermodynamic driving force for this reaction. This ligation strategy has been used for glycan profiling on live cell surfaces and in live animals including *Caenorhabditis elegans*, zebrafish, and mice [82]. SPAAC has a lower rate of reaction compared with CuAAC; however cyclooctyne reagents have been developed to increase reactivity and retain biocompatibility and stability of the reagents. Some limitations of this ligation method can be attributed to the large size of the functional groups required, which lead to poor water solubility and significant cross-reactions between thiols and cyclooctyne reagents.

3.2.4.4 Diels–Alder Reaction

The cycloaddition reaction between a diene and a dienophile exhibits good selectivity and compatibility in biological conditions, and no additional chemical reagent is needed. The Overkleeft group has successfully used this ligation reaction in ABPP to label endogenous proteasomes in living cells [84]. They synthesized diene-containing ABPs based on epoxomicin, a proteasome inhibitor, which could be ligated to dienophile-functionalized fluorescent tags for visualization. Similarly, an inverse electron-demand Diels–Alder (IEDDA) ligation has also been applied in ABPP by introducing a strained, electron-deficient alkene handle, such as a norbornene, into the warhead [85]. This was later coupled with a tetrazine-functionalized tag. Recently, van der Stelt and co-workers have synthesized a norbornene-modified diacylglycerol lipase (DAGL) inhibitor to label DAGLs in living cells. This was used in combination with fluorogenic BODIPY-tetrazine, and the probe-DAGL adducts were detected by in-gel fluorescence [98]. Limitations of the Diels–Alder reactions can include cross-reactivity with biological nucleophiles, metabolic instability, solubility, and the large size of the chemical tag, leading to low labelling efficiency and selectivity.

3.3 Chemical Proteomic Workflow

To identify and quantify proteins, ABPs must be used in conjunction with proteomics using MS techniques. This section focuses on the two-step labelling chemical proteomic workflow used by the Tate group for ABPP and related profiling approaches [23, 24, 72, 74, 75, 81], shown in Figure 3.3.

Initially, cells modelling the biological system of interest are incubated with an alkyne-tagged ABP. For inhibitor screening or profiling, cells are pre-treated with varying concentrations of inhibitor for a competition assay. Protein targets are then covalently linked to the ABP via mechanism-based or photoactivatable tagging, resulting in protein–probe adducts. Following cell lysis, protein–probe adducts are 'clicked' to azide-containing reporter tags via a CuAAC reaction as described in Section 3.2.4.2. These reporter tags also contain fluorescent and/or biotin affinity moieties. Direct visualization of labelled proteins by in-gel fluorescence enables optimization of crosslinking or tagging prior to MS experiments.

For subsequent proteomic analysis, the probe-labelled proteins are enriched or isolated from the protein pool using neutravidin-conjugated beads. Enriched proteins then undergo on-bead digestion by the enzyme trypsin, which cleaves

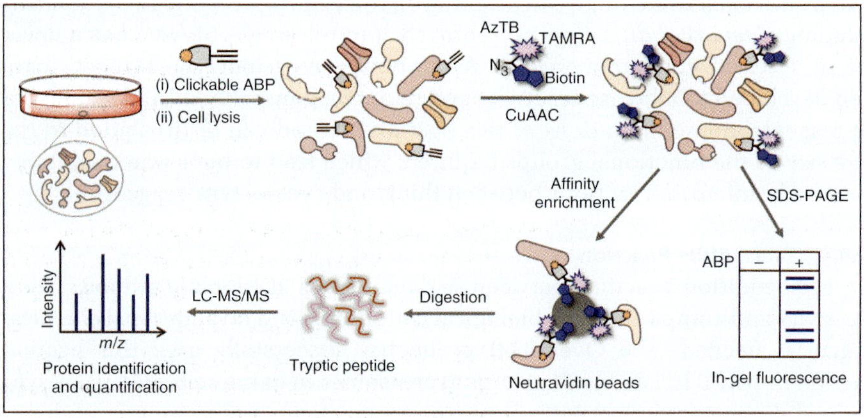

Figure 3.3 General chemical proteomic workflow using two-step labelling. Cells are treated with a clickable ABP in the first step of labelling. In this example we use an alkyne probe. Additional treatments with inhibitors or activating agents can also be performed at this stage. The cells are lysed, and probe-labelled proteins are labelled with an azide-TAMRA-biotin (AzTB) capture reagent via CuAAC. AzTB allows for both gel-based fluorescence analysis and affinity enrichment by utilizing the strong binding between biotin-labelled proteins and neutravidin-conjugated beads. The enriched proteins undergo on-bead trypsinization into their constituent peptides and are subsequently analysed by LC-MS/MS for protein identification and quantification.

the proteins specifically after each lysine (K) or arginine (R) residue into their constituent peptides. These peptides are analysed by liquid chromatography followed by tandem mass spectrometry (LC-MS/MS) to facilitate protein identification and quantification. Different techniques have been developed to enable quantitation, such as label-free, chemical labelling, and metabolic labelling quantification approaches, discussed below.

3.3.1 Quantitative Proteomics by Mass Spectrometry

Analysing changes in protein expression levels in response to different conditions is one of the most complex steps of the chemical proteomic workflow but is critical to enable objective and quantitative analysis of labelling (and thus of activity). Quantitative analysis of proteins is performed at the peptide level using MS and uses one of several quantification methods [99, 100]. These methods include label-free quantification (LFQ), chemical labelling, and metabolic labelling, shown in Figure 3.4.

3.3.1.1 Label-Free Quantification (LFQ)

LFQ is a relative quantification method that compares the ion intensity or the signal (spectral counts) between two or more samples, which have been separately analysed by MS [101–104]. The sample preparation of LFQ is simpler, faster, and cheaper than other labelling methods and can be used with an unlimited number of compared samples. This method is therefore suitable for large animal or biomarker studies [105, 106]. In addition, the simplicity of LFQ samples maximizes the protein coverage of the MS runs. However, some limitations of this method arise from variation in the sample preparation, which leads to a lower level of accuracy and reproducibility. The MS processing time is also longer than for labelled methods, as only one sample can be run at a time [107]. Nonetheless, the LFQ method has been used in combination with ABPP by many groups [92, 108–110].

3.3.1.2 Chemical Labelling Quantification

Chemical labelling quantification is a method that labels specific reactive groups on peptides, such as cysteines and primary amines. These chemical tags utilize isotopic and isobaric groups that result in different masses in MS analysis that are used to quantify the relative amount of each associated peptide/protein. In isotope-coded affinity tag (ICAT) labelling, the tags can directly label protein or peptide samples using the reactivity of the amino acid side chains to incorporate both an isotopically coded linker and a handle for affinity purification [111]. The advantages of this labelling method are high reaction yield, high reproducibility, and low cost. However, the analysis of the MS data from these stable isotope labelling methods can be complicated due to the increased complexity of the overall protein mixture, which leads to the reduction of protein coverage. In contrast, isobaric tags such as iTRAQ [112] and tandem mass tag (TMT) [113–115] are designed so that the different tags have identical masses at the MS^1 level, which does not increase peptide complexity. Then, during fragmentation at the MS^2 level, tag-modified peptides generate

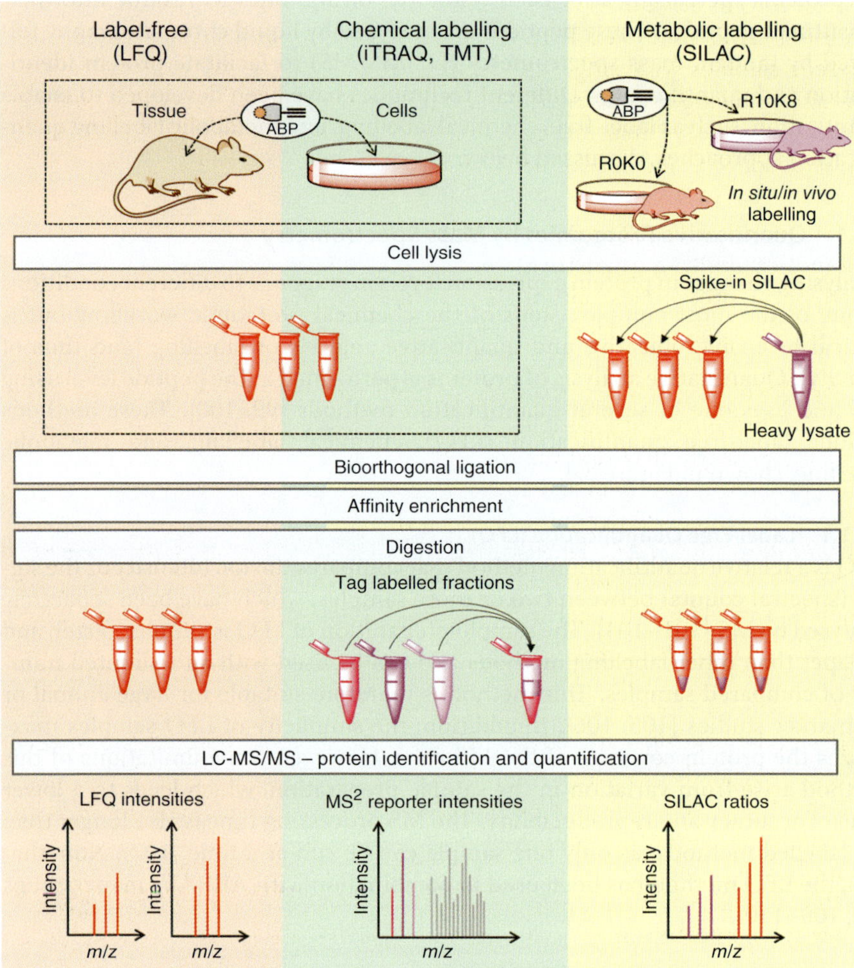

Figure 3.4 An overview workflow of quantitative proteomic approaches by mass spectrometry. **Label-free (LFQ)**: untreated/treated tissues or cells of interest are lysed and coupled with a suitable reporter tag. Labelled proteins are then purified and proteolytically digested, yielding an enriched pool of peptides from the labelled proteins. The enriched peptides are directly analysed by LC-MS/MS, with the intensity of each peptide being recorded in each MS run, allowing for comparative approximation of protein quantification. **Chemical labelling (iTRAQ, TMT)**: samples are prepared as for LFQ, but with a quantifying labelling step at the peptide level. Peptides are labelled with TMT or iTRAQ reagents and then pooled and analysed by LC-MS/MS. The relative quantity of a peptide (and by inference, protein) in each sample is given by the relative MS2 reporter ion intensities derived from each isobaric label. **Metabolic labelling (SILAC)**: cells are cultured in media containing either isotopically light or heavy amino acids. After cell lysis, the heavy- and light-labelled lysates are combined, and the chemical proteomic workflow is performed as already described. The relative intensities of heavy versus light peptides provide information regarding the change in protein levels between the two samples. While this is restricted to pairwise comparisons, an alternative approach exists where the heavy-labelled lysate can be 'spiked in' to light-labelled lysates of interest, acting as an internal standard for comparative quantification.

reporter ions of different masses that are used to quantify peptide levels in each condition. TMT multiplex reagents can be used to quantify up to 10 (or more) different samples in a single LC-MS/MS run, eliminating variation between runs and reducing processing time and running costs. However, TMT reagents are more expensive than other labelling reagents, and quantification can be challenging due to ion contamination in MS^2 analysis [116–118].

3.3.1.3 Metabolic Labelling Quantification

Metabolic labelling quantification is a widely used quantification technique in chemical proteomics, although it is not generally applicable to systems that are challenging to label metabolically (e.g. clinical samples and many *in vivo* systems). *S*table *I*sotope *L*abelling by/with *A*mino acids in *C*ell culture (SILAC) involves metabolic incorporation of heavy ^{13}C- and ^{15}N-labelled amino acids into proteins. For example, cells are cultured in media containing heavy (Arg10Lys8), medium (Arg6Lys4), or light (Arg0Lys0) isotopically labelled amino acids [119, 120]. These labelled amino acids are used as protein building blocks by the cell and generally require at least five full cell cycles for >99% metabolic incorporation. In SILAC, labelled samples are combined at the beginning of sample preparation, and the combined lysate is continually treated as one sample until LC-MS/MS analysis, increasing accuracy by removing variation in sample handling. For protein quantification, the ratio of light- to heavy-modified peptides can be used to infer the relative protein abundance in each sample. SILAC has been widely performed in cell experiments [121–123] and in select *in vivo* models in which animals are fed heavy or light amino acids; however the latter is associated with a high financial cost [124–127].

The main limitation of SILAC, aside from the need for metabolic activity, is that the number of samples that can be run together in a classical SILAC experiment is limited by typically three combinations of isotopically labelled amino acids. Alternatively, in 'spike-in SILAC' methodologies, a heavy isotopically labelled sample, usually the control sample, is 'spiked' into every light-labelled condition as an internal standard or reference proteome [23, 24, 128, 129]. The combined lysate is then analysed by LC-MS/MS, and proteins are quantified relative to the internal standard to give difference ratios between the analysed and reference proteomes. A broad limitation of all SILAC approaches is that some organisms or samples cannot efficiently incorporate isotope labelled amino acids, for example, many microbes (due to lack of relevant auxotrophy), non-proliferating cells, or tissue lysates. To address this limitation, chemical labelling as described above provides a way to label the sample at the protein or peptide levels. However, the lysates must be processed separately, meaning that the benefit of consistency in sample preparation is lost.

3.4 ABPP Applications and Case Studies

The ABPP strategy has become more popular in recent decades as a result of extensive development around the design and applications of ABPs. Probes have been applied in several cases related to drug discovery including protein/enzyme profiling, inhibitor screening, target ID, and protein imaging (Figure 3.5). Protein activity profiling is the main application of conventional ABPs, identifying new biomarkers or therapeutic targets in different stages of a disease. The enzyme classes being profiled are targeted depending on both the warhead and the specific linkers included in the ABP. For example, the serine hydrolase family is targeted by well-established fluorophosphonate (FP) probes [27, 29, 130], while the cysteine protease family is targeted by probes with vinyl ketone [42] or epoxide [39] warheads.

Given that well-designed ABPs can deliver broad-spectrum protein profiling of a particular enzyme class, it is possible to perform inhibitor screening using these probes. In a so-called competition experiment, the biological sample is pre-incubated with the inhibitor and then treated with the ABP; potent and selective inhibitors can be identified by comparing the labelling profile of probe in the competed sample against the sample with no inhibitor pre-treatment (Figure 3.5). Key advantages of this competitive ABPP strategy include inhibitor screening against a range of proteins instead of a single target protein and that this profiling occurs inside a living cell [23, 24, 73, 81].

A further application of ABPP is to determine the on- and off-targets of a specific inhibitor molecule across the whole cellular proteome, potentially uncovering the associated mode(s) of action and investigating any undesirable side effects. In these instances, the ABP (or AfBP) warhead is based around the specific structure of the inhibitor. This ABP can be used to label the target protein(s) of the inhibitor, and the ABP–protein complex can be visualized by the chemical proteomic workflow as previously described. However, competition-based ABPP using the parent inhibitor molecule is still necessary to uncouple true targets of the parent inhibitor from false protein hits resulting from chemical modifications made to the probe (e.g. to enable bioorthogonal ligation, visualization, and/or enrichment) or from non-specific enrichment on an affinity resin. This strategy

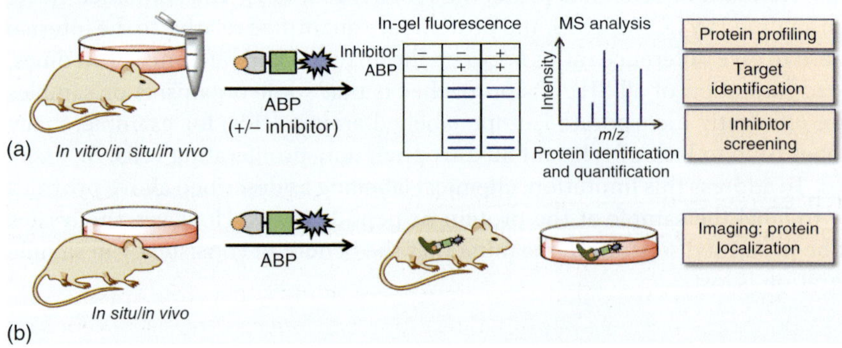

Figure 3.5 Highlighted applications of ABPs. (a) ABPs combined with gel-based and MS-based proteomic identification methods are widely used *in vitro*, *in situ*, and *in vivo* for protein profiling, target identification, and inhibitor screening. (b) Fluorescence microscopy imaging with fluorescently tagged or fluorescence-quenched ABPs allows active proteome imaging in live cells and in animal models.

has been extensively used in drug discovery in order to minimize the cost and time in the drug discovery pipeline and to identify the possible off-target proteins that may lead to clinical failure of a molecule [16–18, 131, 132].

Aside from their use as tools for drug development, fluorescently tagged ABPs have been developed for real-time monitoring of enzyme activity *in situ* or *in vivo* in order to study enzyme localization and to monitor different stages of disease (Figure 3.5) [10, 19, 133]. However, fluorescent ABPs are often limited for imaging applications by a strong fluorescent signal in both the control samples and when interacting with the target enzyme(s) that is not always readily removed by washing. To overcome this, quenched fluorescent activity-based probes (qABPs) have been developed for real-time localization studies and analysis of enzyme activity *in situ* and *in vivo* [9, 20, 134–136]. The fluorescent signal of a qABP is only generated in the reaction between the active enzyme and the qABP, resulting in the reduction or elimination of background signal from free probe.

We describe below five recent case studies that highlight applications of ABPs. In the first case study, ABPP has been used as a tool to profile undiscovered serine hydrolases in the Archaea domain [137]. These broad-spectrum ABPs that target serine hydrolases are further used in the second case study, identifying on- and off-targets of BIA 10-2474, a drug that failed at phase I clinical trials [2]. In the third case study, we look at two papers from the Tate group where natural product-derived ABPs have been used to selectively label the target protein [24, 81]. The fourth case study uses fragment-based ligand discovery in combination with MS-based analysis to search for new fragment–protein interactions [15], while the final case study uses a qABP to study protein localization in live cells and *in vivo* [135].

3.4.1 Case Study 1: Activity-Based Protein Profiling as a Robust Method for Enzyme Identification and Screening in Extremophilic Archaea

As the search for new medicines broadens, scientists are increasingly stretching further afield for novel pathways, enzymes, and metabolites to provide inspiration for next-generation drug design. The Kaiser and Siebers groups have recently used ABPP to investigate undiscovered enzymology within the Archaea domain, focusing on extremophilic species with highly individual biochemical pathways [137]. Any new enzymes discovered could also be adapted into useful biocatalytic tools.

Archaea represent a distinct domain of life, separate from the eukaryotic and prokaryotic branches, with alternative metabolic pathways to these other domains. Some of these pathways involve enzymes that are completely distinct from, or only weakly related to, their equivalents found in bacterial or eukaryotic cells [138]. Many Archaea possess interesting and unusual cellular properties, such as atypical membrane lipids and a different cell wall structure [139, 140]. Some Archaea have adapted to their extreme living conditions, such as high and low temperatures, pH, and salinity, widening the scope of cellular properties. However, despite this intriguing pool of discoveries, research into the different species of Archaea is limited by these same extreme environmental conditions and by difficulties in cultivation. Archaeal enzymes are most commonly studied after expression in *Escherichia coli*; however this affects protein folding and omits any native PTMs. Further complications arise from the difference in archaeal promoter sequences to those present in bacteria, making it difficult to identify archaeal enzymes in bacterial host-based screens.

Kaiser and Siebers chose ABPP as a technique to study archaeal enzyme activity because, used *in vivo*, the probes provide a sensitive, simple method to identify and study these enzymes in their native host cell. Prior to this paper, no groups had used ABPs in *in vivo* Archaea experiments. The initial challenge was to choose a probe and Archaea species pairing which could be used in the same extreme conditions. Phosphonate-based serine hydrolase probes are particularly well-characterized probes that display strong labelling, and so these probes were chosen as a starting point. These probes contain a phosphonate warhead, which reacts with the active site of the enzyme, a linker, and an alkyne reporter tag for visualization, detection, or enrichment of labelled proteins using click chemistry (Figure 3.6).

An Archaea species, *Sulfolobus acidocaldarius*, was chosen based on its capacity for facile genetic modification. This species was discovered in Yellowstone National Park in an acidic hot spring and can be grown in culture at 75–80 °C in pH 2–3. Additionally, two more species were investigated to demonstrate the versatility of this technique: a closely related species, *Sulfolobus solfataricus*, which has a larger genome and greater metabolic diversity, and a more distant species, *Haloferax volcanii*, which grows optimally in high salt levels and at temperatures between 30 and 55 °C.

Kaiser and Siebers initially labelled *S. acidocaldarius* lysates with five different probes, performed click chemistry with rhodamine-azide (Rho-N_3), and compared the results via in-gel fluorescence, demonstrating that labelling with each probe was comparable when performed at 25 and 78 °C at pH 8.0. The first probe was a FP-type probe [141], with an FP warhead. This probe was adapted with a nitrophenol ethyl leaving group to give a second probe with a lower activity (Figure 3.6). Two further nitrophenol phosphonate probes were developed with hydrophobic warheads, a phthalylalkyl group and a heptanyl chain, respectively. The final probe was a negative control probe derived from the nitrophenol ethyl probe, which lacked a leaving group, therefore rendering it inactive. They chose two of the probes, the most selective nitrophenol ethyl phosphonate probe (NP) and the probe with the most labelling, fluorophosphonate-based probe (FP), for further experiments.

The authors went on to show that the extreme pH *in vivo* did not affect the labelling profile, again using *S. acidocaldarius*, but this time in cultures at pH 3.0, with click chemistry to rhodamine-biotin-azide (Rh-Biot-N_3). Following enrichment with avidin-conjugated beads and subsequent in-gel fluorescence, key bands at 38 and 140 kDa were identified as serine hydrolases through in-gel digestion and MS. This was confirmed through the production of deletion mutants and complementation analysis. In total, 10 out of the predicted 17 serine hydrolases were identified through ABPP.

To demonstrate the robustness of this method, ABPP was further performed in additional archaeal species. *S. solfataricus* was used in the same workflow under

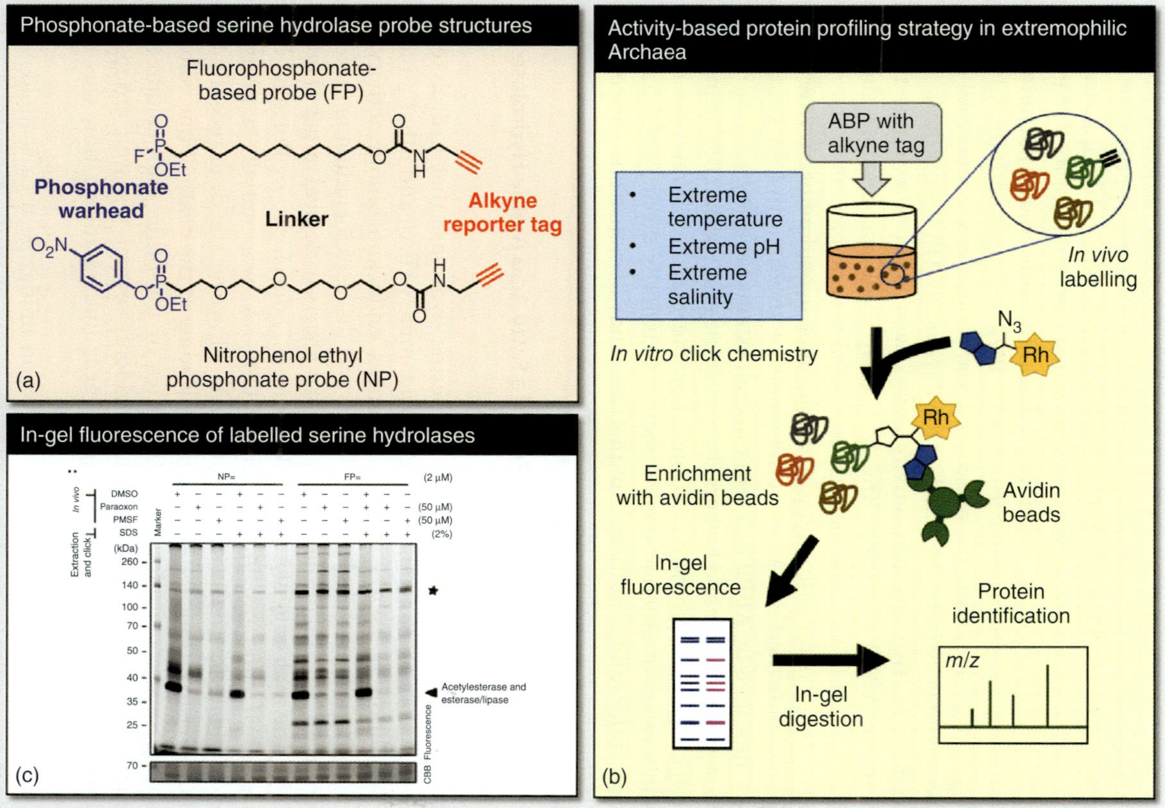

Figure 3.6 (a) Structure of FP and NP probes used, with phosphonate warheads highlighted in blue and alkyne tag in red. (b) ABPP strategy in extremophilic Archaea: Archaea are cultured in extreme conditions with alkyne-tagged probe. Lysates are 'clicked' to reporter tag Rh-Biot-N_3 via CuAAC chemistry and enriched using avidin beads before in-gel fluorescence, in-gel digestion, and proteomic analysis for protein identification. (c) An example in-gel fluorescence readout with NP and FP probes. Both probes label proteins at 140 and 38 kDa, which were later identified as serine hydrolases. Source: This image is a derivative of Figure 2 from [137] (https://www.nature.com/articles/ncomms15352), licensed under CC BY 4.0 (https://creativecommons.org/licenses/by/4.0/legalcode).

the same thermoacidophilic conditions. Again, strong labelling was observed, and 10 out of a predicted 18 serine hydrolases were identified. To study the effect of salinity of the labelling efficiency, *H. volcanii* was used for equivalent experiments, in high salt conditions and at 45 °C. Five serine hydrolases were successfully identified out of the predicted 22, despite little optimization.

Kaiser and Siebers went on to show that heterologously expressed bacterial serine hydrolases could be detected using ABPP. They used a deletion mutant of *S. acidocaldarius* expressing bacterial enzymes LipT and LipS, two thermophilic serine esterases identified from a metagenomic library [142], which are distinct from esterases present in Archaea. In addition, the bacterial serine hydrolase from *Thermotoga maritima*, TM_1022, was cloned into the mutant *S. acidocaldarius*, including the native bacterial promoter sequence. All of these proteins were successfully identified by the developed ABPP workflow.

Following this, two enzyme activity assays were used to evaluate the sensitivity of the ABPP approach. The first assay used opaque lipid substrates embedded in agar to visualize esterase activity. A second biochemical assay with *para*-nitrophenol octanoate ester gave a colorimetric readout of enzyme activity. Both assays confirmed the ABPP results: mutant strains with knockouts of the esterases identified by ABPP had lower overall esterase activity.

Taken together, Kaiser and Siebers showed an elegant use of ABPP using serine hydrolase probes in extreme conditions to profile enzymes in multiple Archaea species in a range of different environments. Classically these probes have only been used under mild conditions, but this case study demonstrates the versatility of this technique for enzyme identification and screening.

3.4.2 Case Study 2: Failed Clinical Trial of a Fatty Acid Amide Hydrolase (FAAH) Inhibitor

Fatty acid amide hydrolase (FAAH) is a serine hydrolase that hydrolyses the amide bond of endocannabinoids, e.g. anandamide (AEA), and other amidated lipids. Inhibition of FAAH activity enhances endocannabinoid activity, and this is a potentially useful treatment for several diseases including neurological disorders, pain, and inflammation, making it a pharmacological target of interest [143, 144]. The molecule BIA 10-2474 (Figure 3.7) developed by Portugal-based pharmaceutical company Bial-Portela & CA. SA. was initially a promising clinical candidate for the inhibition of FAAH. However the drug recently failed in the first phase of clinical trials, tragically leading to the death of one volunteer and causing severe neurological deficiencies in the other four volunteers in the same group [145, 146]. Since this incident, several research groups and regulatory bodies have been working towards understanding how this could have occurred [2].

The structure of BIA 10-2474 is based on an imidazole-urea scaffold, which is thought to covalently react with the active site of serine hydrolases. ABPP presents a powerful approach to characterize the target protein profile of this molecule, helping to further understand its mechanisms of action and any off-targets that may have led to this outcome. In this international study by the van der Stelt and Kushner groups, alkyne analogues of BIA 10-2474 were synthesized to first confirm the mode of action [2]. These alkyne analogues

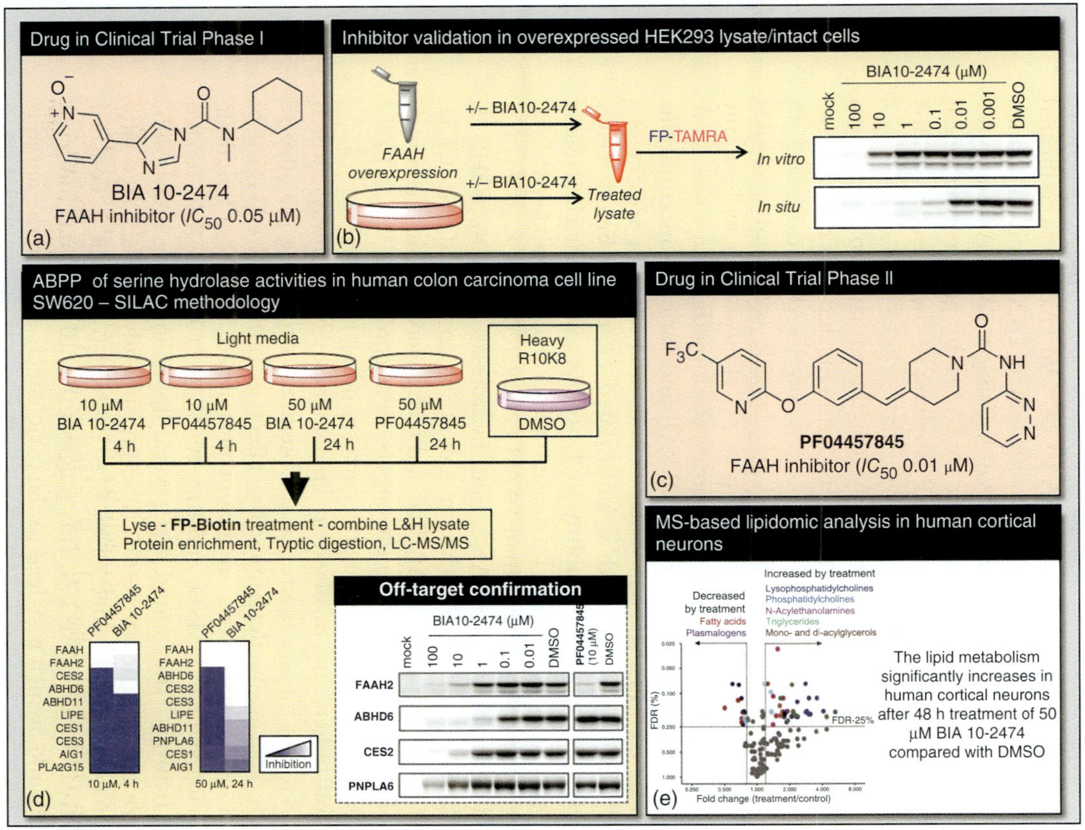

Figure 3.7 Identification of the on- and off-targets of the FAAH inhibitor BIA 10-2474 using ABPP. (a) Structure of BIA 10-2474, a proposed FAAH inhibitor that failed in phase I clinical trials. (b) Inhibitor validation using ABPP with an in-gel fluorescence approach. FAAH-overexpressed HEK293T lysates and intact cells were pre-incubated with different concentrations of BIA 10-2474 or DMSO control (*in vitro* 30 minutes, *in situ* four hours). The treated samples were subsequently labelled with FP-TAMRA (a broad-spectrum serine hydrolase ABP), and FAAH activity was directly visualized by in-gel fluorescence. (c) Structure of PF04457845, a FAAH inhibitor shown to be safe in phase I and II clinical trials. (d) Competitive ABPP for BIA 10-2474 target identification using a spike-in SILAC approach. The isotopically light SW620 cells were treated with 10 or 50 μM of inhibitors (BIA 10-2474 or PF04457845), and heavy-labelled cells were treated with DMSO as a control. The treated cells were then lysed and labelled with FP-biotin. Following lysate labelling, the combined light and heavy lysates were enriched and digested before analysis by LC-MS/MS. The proteomic heat maps show the top ten serine hydrolases identified in SW620 cells with inhibitor treatment. The off-targets of BIA 10-2474 were confirmed by overexpression of these purported targets in HEK293T cells and competitive labelling using BIA 10-2474 and FP-TAMRA. (e) Human cortical neurons were treated with 50 μM BIA 10-2474 or DMSO for 48 hours and then compared by LC-MS/MS for differences in lipid composition (lipidomics). Source: van Esbroeck et al. 2017 [2]. Reprinted with permission from AAAS.

were first incubated with mouse and human brain lysates. Tagged proteins were then coupled to a fluorescent reporter via click reactions. The alkyne analogues labelled FAAH in these lysates, confirming that BIA 10-2474 is an irreversible covalent inhibitor.

The researchers then used an FP probe (Figure 3.7), a now widely used tool for serine hydrolase inhibitor screening and activity-based profiling of serine hydrolases, in different stages of diseases in order to characterize off-target hydrolases inhibited by BIA 10-2474. The potency of BIA 10-2474 for FAAH was confirmed by co-incubating the FP probe in lysates with added FAAH and in human HEK293T cells artificially overexpressing FAAH. Using a TAMRA-conjugated FP probe, the protein band corresponding to FAAH by gel electrophoresis exhibited a dose-dependent reduction in FP labelling in the presence of BIA 10-2474 (Figure 3.7).

After the validation in the overexpression system, the human colon carcinoma cell line SW620 was chosen for the proteomic experiments due to its documented expression of endogenous serine hydrolases, including FAAH and FAAH2. In this work, BIA 10-2474 was also compared side by side with another FAAH inhibitor, PF04457845, which was tested in phase II clinical trials without any serious side effects [147, 148]. A SILAC quantification methodology was used, treating the cells with Dimethyl sulfoxide (DMSO) and various concentrations of either BIA102474 or PF04457845. After 4 hour and 24 hour treatments, the cells were lysed and treated with a biotinylated FP probe, before heavy and light lysates were combined. Biotinylated proteins were enriched using streptavidin agarose beads, followed by digestion and analysis by LC-MS/MS. The researchers found that while human FAAH is targeted by BIA 10-2474, it has several off-targets including FAAH2, lipid hydrolases (ABHD6, ABHD11, LIPE, and PNPLA6), and xenobiotic drug-metabolizing enzymes (CES1, CES2, and CES3). More than 90% of both ABHD6 and CES2 were inhibited at a high concentration of BIA 10-2474. These off-targets were confirmed by gel-based ABPP in HEK293T cells overexpressing the corresponding protein (Figure 3.7).

Most of the off-targets are involved in lipid metabolism pathways, which are highly expressed in human brain tissue, potentially explaining the adverse neurological side effects. To determine the effect of prolonged exposure of BIA 10-2474 on lipid metabolism, the groups performed MS-based lipidomic analysis, comparing vehicle (DMSO) and BIA 10-2474- or PF04457845-treated human cortical neurons. They found that several lipids, including FAAH substrates, triglycerides, monoacylglycerols, (lyso)phosphatidylcholines, free fatty acids, and plasmalogens, were affected by BIA 10-2474 treatment in contrast to PF04457845 treatment (Figure 3.7). This suggests BIA 10-2474 may interrupt cellular lipid networks, which may lead to the toxic effects seen on the nervous system. Furthermore, the reported inhibition of off-target protein PNPLA6 has previously been shown to be associated with several neurodegenerative disorders [149, 150]. This work is an excellent example of the applications of ABPP in exploring the on- and off-target profile of a clinically relevant inhibitor. It also highlights the critical importance of these studies; had the original researchers working on BIA 10-2474 had this data in hand, they might have prevented the unfortunate events that subsequently occurred.

3.4.3 Case Study 3: Target Identification of Small Molecule Inhibitors

One of the most important applications of ABPP is target protein profiling using inhibitor-based probes in order to better understand the mode of action of these inhibitors or other bioactive compounds. Furthermore, discovery of off-target proteins for these inhibitors may give an indication of the selectivity of the drug and can explain any potential side effects. Recently published research in the Tate group has focused on target ID by the design and synthesis of ABPs based on covalent inhibitor scaffolds. In order to study endogenous protein binding partners in living cells, the probe must be cell permeable and include a small bioorthogonally reactive group such as alkyne or azide, which can allow for conjugation to a clickable reporter tag (or a capture reagent) for downstream manipulation and analysis. Below we describe two recent studies showing target protein profiling of a bioactive small molecule, sulforaphane [24], and an inhibitor of a deubiquitinase enzyme [81].

3.4.3.1 New Target Profiling for Sulforaphane

Sulforaphane is a bioactive compound produced during glucosinolate metabolism in cruciferous vegetables [151]. This compound has been widely reported as a potential drug for cancer therapy, and demonstration that sulforaphane prevents and suppresses tumorigenesis, especially in breast cancer, led to the compound's clinical trial registration [152, 153]. The covalent mode of action of this compound contributes to the compound displaying polypharmacology; it covalently modifies multiple protein targets that are involved in various signalling pathways [154, 155]. Given the lack of knowledge about which proteins are modified, this research aimed to establish a full protein profile for sulforaphane so that the mode of action and any associated off-target effects were better understood [81]. To achieve this, the researchers applied ABPP in combination with quantitative chemical proteomics to identify and profile the target proteins of sulforaphane in two breast cancer cell lines.

The Tate group designed and synthesized an alkyne-modified probe based on the sulforaphane scaffold (Figure 3.8). The isothiocyanate group in the parent compound was replaced with a sulfoxythiocarbamate moiety, with the intention of increasing the stability of the probe and probe–protein adducts, without affecting intrinsic reactivity [156]. Also, the notoriously redox-labile sulfoxide group was replaced with a ketone. For initial target validation, competition of the alkyne-sulforaphane probe with the parent sulforaphane was performed in two human breast cancer cell lines (MCF7 and MDA-MB-231). The cells were pre-treated with various concentrations of sulforaphane and the alkyne-sulforaphane probe. After treatment, the cells were lysed, and the tagged proteins conjugated to a capture reagent (azide-TAMRA-biotin [AzTB]), which allowed for further analysis by gel electrophoresis and fluorescence analysis or enrichment and LC-MS/MS. Several protein bands were labelled by the probe, and most were efficiently outcompeted in response to co-treatment with the parent compound, indicating that this probe is an effective mimetic of the parent sulforaphane. For further target protein identification and

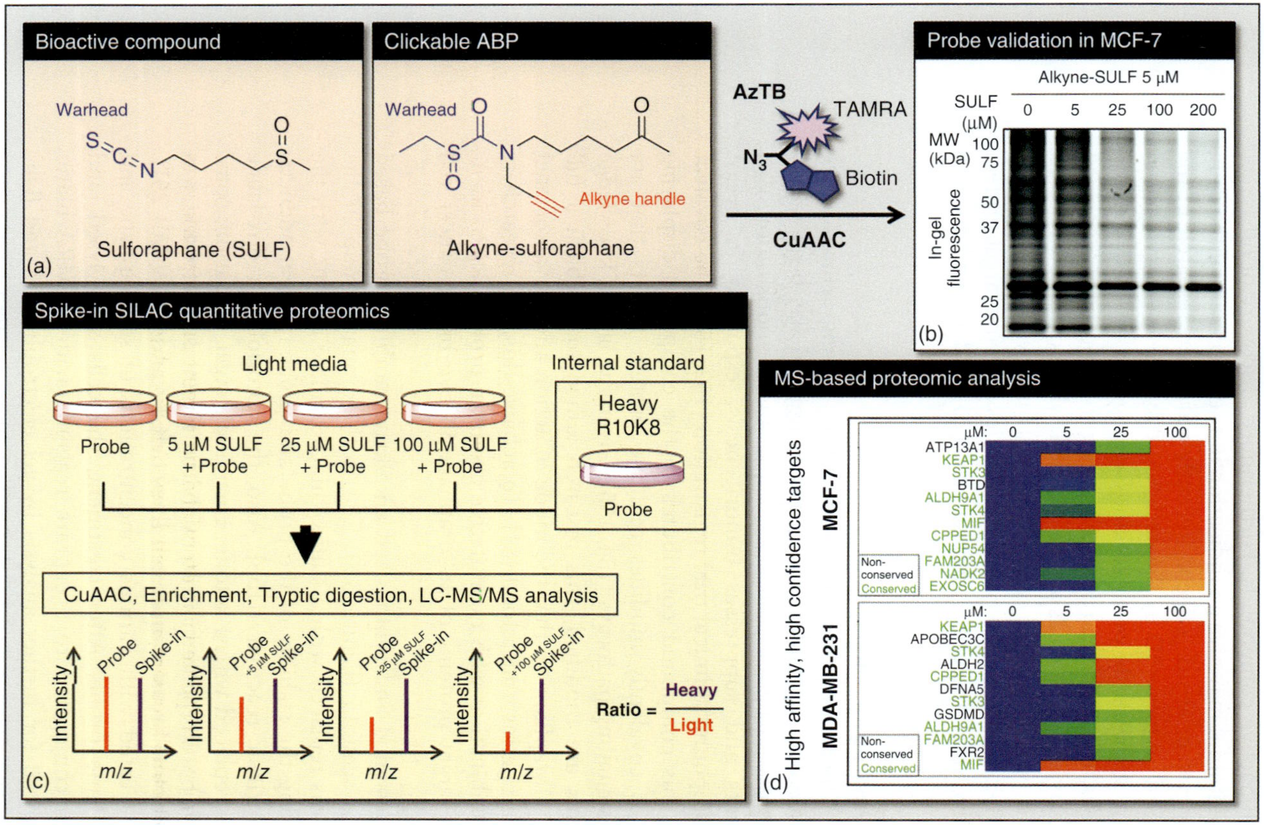

Figure 3.8 Target identification of sulforaphane in breast cancer cells using competitive ABPP and quantitative proteomic approaches. (a) Structure of sulforaphane (parent compound) containing an electrophilic isothiocyanate group. Structure of alkyne-sulforaphane probe (alkyne-SULF) with a sulfoxythiocarbamate group as the warhead. (b) Alkyne-SULF validation in MCF-7 cells using a competitive ABPP approach. The cells were pre-treated with varying concentrations of sulforaphane (parent compound), followed by alkyne-SULF treatment. The cells were then lysed and tagged proteins were clicked to a capture reagent (AzTB) for in-gel visualization. (c) Spike-in SILAC workflow: light-labelled cells were pre-treated with different concentrations of sulforaphane followed by the alkyne-SULF probe. Heavy (R10K8)-labelled cells were treated with the alkyne-SULF probe only. Both light- and heavy-labelled cells were lysed, and the R10K8-labelled lysate was spiked into the light lysates as an internal standard to quantify any depletion in protein labelling in the light-labelled samples caused by incubation with the parent sulforaphane. CuAAC reporter ligation, enrichment, digestion, and LC-MS/MS analysis were then performed, and quantification was achieved by calculating the ratio between heavy/light peptide signals. (d) Heat maps representing high confidence target proteins responding to sulforaphane at different concentrations. Blue: no competition, red: high competition. Source: This image is a derivative of figures from [24] (https://pubs.rsc.org/en/content/articlehtml/2017/cc/c6cc08797c) – Published by The Royal Society of Chemistry, licensed under CC BY 3.0 (https://

quantification, the Tate group applied the 'spike-in SILAC' approach combined with competition-based chemical proteomics as shown in Figure 3.8.

Using this approach, more than 120 proteins were identified as high confidence targets of sulforaphane, with 56 proteins identified in both cell lines. Several targets were labelled by sulforaphane even at low concentrations while in the presence of the probe, suggesting a high binding potency for sulforaphane. These proteins include macrophage migration inhibitory factor (MIF) and Kelch-like ECH-associated protein 1 (KEAP1), which have been reported previously as sulforaphane targets [156–158], validating ABPP for sulforaphane target ID.

The Tate group also applied the bioinformatics platform Ingenuity® Pathway Analysis (IPA) to classify the biological roles of the targets. From IPA analysis of the dose-responsive proteins in both cell lines, the major canonical pathway of protein up-regulation was apoptosis signalling [159], exemplified by the identification of a target common to both cell lines, NF-kB, a transcription factor linked to cancer cell survival [160]. The major pathways down-regulated by sulforaphane in a dose-dependent manner were growth hormone and ERK/MAP kinase signalling pathways [161, 162]. These pathways have common upstream mediators, the signal transducer and activator of transcription (STAT) 1 and 3 proteins. STAT1 and STAT3 were identified as direct targets of sulforaphane in both cell lines, indicating that the likely mode of action for sulforaphane is down-regulation of these pathways [163]. Indeed, STAT1/3 were verified as *bona fide* targets of sulforaphane by complementary western blot approaches.

By designing and synthesizing an ABP and applying it in competition-based chemical proteomic studies, this work delivers a comprehensive target profile of sulforaphane in living cells. This data will be useful for clinical studies involving sulforaphane treatment and for drug discovery and development around the identified target proteins. Additionally, the developed probe may be used as a chemical tool for future inhibitor screening of the aforementioned target proteins.

3.4.3.2 Profiling USP Inhibitors in Human Cell Lines as Potential Therapeutic Molecules

In a recent paper from the Tate group, we reported the first cell-permeable small molecule ABP for the ubiquitin-specific protease (USP) family of DUBs [81]. Ubiquitination is the PTM of a protein by the attachment of one or more ubiquitin (Ub) protein(s), the most common consequence being the degradation of the tagged protein [164]. The reverse process, termed deubiquitination, is catalysed by DUBs, which have been reported as potential drug targets and biomarkers in several diseases including cancers and neurodegenerative diseases [165–167]. To profile the activity of DUBs, Ub-modified ABPs such as HA-ubiquitin vinyl methyl ester (HA-UbVME) and HA-ubiquitin bromoethyl (HA-UbBr2) have been widely used. These probes covalently bind to a cysteine residue in the active site of the DUBs and therefore subsequently label the enzyme [43, 168]. DUB profiling allows researchers to quantify the potency and selectivity of potential DUB inhibitors [50, 51]; however, these Ub-based probes have been limited to lysate screening due to the probes' lack of membrane permeability, in part due to their large size.

To address this limitation, the Tate group reported a small molecule ABP for the USP family of DUBs in intact cancer cells. From an initial high-throughput screen (HTS) of USP inhibitors, a 4-chloroacetylpyrrole derivative was discovered as a potent covalent inhibitor for USP4 and USP11. The potency of this inhibitor was assessed in both *in vitro* biochemical assays and in human osteosarcoma (U2OS) lysate using the aforementioned HA-UbVME probe. In order to investigate USP activity in living cells, the Tate group synthesized an alkyne-tagged derivative of USP inhibitors (Figure 3.9). This alkyne-ABP was validated in U2OS cells using an in-house chemical proteomic workflow as described in Section 3.3. The co-incubation and resulting competition of the parent compound with the alkyne probe revealed a dose-dependent reduction in labelling of various protein targets via in-gel fluorescence, leading to further analysis by LC-MS/MS. Once again, we applied the 'spike-in SILAC' approach combined with competition-based chemical proteomics as shown in Figure 3.9.

Twelve USPs were enriched and subsequently identified by the alkyne-ABP with high selectivity. When competed with the parent compound as above, the two most potent targets were identified as USP16 and USP33, not USP4 and USP11 as expected from the HTS. While USP4 did show significant competition, USP11 was relatively weakly competed. These competitive target engagement results were validated using western blotting with both alkyne-ABP and HA-UbVME labelling experiments. USP33, a novel target of the 4-chloroacetylpyrrole derivative HTS hit, has been reported as the DUB and genomic stabilizer for centriolar coiled-coil protein of 110 kDa (CP110) [169]. In this work we further demonstrated a reduction in CP110 protein level following USP33 inhibition by the USP inhibitor parent compound (Figure 3.9).

This work reports the first cell-permeable small molecule ABP to selectively target USPs. A quantitative chemical proteomic methodology was used to profile USP activity and identify a novel target of this USP inhibitor, USP33, which may be useful for future drug discovery programmes. Moreover, these inhibitor-based probes provide potential on-/off-target information that might assist in the explanation of any possible side effects of the parent compound.

3.4.4 Case Study 4: Fragment-Based Ligand Discovery Aided by Photoaffinity Labelling

Photoaffinity labelling (PAL) is traditionally used to interrogate the cellular protein profile of a particular compound of interest in the hope of learning more about both the mechanism of action and any associated off-target interactions that may compromise their utility as chemical probes and/or potential therapeutics [52]. A recent report from the Cravatt laboratory at the Scripps Research Institute has extended this concept to profiling the in-cell protein interactions of a set of biologically relevant drug fragments, with the goal of identifying new fragment–target interactions that could stimulate the development of new tool molecules [15].

Fragment-based screening has been a mainstay of drug discovery programmes in recent decades; however the approach requires the protein target to be known, the protein, or a constituent part, to be synthesized in an appreciable quantity and

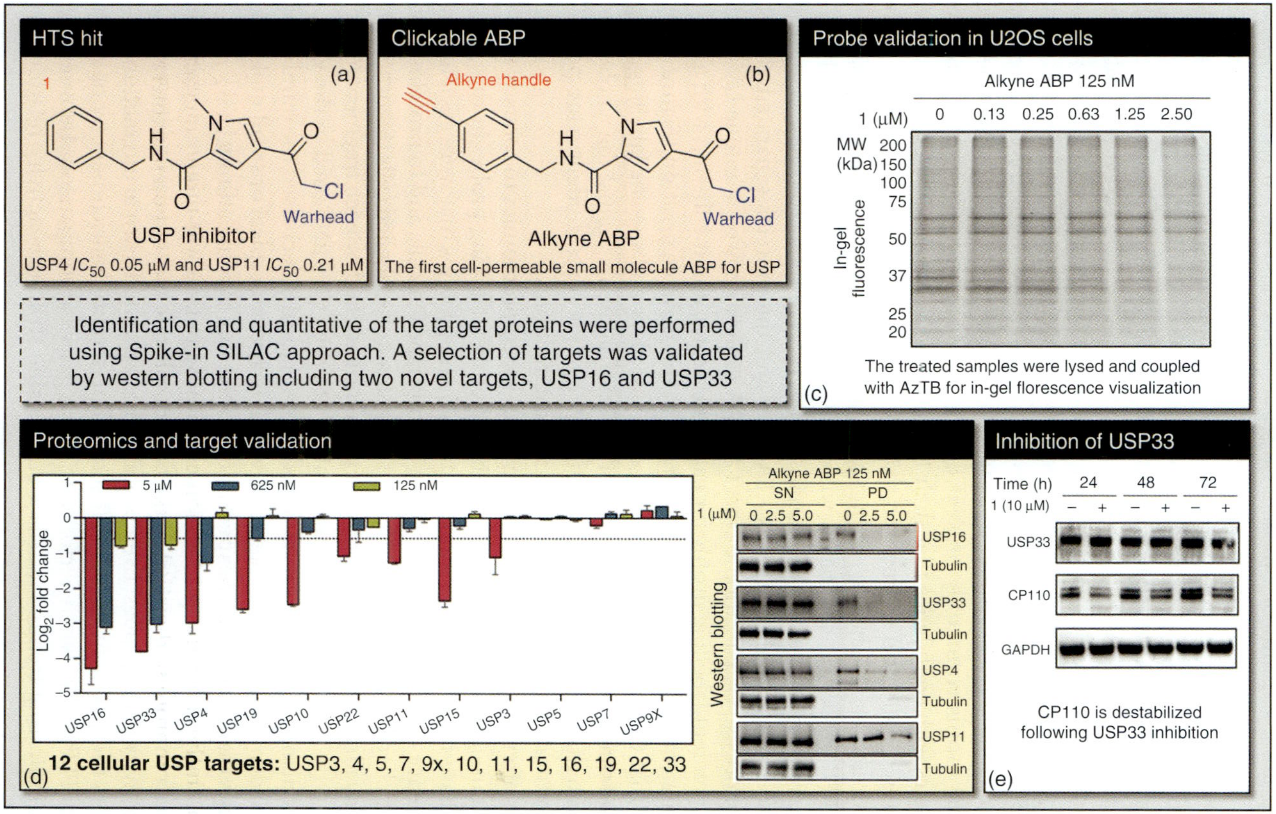

Figure 3.9 USP profiling using competitive ABPP that quantitative proteomic approaches. (a) Structure of USP inhibitor(**1**) that exhibits low micromolar inhibition of USP4 and USP11. (b) The novel alkyne-modified USP inhibitor used herein for ABPP studies. (c) In-gel fluorescence analysis after in-cell competition-based ABPP of USP inhibitor (parent compound) and the alkyne probe. (d) Dose-dependent depletion of probe labelling can be seen for proteins that are targets of the parent inhibitor. Histogram identifying and quantifying the specific USPs that are labelled by the alkyne-ABP and subsequently have that labelling depleted by increasing concentrations of the parent compound. (e) Identification and quantification were performed using competitive ABPP combined with the spike-in SILAC approach, as described in Section 3.3. The target proteins identified from MS analysis were validated by western blotting using a similar competitive ABPP and enrichment approach. SN: supernatant from enrichment process, PD: enriched fraction (pull down). The downstream effect of USP33 inhibition as analysed by western blotting. Source: Ward et al. 2016 [81]. Reprinted with permission from ACS.

purity for *in vitro* assays and to have an associated crystal structure to assist with the structure-aided diversification of the hit fragment(s) into a lead compound [170]. Furthermore, the standard methodology only allows for the screening of a fragment library against one protein target at a time, and the target is removed from its native cellular environment, neglecting the effect of the complex biological system on the fragment–protein interaction, potentially leading to problems further down the costly drug development pipeline.

In this article, the Cravatt group screened a small library of fragments against the whole cellular proteome, as opposed to just one protein target, compiling a list of interacting protein partners for each molecule. In order to achieve this, a set of 14 fully functionalized fragment (FFF) probes were synthesized, consisting of a minimal clickable photocrosslinking moiety coupled to a variety of small molecule fragments (Figure 3.10). The fragments selected were based on structural motifs commonly present in existing drug molecules, providing the researchers with confidence that their FFF probes should non-covalently engage proteins in a biological setting and that any interactions of the fragments with targets already established in the literature could be independently verified.

Each FFF probe was incubated with HEK293T cells and irradiated with UV light to crosslink any engaged protein targets to the probe. The cells were subsequently lysed and 'clicked' to N_3-TAMRA and the proteins separated via gel electrophoresis. Visualization of the TAMRA moiety showed a unique UV- and dose-dependent labelling profile for each FFF probe, and incubation with a control probe containing only a methyl group in the variable position (Figure 3.10) showed that the fragment group is required for clear and specific labelling. This suggested that it was possible to screen various fragments against the whole proteome simultaneously, and in a biologically relevant context, identifying potentially new and interesting fragment–target interactions.

PAL is often coupled with quantitative MS-based proteomics to robustly identify the target proteins associated with a photocrosslinking probe. In this case, SILAC-based quantification was used to compare proteins that were enriched in the presence of an FFF probe in heavy isotope labelled cells and to proteins that were enriched by the control FFF probe in light isotope labelled cells (Figure 3.10). This study identified a large number of proteins enriched by each fragment, owed in part to the relatively high concentration of probe (200 μM) used in the workflow. Reducing the concentration of probe dramatically decreased the number of proteins identified for each fragment, which is a result typical of small molecule fragments that are generally expected to exhibit low binding affinity [171].

Importantly, the target profile of each of these probes was unique, suggesting that the structural composition of the target molecule was crucial in determining the selectivity of the probes. Even proteins that exhibited a broad interaction profile across the fragment library still showed preferential enrichment by one or a subset of FFF probes when performing direct pairwise comparisons between the probes, indicating trends towards a quantifiable structure–activity relationship (SAR).

The range of proteins targeted by these FFF probes is impressive; more soluble proteins were enriched than membrane proteins, but this could in part be due to the lower abundance of membrane proteins in the cellular proteome

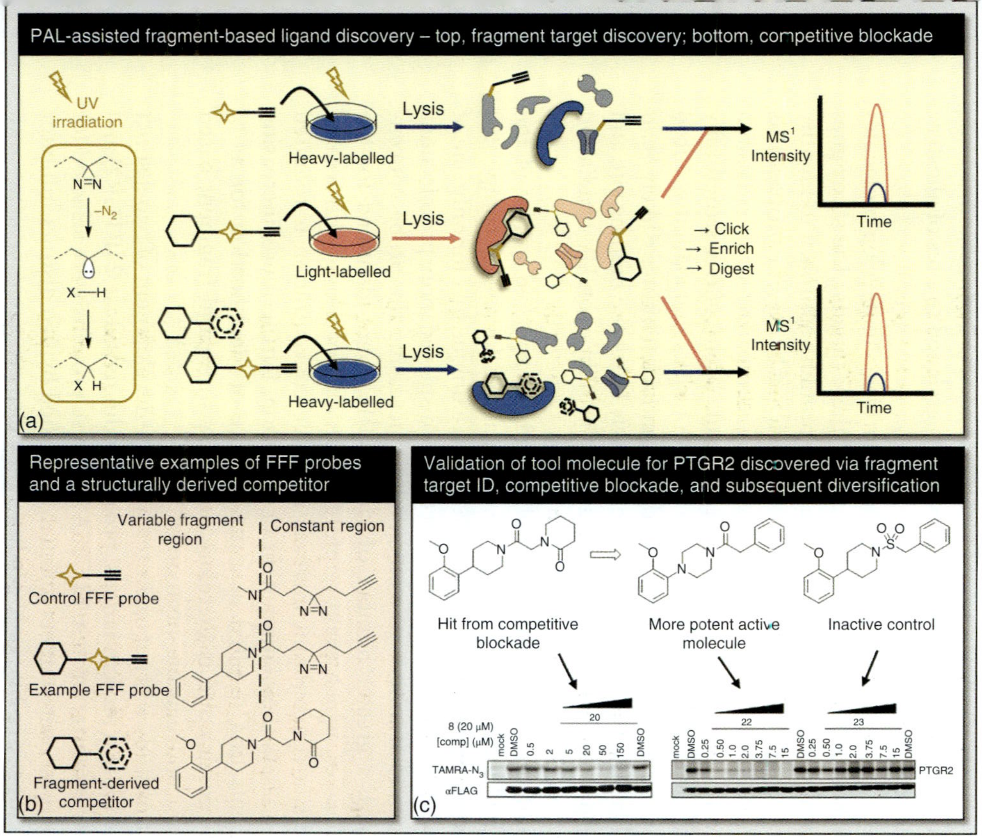

Figure 3.10 (a) Photoaffinity labelling workflow: SILAC light-labelled HEK293T cells were incubated with an FFF probe (middle pink), and heavy-labelled cells were treated with either the control probe (top blue – fragment-based target discovery) or the same probe plus a structurally similar competitor molecule (bottom blue – competitive blockade). UV irradiation transforms non-covalent protein–ligand interactions into an irreversible covalent linkage by the formation of a highly reactive carbene intermediate (left sub-panel). The cells are lysed, and heavy- and light-labelled samples are combined. Tagged proteins are clicked to azide-biotin, enriched using streptavidin on a solid support, and digested to peptides that can be analysed by MS-based proteomics. Relative enrichment indicated whether targets were specifically engaged by the FFF probe versus control (top) and successfully depleted by co-incubation with an active competitor (bottom). (b) Examples of some of the fully functionalized fragment (FFF) probes synthesized for this project, including a control probe to interrogate the background proteins enriched by this method, an FFF probe of interest, and a competitor molecule derived from the same fragment. (c) Competitive blockade studies identified a hit ligand for PTGR2 using the FFF probe displayed in the panel to the left. Further screening identified both a more potent, selective inhibitor of PTGR2 and a structurally related yet inactive control molecule. The more potent molecule could effectively deplete FFF-probe labelling of recombinant epitope-tagged PTGR2 at lower concentrations than the original hit by gel-based competition assays. The inactive control failed to deplete FFF-probe labelling over the same concentration range. Source: Reprinted with permission of Parker et al. 2017 [15]. Copyright 2017, Elsevier.

and the difficulty in processing and analysis of the more hydrophobic peptide fragments [172]. The target class of proteins enriched by the probes included enzymes, but also extended to structural proteins, transcriptomic and genomic regulators, and as yet uncategorized protein targets. Of all of these proteins, less than 20% were proteins with pre-confirmed ligands in the DrugBank, meaning that many new targets, even so-called 'undruggable' proteins, have been discovered to have potential fragment binding partners by this methodology. Of those with known binding partners, when interrogating enrichment at the peptide level, ~80% of fragment-modified peptides corresponded to a confirmed binding pocket in the protein of interest, with the rest being assigned to sites of allostery or protein–protein interactions.

These discoveries could lead to the initiation of projects to develop molecules that could be elaborated into inhibitors for any of these targets. The study goes further however by extending this proteome-wide profiling approach to identify potential new inhibitors for the various proteins enriched by the FFF probes. This is achieved using SILAC-based proteomic profiling, comparing samples treated with an FFF probe to samples treated with the same probe *plus* a structurally related but larger drug-like molecule. Those protein targets that exhibit reduced probe-based enrichment in the presence of the potential inhibitor are likely *bona fide* targets of this molecule, as it is able to effectively block the binding site and prevent the FFF probe from covalently tagging the protein upon UV irradiation (Figure 3.10).

Using 20 μM of three different FFF probes and an eightfold excess of the structurally related inhibitor, 100 targets were identified for the 17 competitor molecules tested. Around 60% of these proteins were unique hits for only one of these inhibitors, while the rest of the protein targets displayed more promiscuous binding to the panel of inhibitors tested. When increasing the probe concentration to 200 μM, a greater number of targets (215) were identified for the competitor molecules, which again reinforces that when working with weaker fragment binders, a concomitant increase in probe concentration is required to quantitatively assess their enrichment or depletion. Furthermore, increasing the probe concentration resulted in a greater rate of identification for as of yet unliganded proteins and is therefore necessary to expand fragment-based screening into the 'undruggable' proteome.

The utility of this study was put to the test with the development of two distinct chemical probes for two protein targets, prostaglandin reductase 2 (PTGR2) and the membrane transporter protein SLC25A20. These proteins were selected for further study as these were targets uniquely identified by two distinct inhibitor molecules in competitive blockade studies. They also represent proteins with important roles in cellular metabolism yet currently lack any chemical probes that effectively and selectively modulate their biomolecular activity.

Taking the case of PTGR2, an initial hit molecule was discovered by the above competitive blockade experiment and was verified by both gel-based competition studies (Figure 3.10) and an *in vitro* inhibition assay, which delivered an IC_{50} value of 79 μM. It was envisaged that this could be improved by screening further molecules that were structurally similar to this competitor. This resulted in the identification of an inhibitor of PTGR2 with an IC_{50} value of around 0.7 μM, a remarkable 100-fold increase in potency. This tool molecule was able to block the labelling of recombinant and endogenous PTGR2 by the corresponding FFF probe (Figure 3.10) and furthermore was able to inhibit the reduction of the cellular substrate of PTGR2. A structurally similar molecule was also screened and found to be inactive against PTGR2; as such, this method has effectively discovered a new tool molecule and a homologous inactive control for a previously unliganded protein of metabolic interest.

Finally, a further fragment library of 465 probes was synthesized, with an increase in average molecular weight of the variable recognition element of ~100 Da from the previous library. The idea was to screen this library of compounds against a particular phenotype and then take the key hits forward in PAL proteomic studies. The researchers screened for agonists of adipogenesis, the maturation of proadipocytes to adipocytes, using a lipid accumulation assay as a readout. From the library, nine probes stimulated adipogenesis in human mesenchymal stem cells, with one active at concentrations of 10 μM.

As such, the hit probe was taken forward into proteomic-based target ID studies using effective comparisons between both inactive probes and also co-incubations with active (hit FFF probe without minimal photocrosslinker) and inactive competitor molecules, all generated from the early phenotypic screen. These experiments identified progesterone receptor membrane component 2 (PGRMC2) as a *bona fide* target of both the FFF probe and the active competitor in proteomic studies, and this was subsequently verified by gel-based studies; shRNA-mediated knockdown of PGRMC2 was also sufficient to block adipogenesis induced by the hit probe. While further modification of this probe might be necessary to generate a more potent tool molecule, this study has been effective in not only identifying a probe for adipogenesis but also in uncovering PGRMC2 as a promoter of adipogenesis, something that had not been previously reported in the literature.

This report clearly represents a massive synthetic effort, with approximately 1000 molecules synthesized to generate all the data presented in this article. This may be a barrier to wider application of this technique. However recent advances in multicomponent reactions for the synthesis of photocrosslinking probes may go some way to ameliorate this issue, providing potentially facile synthetic routes to diverse probe libraries [173, 174]. Nonetheless, the application of these probes is impressive; in a singular study the Cravatt group has pioneered a new methodology of fragment-based screening, extending the concept from single- to multi-target interrogation. They have identified new fragment–protein interactions and extended this concept to developing probes for two previously unliganded but important drug targets, indicating this may be a powerful technique to identify previously under represented proteins with pharmaceutical relevance. Finally, they expanded their probe library dramatically to include more complex fragment groups and applied them in a phenotypic screen against adipogenesis. Proteomic-based target ID with a hit probe revealed an as of yet uncharacterized promoter of adipogenesis, once again demonstrating the power of PAL in target ID studies. ABPP has long been an effective technique to globally profile reactive molecules throughout the cellular proteome, and this study by the Cravatt group represents the first serious step towards achieving the same for molecules that interact with the proteome in a non-covalent, reversible manner.

3.4.5 Case Study 5: Quenched Fluorescent Activity-Based Probe (qABP) Design and Application in Protein Localization

A qABP is a covalent ABP in which the warhead is conjugated with a leaving group, which is also a fluorescence quencher (Figure 3.11). The qABP without activity from its target enzyme is in the 'off' or 'dark' state; the fluorescence is quenched. Displacement of the quencher by the target enzyme generates a real-time fluorescent signal based upon the enzyme's activity [10, 20]. The applications of fluorescent ABPs, including qABPs, have been widely developed particularly by the Bogyo group and have been used for in-cell fluorescence microscopy and *in vivo* fluorescence imaging [134, 175].

Cysteine cathepsins are a class of clan CA proteases that play many important roles in biological systems, mainly in proteolytic degradation in lysosomes and regulation of both normal and disease physiological conditions including inflammatory disease and cancer [176, 177]. Cathepsin S is unusual as its expression is almost entirely restricted to antigen-presenting cells (APCs), such as dendritic cells (DCs) and B cells, indicating specificity in its function [178]. Increased expression of cathepsin S often correlates with disease states such as tumour development [179, 180], TRPV-mediated inflammatory pain [181, 182], and cystic fibrosis [183]. Although cathepsin S is clearly a potential biomarker and therapeutic target, the biological mechanism of this protease is still unclear. To clearly understand the function and localization of cathepsin S, the Bogyo group reported a near-infrared (IR) qABP that allowed for direct visualization in living cells and in mouse models [135].

To develop a qABP that selectively targets cathepsin S, two previously reported qABPs for cathepsin profiling from the same research group were used as scaffolds [134, 175, 184]. The synthesized probes were validated using

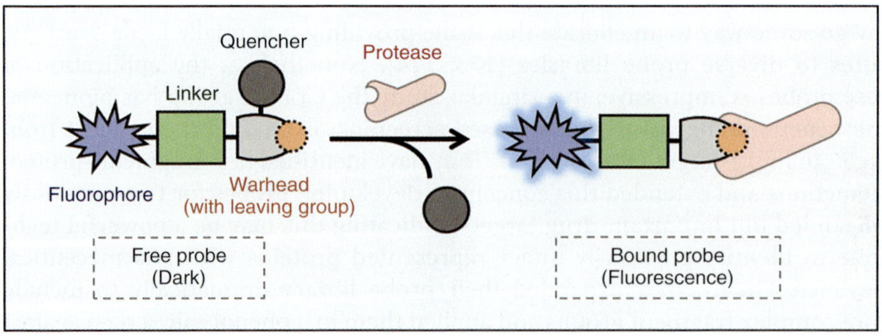

Figure 3.11 The quenched fluorescent activity-based probe (qABP) consists of four key components: a fluorophore, a selective linker, an electrophilic warhead, and a quencher. The qABP is in the 'off' state when free in solution due to fluorescence suppression by the quencher group. In the presence of a specific protease, the qABP binds to the enzyme's active site, and the quencher is cleaved off, restoring the fluorescent signal.

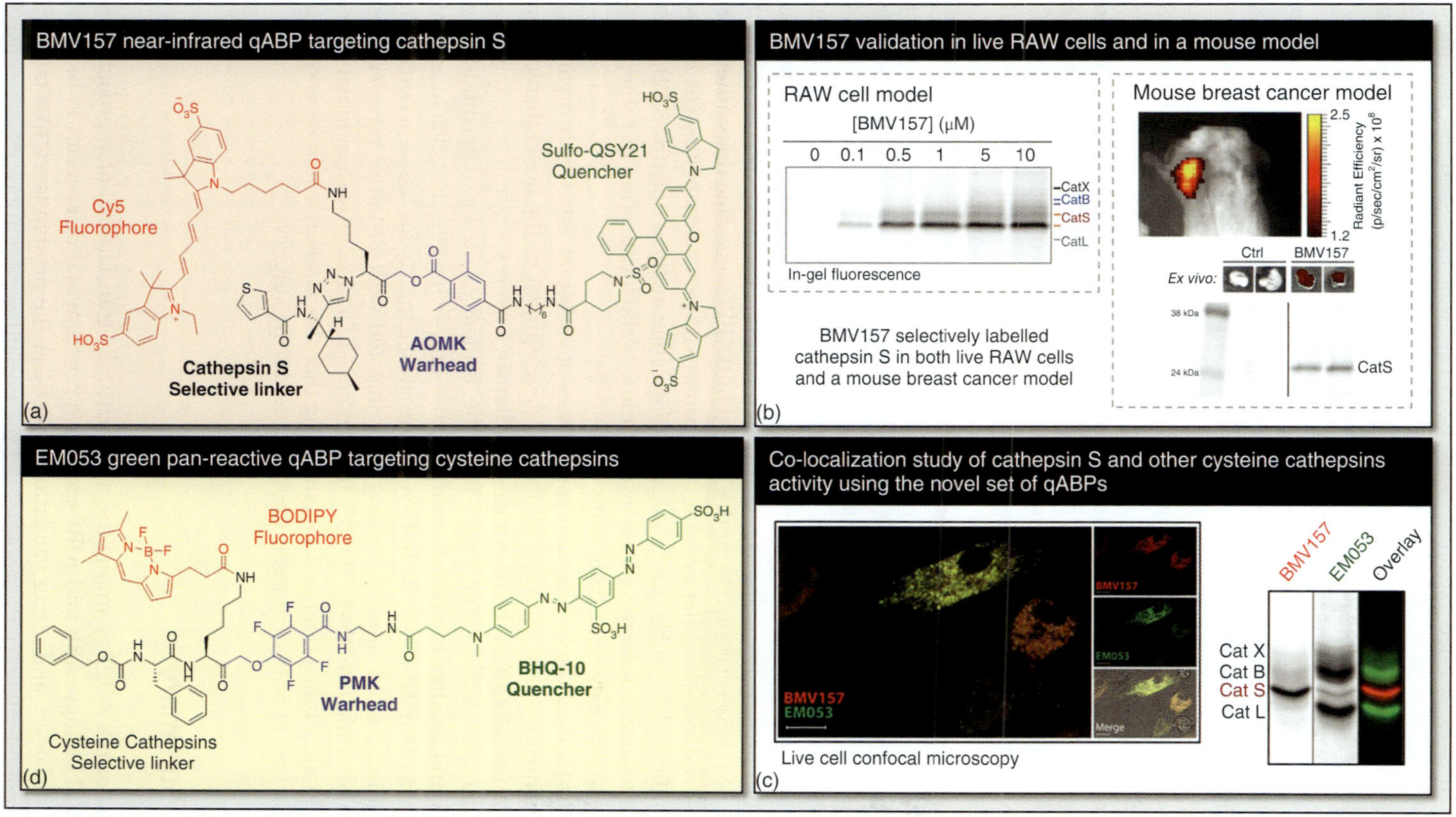

Figure 3.12 Selective qABPs for imaging cathepsin activity in live RAW cells and a mouse breast cancer model. (a) Structure of cathepsin S selective qABP (BMV157) incorporating a selective linker (black), a cysteine protease specific acyloxymethyl ketone (AOMK) warhead (blue), a sulfo-QSY21 quencher (green), and a Cy5 fluorophore. (b) Validation of BMV157 in live RAW cells and a mouse breast cancer model shows the concentration-dependent labelling profile of cathepsin S and live imaging of a tumour, respectively. The fluorescently labelled tumour was analysed *ex vivo*, and cathepsin S labelling was confirmed by gel-based fluorescence analysis. (c) Real-time confocal microscopy images of primary mouse bone marrow-derived macrophages show the dual labelling with both BMV157 (red) and EM053 (green); the dual-probe treated cells were lysed and analysed by gel-based fluorescence. (d) Structure of pan-reactive cathepsin probe (EM053) incorporating a general selective cysteine cathepsin linker (black), a tetrafluoro-substituted PMK electrophile (blue), a BHQ10 quencher (green), and a BODIPY fluorophore. Source: Oresic Bender et al. 2015 [135]. Copyright 2015, American Chemical Society.

gel-based fluorescence labelling, and BMV157 was identified as the most selective and potent qABP for cathepsin S (Figure 3.12). BMV157 contains a *trans*-4-methylcyclohexyl group as part of the selective linker, which had been known to target cathepsin S, and a bulky electrophilic acyloxymethyl ketone (AOMK) group, used as a specific cysteine protease warhead. Additionally, the quencher (sulfo-QSY21) also acts to increase the hydrophilicity of the qABP. BMV157 was subsequently applied *in vivo* for imaging breast tumours in mice, showing a clear tumour area with excellent contrast against the surrounding healthy tissue. Subsequent extraction of breast tissue and *ex vivo* analysis of the fluorescence labelling profile confirmed the qABP's selectivity for cathepsin S (Figure 3.12).

To compare the activity and localization of cathepsin S to the other cysteine cathepsins, a green-fluorescent qABP (EM053), broad spectrum against the cysteine cathepsin family, was synthesized as a complementary tool to BMV157. The conditions and concentrations of both probes were carefully optimized to achieve visible labelling of the cysteine cathepsins (cathepsins X, B, and L) with EM053 (BODIPY fluorophore) while also achieving concomitant labelling of cathepsin S with BMV157 (Cy5 fluorophore), which will also be a target of the broad-spectrum probe. After this optimization, the qABPs were used as imaging tools to study the degree of co-localization between cathepsin S and the other cysteine cathepsins in primary bone marrow-derived macrophages (BMMs) visualized by confocal microscopy. Following a two hour incubation with both probes, live cell imaging revealed that the vesicular compartment of mouse BMMs was labelled by both Cy5 and BODIPY, suggesting that cathepsin S co-localized with the other cysteine cathepsins in BMMs, and labelling specificity was confirmed by subsequent in-gel fluorescence analysis (Figure 3.12). This novel dual-probe strategy allows visualization of the localization of cathepsin S relative to other cysteine cathepsins in live cells.

Understanding the localization and activity of cathepsin S in whole organisms would provide useful information for the development of the novel therapeutic drugs, especially given the relevance of cathepsin S overexpression in certain disease states. BMV157, being a near-IR probe, is ideally suited to determining the activity and localization of cathepsin S in not only living cells but also in animal models, as near-IR wavelengths have the greatest capacity for tissue penetration. Optical imaging of tumour-bearing mice injected with BMV157 revealed that this qABP could effectively identify the presence of a tumour with minimal background interference (Figure 3.12), meaning that this strategy could be used as a contrast tool in both diagnostic imaging and during surgery.

3.5 Summary

In conclusion, ABPP is among the most naturally translational of approaches in chemical biology. ABP and AfBP can drive fundamental discoveries in biology, target discovery and target validation directly at the protein level, in a manner highly complementary to genomics. At the same time, A(f)BP probes employed for discovery can be seamlessly adapted into tools for assay development, inhibitor discovery, on- and off-target characterization, biomarker analysis, and bioimaging by simple modification with innovative chemical labelling technologies.

In this chapter we have introduced some of the most commonly applied approaches in ABPP and AfBPP, from probe design to quantitative proteomic analysis, and described some cutting-edge applications of this technology, from target ID and *de novo* ligand discovery to biomedical imaging. However, these examples illustrate just a small part of the remarkable and growing impact of ABPP on bioscience, biomedicine, and industry, thanks to a vibrant and international community of researchers driving innovative chemistry and chemical biology in this field. Among many recent innovations, particularly notable are the applications of ABPP to immunology (e.g. antigen presentation [185] and immunoproteasome activity [186]), glycosidase biology [187], natural product target ID [23, 25, 63], herbicide toxicology [188], high-throughput screening [189], small ubiquitin-like modifier (SUMO) proteases [190], and ubiquitin ligase biology [191–193], to mention but a few. The authors would like to apologize for the omission of discussion of these and other innovations by our esteemed colleagues in chemical biology, for which space precludes detailed analysis.

References

1 Schenone, M., Dancik, V., Wagner, B.K., and Clemons, P.A. (2013). Target identification and mechanism of action in chemical biology and drug discovery. *Nat. Chem. Biol.* 9 (4): 232–240.

2 van Esbroeck, A.C.M., Janssen, A.P.A., Cognetta, A.B. et al. (2017). Activity-based protein profiling reveals off-target proteins of the FAAH inhibitor BIA 10-2474. *Science* 356 (6342): 1084–1087.

3 Cravatt, B.F., Simon, G.M., Yates, I.I.I., and R, J. (2007). The biological impact of mass-spectrometry-based proteomics. *Nature* 450: 991.

4 Cravatt, B.F., Wright, A.T., and Kozarich, J.W. (2008). Activity-based protein profiling: from enzyme chemistry to proteomic chemistry. *Annu. Rev. Biochem.* 77: 383–414.

5 Heal, W.P., Dang, T.H., and Tate, E.W. (2011). Activity-based probes: discovering new biology and new drug targets. *Chem. Soc. Rev.* 40 (1): 246–257.

6 Serim, S., Haedke, U., and Verhelst, S.H. (2012). Activity-based probes for the study of proteases: recent advances and developments. *ChemMedChem* 7 (7): 1146–1159.

7 Benns, H.J., Tate, E.W., and Child, M.A. (2018). Activity-based protein profiling for the study of parasite biology. *Curr. Top. Microbiol. Immunol.* https://doi.org/10.1007/82_2018_123.

8 Niphakis, M.J. and Cravatt, B.F. (2014). Enzyme inhibitor discovery by activity-based protein profiling. *Annu. Rev. Biochem.* 83: 341–377.

9 Edgington-Mitchell, L., Bogyo, M., and Verdoes, M. (2017). Live cell imaging and profiling of cysteine cathepsin activity using a quenched activity-based

probe. In: *Activity-Based Proteomics: Methods and Protocols* (eds. H.S. Overkleeft and B.I. Florea). New York, NY: Springer New York.

10 Edgington, L.E., Verdoes, M., and Bogyo, M. (2011). Functional imaging of proteases: recent advances in the design and application of substrate-based and activity-based probes. *Curr. Opin. Chem. Biol.* 15 (6): 798–805.

11 Evans, M.J. and Cravatt, B.F. (2006). Mechanism-based profiling of enzyme families. *Chem. Rev.* 106: 3279.

12 Galmozzi, A., Dominguez, E., Cravatt, B.F., and Saez, E. (2014). Chapter 8 – Application of activity-based protein profiling to study enzyme function in adipocytes. *Methods Enzymol.* 538: 151–169.

13 Bar-Peled, L., Kemper, E.K., Suciu, R.M. et al. (2017). Chemical proteomics identifies druggable vulnerabilities in a genetically defined cancer. *Cell* 171 (3): 709.e23.

14 Leung, D., Hardouin, C., Boger, D.L., and Cravatt, B.F. (2003). Discovering potent and selective reversible inhibitors of enzymes in complex proteomes. *Nat. Biotechnol.* 21 (6): 687–691.

15 Parker, C.G., Galmozzi, A., Wang, Y. et al. (2017). Ligand and target discovery by fragment-based screening in human cells. *Cell* 168 (3): 541.e29.

16 Nomura, D.K. and Maimone, T.J. (2018). Target identification of bioactive covalently acting natural products. *Curr. Top. Microbiol. Immunol.* https://doi.org/10.1007/82_2018_121.

17 Pichler, C.M., Krysiak, J., and Breinbauer, R. (2016). Target identification of covalently binding drugs by activity-based protein profiling (ABPP). *Bioorg. Med. Chem.* 24 (15): 3291–3303.

18 Su, Y., Ge, J., Zhu, B. et al. (2013). Target identification of biologically active small molecules via in situ methods. *Curr. Opin. Chem. Biol.* 17 (5): 768–775.

19 Vizovisek, M., Vidmar, R., Drag, M. et al. (2018). Protease specificity: towards in vivo imaging applications and biomarker discovery. *Trends Biochem. Sci.* 43 (10): 829–844.

20 Fernandez, A. and Vendrell, M. (2016). Smart fluorescent probes for imaging macrophage activity. *Chem. Soc. Rev.* 45 (5): 1182–1196.

21 Shi, H., Liu, K., Xu, A., and Yao, S.Q. (2009). Small molecule microarray-facilitated screening of affinity-based probes (AfBPs) for gamma-secretase. *Chem. Commun. (Cambridge)* (33): 5030–5032.

22 Murale, D.P., Hong, S.C., Haque, M.M., and Lee, J.S. (2017). Photo-affinity labeling (PAL) in chemical proteomics: a handy tool to investigate protein-protein interactions (PPIs). *Proteome Sci.* 15: 3. eCollection 2016.

23 Kalesh, K.A., Clulow, J.A., and Tate, E.W. (2015). Target profiling of zerumbone using a novel cell-permeable clickable probe and quantitative chemical proteomics. *Chem. Commun. (Cambridge)* 51 (25): 5497–5500.

24 Clulow, J.A., Storck, E.M., Lanyon-Hogg, T. et al. (2017). Competition-based, quantitative chemical proteomics in breast cancer cells identifies new target profiles for sulforaphane. *Chem. Commun. (Cambridge)* 53 (37): 5182–5185.

25 Wright, M.H., Tao, Y., Drechsel, J. et al. (2017). Quantitative chemoproteomic profiling reveals multiple target interactions of spongiolactone

derivatives in leukemia cells. *Chem. Commun. (Cambridge)* 53 (95): 12818–12821.
26 Liu, Y., Patricelli, M.P., and Cravatt, B.F. (1999). Activity-based protein profiling: the serine hydrolases. *Proc. Natl. Acad. Sci. U. S. A.* 96 (26): 14694–14699.
27 Jessani, N., Niessen, S., Wei, B.Q. et al. (2005). A streamlined platform for high-content functional proteomics of primary human specimens. *Nat. Methods* 2 (9): 691–697.
28 Kidd, D., Liu, Y., and Cravatt, B.F. (2001). Profiling serine hydrolase activities in complex proteomes. *Biochemistry* 40 (13): 4005–4015.
29 Okerberg, E.S., Wu, J., Zhang, B. et al. (2005). High-resolution functional proteomics by active-site peptide profiling. *Proc. Natl. Acad. Sci. U. S. A.* 102 (14): 4996–5001.
30 Jessani, N., Young, J.A., Diaz, S.L. et al. (2005). Class assignment of sequence-unrelated members of enzyme superfamilies by activity-based protein profiling. *Angew. Chem. Int. Ed.* 44 (16): 2400–2403.
31 Abuelyaman, A.S., Hudig, D., Woodard, S.L., and Powers, J.C. (1994). Fluorescent derivatives of diphenyl [1-(*N*-peptidylamino)alkyl]phosphonate esters: synthesis and use in the inhibition and cellular localization of serine proteases. *Bioconjug. Chem.* 5 (5): 400–405.
32 Edgington-Mitchell, L.E., Barlow, N., Aurelio, L. et al. (2017). Fluorescent diphenylphosphonate-based probes for detection of serine protease activity during inflammation. *Bioorg. Med. Chem. Lett.* 27 (2): 254–260.
33 Pan, Z., Jeffery, D.A., Chehade, K. et al. (2006). Development of activity-based probes for trypsin-family serine proteases. *Bioorg. Med. Chem. Lett.* 16 (11): 2882–2885.
34 Kam, C.M., Abuelyaman, A.S., Li, Z. et al. (1993). Biotinylated isocoumarins, new inhibitors and reagents for detection, localization, and isolation of serine proteases. *Bioconjug. Chem.* 4 (6): 560–567.
35 Haedke, U., Götz, M., Baer, P., and Verhelst, S.H.L. (2012). Alkyne derivatives of isocoumarins as clickable activity-based probes for serine proteases. *Bioorg. Med. Chem.* 20 (2): 633–640.
36 Arastu-Kapur, S., Ponder, E.L., Fonović, U.P. et al. (2008). Identification of proteases that regulate erythrocyte rupture by the malaria parasite Plasmodium falciparum. *Nat. Chem. Biol.* 4: 203.
37 Kato, D., Boatright, K.M., Berger, A.B. et al. (2005). Activity-based probes that target diverse cysteine protease families. *Nat. Chem. Biol.* 1 (1): 33–38.
38 Garenne, T., Saidi, A., Gilmore, B.F. et al. (2015). Active site labeling of cysteine cathepsins by a straightforward diazomethylketone probe derived from the N-terminus of human cystatin C. *Biochem. Biophys. Res. Commun.* 460 (2): 250–254.
39 Greenbaum, D., Medzihradszky, K.F., Burlingame, A., and Bogyo, M. (2000). Epoxide electrophiles as activity-dependent cysteine protease profiling and discovery tools. *Chem. Biol.* 7 (8): 569–581.
40 Kato, D., Verhelst, S.H., Sexton, K.B., and Bogyo, M. (2005). A general solid phase method for the preparation of diverse azapeptide probes directed against cysteine proteases. *Org. Lett.* 7 (25): 5649–5652.

41 Roiban, G.D., Matache, M., Hadade, N.D., and Funeriu, D.P. (2012). A general solid phase method for the synthesis of sequence independent peptidyl-fluoromethyl ketones. *Org. Biomol. Chem.* 10 (23): 4516–4523.

42 Yang, Z., Fonovic, M., Verhelst, S.H. et al. (2009). Evaluation of alpha,beta-unsaturated ketone-based probes for papain-family cysteine proteases. *Bioorg. Med. Chem.* 17 (3): 1071–1078.

43 Borodovsky, A., Ovaa, H., Kolli, N. et al. (2002). Chemistry-based functional proteomics reveals novel members of the deubiquitinating enzyme family. *Chem. Biol.* 9 (10): 1149–1159.

44 Wang, G., Mahesh, U., Chen, G.Y., and Yao, S.Q. (2003). Solid-phase synthesis of peptide vinyl sulfones as potential inhibitors and activity-based probes of cysteine proteases. *Org. Lett.* 5 (5): 737–740.

45 Greenbaum, D., Baruch, A., Hayrapetian, L. et al. (2002). Chemical approaches for functionally probing the proteome. *Mol. Cell. Proteomics* 1 (1): 60–68.

46 Joyce, J.A., Baruch, A., Chehade, K. et al. (2004). Cathepsin cysteine proteases are effectors of invasive growth and angiogenesis during multistage tumorigenesis. *Cancer Cell.* 5 (5): 443–453.

47 Blum, G., Mullins, S.R., Keren, K. et al. (2005). Dynamic imaging of protease activity with fluorescently quenched activity-based probes. *Nat. Chem. Biol.* 1 (4): 203–209.

48 Sexton, K.B., Kato, D., Berger, A.B. et al. (2007). Specificity of aza-peptide electrophile activity-based probes of caspases. *Cell Death Differ.* 14 (4): 727–732.

49 Rolen, U., Kobzeva, V., Gasparjan, N. et al. (2006). Activity profiling of deubiquitinating enzymes in cervical carcinoma biopsies and cell lines. *Mol. Carcinog.* 45 (4): 260–269.

50 Altun, M., Kramer, H.B., Willems, L.I. et al. (2011). Activity-based chemical proteomics accelerates inhibitor development for deubiquitylating enzymes. *Chem. Biol.* 18 (11): 1401–1412.

51 de Jong, A., Merkx, R., Berlin, I. et al. (2012). Ubiquitin-based probes prepared by total synthesis to profile the activity of deubiquitinating enzymes. *ChemBioChem* 13 (15): 2251–2258.

52 Smith, E. and Collins, I. (2015). Photoaffinity labeling in target- and binding-site identification. *Future Med. Chem.* 7 (2): 159–183.

53 Preston, G.W. and Wilson, A.J. (2013). Photo-induced covalent cross-linking for the analysis of biomolecular interactions. *Chem. Soc. Rev.* 42 (8): 3289–3301.

54 Dubinsky, L., Krom, B.P., and Meijler, M.M. (2012). Diazirine based photoaffinity labeling. *Bioorg. Med. Chem.* 20 (2): 554–570.

55 Li, Z., Hao, P., Li, L. et al. (2013). Design and synthesis of minimalist terminal alkyne-containing diazirine photo-crosslinkers and their incorporation into kinase inhibitors for cell- and tissue-based proteome profiling. *Angew. Chem. Int. Ed.* 52 (33): 8551–8556.

56 Lapinsky, D.J. (2012). Tandem photoaffinity labeling-bioorthogonal conjugation in medicinal chemistry. *Bioorg. Med. Chem.* 20 (21): 6237–6247.

57 Li, Y.M., Xu, M., Lai, M.T. et al. (2000). Photoactivated gamma-secretase inhibitors directed to the active site covalently label presenilin 1. *Nature* 405 (6787): 689–694.
58 Chan, E.W., Chattopadhaya, S., Panicker, R.C. et al. (2004). Developing photoactive affinity probes for proteomic profiling: hydroxamate-based probes for metalloproteases. *J. Am. Chem. Soc.* 126 (44): 14435–14446.
59 Sieber, S.A., Niessen, S., Hoover, H.S., and Cravatt, B.F. (2006). Proteomic profiling of metalloprotease activities with cocktails of active-site probes. *Nat. Chem. Biol.* 2 (5): 274–281.
60 Saghatelian, A., Jessani, N., Joseph, A. et al. (2004). Activity-based probes for the proteomic profiling of metalloproteases. *Proc. Natl. Acad. Sci. U. S. A.* 101 (27): 10000–10005.
61 Hulce, J.J., Cognetta, A.B., Niphakis, M.J. et al. (2013). Proteome-wide mapping of cholesterol-interacting proteins in mammalian cells. *Nat. Methods* 10 (3): 259–264.
62 Cisar, J.S. and Cravatt, B.F. (2012). Fully functionalized small-molecule probes for integrated phenotypic screening and target identification. *J. Am. Chem. Soc.* 134 (25): 10385–10388.
63 Wright, M.H., Fetzer, C., and Sieber, S.A. (2017). Chemical probes unravel an antimicrobial defense response triggered by binding of the human opioid dynorphin to a bacterial sensor kinase. *J. Am. Chem. Soc.* 139 (17): 6152–6159.
64 Mahrus, S. and Craik, C.S. (2005). Selective chemical functional probes of granzymes A and B reveal granzyme B is a major effector of natural killer cell-mediated lysis of target cells. *Chem. Biol.* 12 (5): 567–577.
65 Verhelst, S.H., Fonovic, M., and Bogyo, M. (2007). A mild chemically cleavable linker system for functional proteomic applications. *Angew. Chem. Int. Ed.* 46 (8): 1284–1286.
66 Yang, Y.Y., Grammel, M., Raghavan, A.S. et al. (2010). Comparative analysis of cleavable azobenzene-based affinity tags for bioorthogonal chemical proteomics. *Chem. Biol.* 17 (11): 1212–1222.
67 Gartner, C.A., Elias, J.E., Bakalarski, C.E., and Gygi, S.P. (2007). Catch-and-release reagents for broadscale quantitative proteomics analyses. *J. Proteome Res.* 6 (4): 1482–1491.
68 Yang, Y., Hahne, H., Kuster, B., and Verhelst, S.H. (2013). A simple and effective cleavable linker for chemical proteomics applications. *Mol. Cell. Proteomics* 12 (1): 237–244.
69 Kim, H.Y., Tallman, K.A., Liebler, D.C., and Porter, N.A. (2009). An azido-biotin reagent for use in the isolation of protein adducts of lipid-derived electrophiles by streptavidin catch and photorelease. *Mol. Cell. Proteomics* 8 (9): 2080–2089.
70 Truong, T.H., Garcia, F.J., Seo, Y.H., and Carroll, K.S. (2011). Isotope-coded chemical reporter and acid-cleavable affinity reagents for monitoring protein sulfenic acids. *Bioorg. Med. Chem. Lett.* 21 (17): 5015–5020.
71 Speers, A.E. and Cravatt, B.F. (2005). A tandem orthogonal proteolysis strategy for high-content chemical proteomics. *J. Am. Chem. Soc.* 127 (28): 10018–10019.

72 Broncel, M., Serwa, R.A., Ciepla, P. et al. (2015). Multifunctional reagents for quantitative proteome-wide analysis of protein modification in human cells and dynamic profiling of protein lipidation during vertebrate development. *Angew. Chem. Int. Ed.* 54 (20): 5948–5951.

73 Weerapana, E., Wang, C., Simon, G.M. et al. (2010). Quantitative reactivity profiling predicts functional cysteines in proteomes. *Nature* 468 (7325): 790–795.

74 Wright, M.H., Clough, B., Rackham, M.D. et al. (2014). Validation of N-myristoyltransferase as an antimalarial drug target using an integrated chemical biology approach. *Nat. Chem.* 6 (2): 112–121.

75 Thinon, E., Serwa, R.A., Broncel, M. et al. (2014). Global profiling of co- and post-translationally N-myristoylated proteomes in human cells. *Nat. Commun.* 5: 4919.

76 Verdoes, M., Florea, B.I., Hillaert, U. et al. (2008). Azido-BODIPY acid reveals quantitative Staudinger-Bertozzi ligation in two-step activity-based proteasome profiling. *ChemBioChem* 9 (11): 1735–1738.

77 Hang, H.C., Loureiro, J., Spooner, E. et al. (2006). Mechanism-based probe for the analysis of cathepsin cysteine proteases in living cells. *ACS Chem. Biol.* 1 (11): 713–723.

78 Ovaa, H., van Swieten, P.F., Kessler, B.M. et al. (2003). Chemistry in living cells: detection of active proteasomes by a two-step labeling strategy. *Angew. Chem. Int. Ed.* 42 (31): 3626–3629.

79 Speers, A.E. and Cravatt, B.F. (2004). Profiling enzyme activities in vivo using click chemistry methods. *Chem. Biol.* 11 (4): 535–546.

80 Speers, A.E., Adam, G.C., and Cravatt, B.F. (2003). Activity-based protein profiling in vivo using a copper(i)-catalyzed azide-alkyne [3 + 2] cycloaddition. *J. Am. Chem. Soc.* 125 (16): 4686–4687.

81 Ward, J.A., McLellan, L., Stockley, M. et al. (2016). Quantitative chemical proteomic profiling of ubiquitin specific proteases in intact cancer cells. *ACS Chem. Biol.* 11 (12): 3268–3272.

82 Debets, M.F., Van, d.D., Rutjes, F.P.J.T., and Van Delft, F.L. (2010). Azide: a unique dipole for metal-free bioorthogonal ligations. *ChemBioChem* 11: 1168.

83 Ning, X., Guo, J., Wolfert, M.A., and Boons, G.J. (2008). Visualizing metabolically labeled glycoconjugates of living cells by copper-free and fast Huisgen cycloadditions. *Angew. Chem. Int. Ed.* 47: 2253.

84 Willems, L.I., Verdoes, M., Florea, B.I. et al. (2010). Two-step labeling of endogenous enzymatic activities by Diels–Alder ligation. *ChemBioChem* 11 (12): 1769–1781.

85 Oliveira, B.L., Guo, Z., and Bernardes, G.J.L. (2017). Inverse electron demand Diels–Alder reactions in chemical biology. *Chem. Soc. Rev.* 46 (16): 4895–4950.

86 Devaray, N.K., Hilderbrand, S., Upadhyay, R. et al. (2010). Bioorthogonal turn-on probes for imaging small molecules inside living cells. *Angew. Chem. Int. Ed.* 49: 2869.

87 Lang, K. and Chin, J.W. (2014). Bioorthogonal reactions for labeling proteins. *ACS Chem. Biol.* 9 (1): 16–20.

88 Kiick, K.L., Saxon, E., Tirrell, D.A., and Bertozzi, C.R. (2002). Incorporation of azides into recombinant proteins for chemoselective modification by the Staudinger ligation. *Proc. Natl. Acad. Sci. U. S. A.* 99 (1): 19–24.

89 Kolb, H.C., Finn, M.G., and Sharpless, K.B. (2001). Click chemistry: diverse chemical function from a few good reactions. *Angew. Chem. Int. Ed.* 40 (11): 2004–2021.

90 Demko, Z.P. and Sharpless, K.B. (2002). A click chemistry approach to tetrazoles by huisgen 1,3-dipolar cycloaddition: synthesis of 5-sulfonyl tetrazoles from azides and sulfonyl cyanides. *Angew. Chem. Int. Ed.* 41 (12): 2110–2113.

91 Yang, P.Y., Liu, K., Ngai, M.H. et al. (2010). Activity-based proteome profiling of potential cellular targets of Orlistat--an FDA-approved drug with anti-tumor activities. *J. Am. Chem. Soc.* 132 (2): 656–666.

92 Bateman, L.A., Zaro, B.W., Miller, S.M., and Pratt, M.R. (2013). An alkyne-aspirin chemical reporter for the detection of aspirin-dependent protein modification in living cells. *J. Am. Chem. Soc.* 135 (39): 14568–14573.

93 Wang, J., Tan, X.F., Nguyen, V.S. et al. (2014). A quantitative chemical proteomics approach to profile the specific cellular targets of andrographolide, a promising anticancer agent that suppresses tumor metastasis. *Mol. Cell. Proteomics* 13 (3): 876–886.

94 Staub, I. and Sieber, S.A. (2008). Beta-lactams as selective chemical probes for the in vivo labeling of bacterial enzymes involved in cell wall biosynthesis, antibiotic resistance, and virulence. *J. Am. Chem. Soc.* 130 (40): 13400–13409.

95 Ismail, H.M., O'Neill, P.M., Hong, D.W. et al. (2013). Pyrethroid activity-based probes for profiling cytochrome P450 activities associated with insecticide interactions. *Proc. Natl. Acad. Sci. U.S.A.* 110 (49): 19766–19771. https://doi.org/10.1073/pnas.1320185110.

96 Agard, N.J., Prescher, J.A., and Bertozzi, C.R. (2004). A strain-promoted [3 + 2] azide-alkyne cycloaddition for covalent modification of biomolecules in living systems. *J. Am. Chem. Soc.* 126 (46): 15046–15047.

97 Agard, N.J., Baskin, J.M., Prescher, J.A. et al. (2006). A comparative study of bioorthogonal reactions with azides. *ACS Chem. Biol.* 1 (10): 644–648.

98 van Rooden, E.J., Kreekel, R., Hansen, T. et al. (2018). Two-step activity-based protein profiling of diacylglycerol lipase. *Org. Biomol. Chem.* 16 (29): 5250–5253.

99 Bantscheff, M., Lemeer, S., Savitski, M.M., and Kuster, B. (2012). Quantitative mass spectrometry in proteomics: critical review update from 2007 to the present. *Anal. Bioanal. Chem.* 404 (4): 939–965.

100 Ong, S.E. and Mann, M. (2005). Mass spectrometry-based proteomics turns quantitative. *Nat. Chem. Biol.* 1 (5): 252–262.

101 Neilson, K.A., Ali, N.A., Muralidharan, S. et al. (2011). Less label, more free: approaches in label-free quantitative mass spectrometry. *Proteomics* 11 (4): 535–553.

102 Megger, D.A., Bracht, T., Meyer, H.E., and Sitek, B. (2013). Label-free quantification in clinical proteomics. *Biochim. Biophys. Acta* 1834 (8): 1581–1590.

103 Cox, J., Hein, M.Y., Luber, C.A. et al. (2014). Accurate proteome-wide label-free quantification by delayed normalization and maximal peptide ratio extraction, termed MaxLFQ. *Mol. Cell. Proteomics* 13 (9): 2513–2526.

104 Al Shweiki, M.R., Monchgesang, S., Majovsky, P. et al. (2017). Assessment of label-free quantification in discovery proteomics and impact of technological factors and natural variability of protein abundance. *J. Proteome Res.* 16 (4): 1410–1424.

105 Lombard-Banek, C., Reddy, S., Moody, S.A., and Nemes, P. (2016). Label-free quantification of proteins in single embryonic cells with neural fate in the cleavage-stage frog (xenopus laevis) embryo using capillary electrophoresis electrospray ionization high-resolution mass spectrometry (CE-ESI-HRMS). *Mol. Cell. Proteomics* 15 (8): 2756–2768.

106 Itzhak, D.N., Davies, C., Tyanova, S. et al. (2017). A mass spectrometry-based approach for mapping protein subcellular localization reveals the spatial proteome of mouse primary neurons. *Cell. Rep.* 20 (11): 2706–2718.

107 Lai, X., Wang, L., and Witzmann, F.A. (2013). Issues and applications in label-free quantitative mass spectrometry. *Int. J. Proteomics* 2013: 756039.

108 Yang, P.Y., Liu, K., Zhang, C. et al. (2011). Chemical modification and organelle-specific localization of orlistat-like natural-product-based probes. *Chem. Asian J.* 6 (10): 2762–2775.

109 Wang, J., Zhang, C.J., Zhang, J. et al. (2015). Mapping sites of aspirin-induced acetylations in live cells by quantitative acid-cleavable activity-based protein profiling (QA-ABPP). *Sci. Rep.* 5: 7896.

110 van Rooden, E.J., Florea, B.I., Deng, H. et al. (2018). Mapping in vivo target interaction profiles of covalent inhibitors using chemical proteomics with label-free quantification. *Nat. Protoc.* 13 (4): 752–767.

111 Gygi, S.P., Rist, B., Gerber, S.A. et al. (1999). Quantitative analysis of complex protein mixtures using isotope-coded affinity tags. *Nat. Biotechnol.* 17 (10): 994–999.

112 Wiese, S., Reidegeld, K.A., Meyer, H.E., and Warscheid, B. (2007). Protein labeling by iTRAQ: a new tool for quantitative mass spectrometry in proteome research. *Proteomics* 7 (3): 340–350.

113 Thompson, A., Schäfer, J., Kuhn, K. et al. (2003). Tandem mass tags: a novel quantification strategy for comparative analysis of complex protein mixtures by MS/MS. *Anal. Chem.* 75 (8): 1895–1904.

114 McAlister, G.C., Huttlin, E.L., Haas, W. et al. (2012). Increasing the multiplexing capacity of TMTs using reporter ion isotopologues with isobaric masses. *Anal. Chem.* 84 (17): 7469–7478.

115 McAlister, G.C., Nusinow, D.P., Jedrychowski, M.P. et al. (2014). MultiNotch MS3 enables accurate, sensitive, and multiplexed detection of differential expression across cancer cell line proteomes. *Anal. Chem.* 86 (14): 7150–7158.

116 Karp, N.A., Huber, W., Sadowski, P.G. et al. (2010). Addressing accuracy and precision issues in iTRAQ quantitation. *Mol. Cell. Proteomics* 9 (9): 1885–1897.

117 Shirran, S.L. and Botting, C.H. (2010). A comparison of the accuracy of iTRAQ quantification by nLC-ESI MSMS and nLC-MALDI MSMS methods. *J. Proteomics* 73 (7): 1391–1403.

118 Ting, L., Rad, R., Gygi, S.P., and Haas, W. (2011). MS3 eliminates ratio distortion in isobaric multiplexed quantitative proteomics. *Nat. Methods* 8 (11): 937–940.

119 Ong, S., Blagoev, B., Kratchmarova, I. et al. (2002). Stable isotope labeling by amino acids in cell culture, SILAC, as a simple and accurate approach to expression proteomics. *Mol. Cell. Proteomics* 1 (5): 376–386.

120 Ong, S.E. and Mann, M. (2006). A practical recipe for stable isotope labeling by amino acids in cell culture (SILAC). *Nat. Protoc.* 1 (6): 2650–2660.

121 Ong, S.E., Schenone, M., Margolin, A.A. et al. (2009). Identifying the proteins to which small-molecule probes and drugs bind in cells. *Proc. Natl. Acad. Sci. U. S. A.* 106 (12): 4617–4622.

122 Voigt, T., Gerding-Reimers, C., Ngoc Tran, T.T. et al. (2013). A natural product inspired tetrahydropyran collection yields mitosis modulators that synergistically target CSE1L and tubulin. *Angew. Chem. Int. Ed.* 52 (1): 410–414.

123 Lanning, B.R., Whitby, L.R., Dix, M.M. et al. (2014). A road map to evaluate the proteome-wide selectivity of covalent kinase inhibitors. *Nat. Chem. Biol.* 10 (9): 760–767.

124 Kruger, M., Moser, M., Ussar, S. et al. (2008). SILAC mouse for quantitative proteomics uncovers kindlin-3 as an essential factor for red blood cell function. *Cell* 134 (2): 353–364.

125 Sury, M.D., Chen, J.X., and Selbach, M. (2010). The SILAC fly allows for accurate protein quantification in vivo. *Mol. Cell. Proteomics* 9 (10): 2173–2183.

126 Zanivan, S., Meves, A., Behrendt, K. et al. (2013). In vivo SILAC-based proteomics reveals phosphoproteome changes during mouse skin carcinogenesis. *Cell. Rep.* 3 (2): 552–566.

127 Macleod, A.K., Zang, T., Riches, Z. et al. (2014). A targeted in vivo SILAC approach for quantification of drug metabolism enzymes: regulation by the constitutive androstane receptor. *J. Proteome Res.* 13 (2): 866–874.

128 Geiger, T., Wisniewski, J.R., Cox, J. et al. (2011). Use of stable isotope labeling by amino acids in cell culture as a spike-in standard in quantitative proteomics. *Nat. Protoc.* 6: 147.

129 Lubin, A.S., Rueda-Zubiaurre, A., Matthews, H. et al. (2018). Development of a photo-cross-linkable diaminoquinazoline inhibitor for target identification in plasmodium falciparum. *ACS Infect. Dis.* 4 (4): 523–530.

130 Nomura, D.K., Long, J.Z., Niessen, S. et al. (2010). Monoacylglycerol lipase regulates a fatty acid network that promotes cancer pathogenesis. *Cell* 140 (1): 49–61.

131 Bunnage, M.E., Gilbert, A.M., Jones, L.H., and Hett, E.C. (2015). Know your target, know your molecule. *Nat. Chem. Biol.* 11: 368.

132 Wright, M.H. and Sieber, S.A. (2016). Chemical proteomics approaches for identifying the cellular targets of natural products. *Nat. Prod. Rep.* 33 (5): 681–708.

133 Galande, A.K., Hilderbrand, S.A., Weissleder, R., and Tung, C.H. (2006). Enzyme-targeted fluorescent imaging probes on a multiple antigenic peptide core. *J. Med. Chem.* 49 (15): 4715–4720.
134 Verdoes, M., Oresic Bender, K., Segal, E. et al. (2013). Improved quenched fluorescent probe for imaging of cysteine cathepsin activity. *J. Am. Chem. Soc.* 135 (39): 14726–14730.
135 Oresic Bender, K., Ofori, L., van der Linden, W.A. et al. (2015). Design of a highly selective quenched activity-based probe and its application in dual color imaging studies of cathepsin S activity localization. *J. Am. Chem. Soc.* 137 (14): 4771–4777.
136 Shaulov-Rotem, Y., Merquiol, E., Weiss-Sadan, T. et al. (2016). A novel quenched fluorescent activity-based probe reveals caspase-3 activity in the endoplasmic reticulum during apoptosis. *Chem. Sci.* 7 (2): 1322–1337.
137 Zweerink, S., Kallnik, V., Ninck, S. et al. (2017). Activity-based protein profiling as a robust method for enzyme identification and screening in extremophilic Archaea. *Nat. Commun.* 8: 15352.
138 Brasen, C., Esser, D., Rauch, B., and Siebers, B. (2014). Carbohydrate metabolism in archaea: current insights into unusual enzymes and pathways and their regulation. *Microbiol. Mol. Biol. Rev.* 78 (1): 89–175.
139 Cavicchioli, R. (2011). Archaea – timeline of the third domain. *Nat. Rev. Microbiol.* 9 (1): 51–61.
140 Albers, S.V. and Meyer, B.H. (2011). The archaeal cell envelope. *Nat. Rev. Microbiol.* 9 (6): 414–426.
141 Simon, G.M. and Cravatt, B.F. (2010). Activity-based proteomics of enzyme superfamilies: serine hydrolases as a case study. *J. Biol. Chem.* 285 (15): 11051–11055.
142 Chow, J., Kovacic, F., Dall Antonia, Y. et al. (2012). The metagenome-derived enzymes LipS and LipT increase the diversity of known lipases. *PLoS One* 7 (10): e47665.
143 Kathuria, S., Gaetani, S., Fegley, D. et al. (2003). Modulation of anxiety through blockade of anandamide hydrolysis. *Nat. Med.* 9 (1): 76–81.
144 Long, J.Z., Nomura, D.K., Vann, R.E. et al. (2009). Dual blockade of FAAH and MAGL identifies behavioral processes regulated by endocannabinoid crosstalk in vivo. *Proc. Natl. Acad. Sci. U. S. A.* 106 (48): 20270–20275.
145 Butler, D. and Callaway, E. (2016). Scientists in the dark after French clinical trial proves fatal. *Nature* 529 (7586): 263–264.
146 Eddleston, M., Cohen, A.F., and Webb, D.J. (2016). Implications of the BIA-102474-101 study for review of first-into-human clinical trials. *Br. J. Clin. pharmacol.* 81 (4): 582–586.
147 Huggins, J.P., Smart, T.S., Langman, S. et al. (2012). An efficient randomised, placebo-controlled clinical trial with the irreversible fatty acid amide hydrolase-1 inhibitor PF-04457845, which modulates endocannabinoids but fails to induce effective analgesia in patients with pain due to osteoarthritis of the knee. *Pain* 153 (9): 1837–1846.
148 Li, G.L., Winter, H., Arends, R. et al. (2012). Assessment of the pharmacology and tolerability of PF-04457845, an irreversible inhibitor of fatty

acid amide hydrolase-1, in healthy subjects. *Br. J. Clin. Pharmacol.* 73 (5): 706–716.

149 Richardson, R.J., Hein, N.D., Wijeyesakere, S.J. et al. (2013). Neuropathy target esterase (NTE): overview and future. *Chem. Biol. Interact.* 203 (1): 238–244.

150 Topaloglu, A.K., Lomniczi, A., Kretzschmar, D. et al. (2014). Loss-of-function mutations in PNPLA6 encoding neuropathy target esterase underlie pubertal failure and neurological deficits in Gordon Holmes syndrome. *J. Clin. Endocrinol. Metab.* 99 (10): 2067.

151 Yin, T.F., Wang, M., Qing, Y. et al. (2016). Research progress on chemopreventive effects of phytochemicals on colorectal cancer and their mechanisms. *World J. Gastroenterol.* 22 (31): 7058–7068.

152 Ambrosone, C.B., McCann, S.E., Freudenheim, J.L. et al. (2004). Breast cancer risk in premenopausal women is inversely associated with consumption of broccoli, a source of isothiocyanates, but is not modified by GST genotype. *J. Nutr.* 134 (5): 1134–1138.

153 Telang, U., Brazeau, D.A., and Morris, M.E. (2009). Comparison of the effects of phenethyl isothiocyanate and sulforaphane on gene expression in breast cancer and normal mammary epithelial cells. *Exp. Biol. Med. (Maywood)* 234 (3): 287–295.

154 Wang, Z., Fan, J., Liu, M. et al. (2013). Nutraceuticals for prostate cancer chemoprevention: from molecular mechanisms to clinical application. *Expert Opin. Investig. Drugs* 22 (12): 1613–1626.

155 Tortorella, S.M., Royce, S.G., Licciardi, P.V., and Karagiannis, T.C. (2015). Dietary sulforaphane in cancer chemoprevention: the role of epigenetic regulation and HDAC inhibition. *Antioxid. Redox Signal.* 22 (16): 1382–1424.

156 Ahn, Y.H., Hwang, Y., Liu, H. et al. (2010). Electrophilic tuning of the chemoprotective natural product sulforaphane. *Proc. Natl. Acad. Sci. U. S. A.* 107 (21): 9590–9595.

157 Dinkova-Kostova, A.T., Holtzclaw, W.D., Cole, R.N. et al. (2002). Direct evidence that sulfhydryl groups of Keap1 are the sensors regulating induction of phase 2 enzymes that protect against carcinogens and oxidants. *Proc. Natl. Acad. Sci. U. S. A.* 99 (18): 11908–11913.

158 Cross, J.V., Rady, J.M., Foss, F.W. et al. (2009). Nutrient isothiocyanates covalently modify and inhibit the inflammatory cytokine macrophage migration inhibitory factor (MIF). *Biochem. J.* 423 (3): 315–321.

159 Pledgie-Tracy, A., Sobolewski, M.D., and Davidson, N.E. (2007). Sulforaphane induces cell type–specific apoptosis in human breast cancer cell lines. *Mol. Cancer Ther.* 6 (3): 1013–1021.

160 Ben-Neriah, Y. and Karin, M. (2011). Inflammation meets cancer, with NF-kappaB as the matchmaker. *Nat. Immunol.* 12 (8): 715–723.

161 Roy, S.K., Srivastava, R.K., and Shankar, S. (2010). Inhibition of PI3K/AKT and MAPK/ERK pathways causes activation of FOXO transcription factor, leading to cell cycle arrest and apoptosis in pancreatic cancer. *J. Mol. Signal.* 5: 10.

162 Pinz, S., Unser, S., and Rascle, A. (2014). The natural chemopreventive agent sulforaphane inhibits STAT5 activity. *PLoS One* 9 (6): e99391.

163 Aggarwal, B.B., Sethi, G., Ahn, K.S. et al. (2006). Targeting signal-transducer-and-activator-of-transcription-3 for prevention and therapy of cancer: modern target but ancient solution. *Ann. N. Y. Acad. Sci.* 1091: 151–169.

164 Bergink, S. and Jentsch, S. (2009). Principles of ubiquitin and SUMO modifications in DNA repair. *Nature* 458 (7237): 461–467.

165 Jacq, X., Kemp, M., Martin, N.M.B., and Jackson, S.P. (2013). Deubiquitylating enzymes and DNA damage response pathways. *Cell Biochem. Biophys.* 67 (1): 25–43.

166 D'Arcy, P. and Linder, S. (2014). Molecular pathways: translational potential of deubiquitinases as drug targets. *Clin. Cancer Res.* 20 (15): 3908–3914.

167 D'Arcy, P., Wang, X., and Linder, S. (2015). Deubiquitinase inhibition as a cancer therapeutic strategy. *Pharmacol. Ther.* 147: 32–54.

168 Mulder, M.P., El Oualid, F., ter Beek, J., and Ovaa, H. (2014). A native chemical ligation handle that enables the synthesis of advanced activity-based probes: diubiquitin as a case study. *ChemBioChem* 15 (7): 946–949.

169 Li, J., D'Angiolella, V., Seeley, E.S. et al. (2013). USP33 regulates centrosome biogenesis via deubiquitination of the centriolar protein CP110. *Nature* 495 (7440): 255–259.

170 Lamoree, B. and Hubbard, R.E. (2017). Current perspectives in fragment-based lead discovery (FBLD). *Essays Biochem.* 61 (5): 453–464.

171 Davis, B.J. and Erlanson, D.A. (2013). Learning from our mistakes: the 'unknown knowns' in fragment screening. *Bioorg. Med. Chem. Lett.* 23 (10): 2844–2852.

172 Weekes, M.P., Antrobus, R., Lill, J.R. et al. (2010). Comparative analysis of techniques to purify plasma membrane proteins. *J. Biomol. Tech.* 21 (3): 108–115.

173 Kambe, T., Correia, B.E., Niphakis, M.J., and Cravatt, B.F. (2014). Mapping the protein interaction landscape for fully functionalized small-molecule probes in human cells. *J. Am. Chem. Soc.* 136 (30): 10777–10782.

174 Bush, J.T., Walport, L.J., McGouran, J.F. et al. (2013). The Ugi four-component reaction enables expedient synthesis and comparison of photoaffinity probes. *Chem. Sci.* 4 (11): 4115–4120.

175 Blum, G., von Degenfeld, G., Merchant, M.J. et al. (2007). Noninvasive optical imaging of cysteine protease activity using fluorescently quenched activity-based probes. *Nat. Chem. Biol.* 3 (10): 668–677.

176 Turk, V., Stoka, V., Vasiljeva, O. et al. (2012). Cysteine cathepsins: from structure, function and regulation to new frontiers. *Biochim. Biophys. Acta* 1824 (1): 68–88.

177 Turk, B., Turk, D., and Turk, V. (2012). Protease signalling: the cutting edge. *EMBO J.* 31 (7): 1630–1643.

178 Driessen, C., Bryant, R.A.R., Lennon-Duménil, A. et al. (1999). Cathepsin S controls the trafficking and maturation of Mhc class II molecules in dendritic cells. *J. Cell Biol.* 147 (4): 775–790.

179 Small, D.M., Burden, R.E., Jaworski, J. et al. (2013). Cathepsin S from both tumor and tumor-associated cells promote cancer growth and neovascularization. *Int. J. Cancer* 133 (9): 2102–2112.

180 Sevenich, L., Bowman, R.L., Mason, S.D. et al. (2014). Analysis of tumour- and stroma-supplied proteolytic networks reveals a brain-metastasis-promoting role for cathepsin S. *Nat. Cell Biol.* 16 (9): 876–888.
181 Yang, M., Liu, J., Shao, J. et al. (2014). Cathepsin S-mediated autophagic flux in tumor-associated macrophages accelerate tumor development by promoting M2 polarization. *Mol. Cancer* 13 (1): 43.
182 Zhao, P., Lieu, T., Barlow, N. et al. (2014). Cathepsin S causes inflammatory pain via biased agonism of PAR2 and TRPV4. *J. Biol. Chem.* 289 (39): 27215–27234.
183 Weldon, S., McNally, P., McAuley, D.F. et al. (2014). miR-31 dysregulation in cystic fibrosis airways contributes to increased pulmonary cathepsin S production. *Am. J. Respir. Crit. Care Med.* 190 (2): 165–174.
184 Verdoes, M., Edgington, L.E., Scheeren, F.A. et al. (2012). A nonpeptidic cathepsin S activity-based probe for noninvasive optical imaging of tumor-associated macrophages. *Chem. Biol.* 19 (5): 619–628.
185 Pawlak, J.B., Gential, G.P., Ruckwardt, T.J. et al. (2015). Bioorthogonal deprotection on the dendritic cell surface for chemical control of antigen cross-presentation. *Angew. Chem. Int. Ed.* 54 (19): 5628–5631.
186 de Bruin, G., Xin, B.T., Kraus, M. et al. (2016). A set of activity-based probes to visualize human (immuno)proteasome activities. *Angew. Chem. Int. Ed.* 55 (13): 4199–4203.
187 Walvoort, M.T., Kallemeijn, W.W., Willems, L.I. et al. (2012). Tuning the leaving group in 2-deoxy-2-fluoroglucoside results in improved activity-based retaining beta-glucosidase probes. *Chem. Commun. (Cambridge)* 48 (84): 10386–10388.
188 Counihan, J.L., Duckering, M., Dalvie, E. et al. (2017). Chemoproteomic profiling of acetanilide herbicides reveals their role in inhibiting fatty acid oxidation. *ACS Chem. Biol.* 12 (3): 635–642.
189 Bachovchin, D.A., Brown, S.J., Rosen, H., and Cravatt, B.F. (2009). Identification of selective inhibitors of uncharacterized enzymes by high-throughput screening with fluorescent activity-based probes. *Nat. Biotechnol.* 27 (4): 387–394.
190 Mulder, M.P.C., Merkx, R., Witting, K.F. et al. (2018). Total chemical synthesis of SUMO and SUMO-based probes for profiling the activity of SUMO-specific proteases. *Angew. Chem. Int. Ed.* 57 (29): 8958–8962.
191 Mulder, M.P., Witting, K., Berlin, I. et al. (2016). A cascading activity-based probe sequentially targets E1-E2-E3 ubiquitin enzymes. *Nat. Chem. Biol.* 12 (7): 523–530.
192 Pao, K.C., Stanley, M., Han, C. et al. (2016). Probes of ubiquitin E3 ligases enable systematic dissection of parkin activation. *Nat. Chem. Biol.* 12 (5): 324–331.
193 Pao, K., Wood, N.T., Knebel, A. et al. (2018). Activity-based E3 ligase profiling uncovers an E3 ligase with esterification activity. *Nature* 556 (7701): 381–385.

4

Kinobeads: A Chemical Proteomic Approach for Kinase Inhibitor Selectivity Profiling and Target Discovery

Maria Reinecke[1, 2, 3], Stephanie Heinzlmeir[1*], Mathias Wilhelm[1], Guillaume Médard[1], Susan Klaeger[1, 4], and Bernhard Kuster[1, 2, 3, 5]*

[1] *Technical University of Munich, Chair of Proteomics and Bioanalytics, Emil-Erlenmeyer-Forum 5, Freising, 85354, Germany*
[2] *German Cancer Consortium (DKTK), Munich, 80336, Germany*
[3] *German Cancer Research Center (DKFZ), Heidelberg, Germany*
[4] *Broad Institute, Proteomics Platform, 415 Main Street, Cambridge, MA, 02142, USA*
[5] *Technical University of Munich, Bavarian Biomolecular Mass Spectrometry Center, Gregor-Mendel-Strasse 4, Freising, 85354, Germany*

4.1 Kinase Inhibitor Target Deconvolution Using Chemical Proteomics

4.1.1 Polypharmacology of Small Molecule Kinase Inhibitors

Protein Kinases and Their Inhibitors: The human kinome consists of ~500 protein kinases catalysing the transfer of the γ-phosphate group of adenosine triphosphate (ATP) to serine, threonine, or tyrosine residues of their substrate proteins [1, 2] (Figure 4.1a,b). Protein phosphorylation is a versatile biochemical switch leading to changes in the activation state, localization, or protein–protein interactions of the modified substrate proteins. In a cellular background, this mechanism is particularly useful for forwarding external and internal stimuli via complex signalling cascades, ultimately leading to the downstream activation or expression of effector proteins to perform the required cellular response [2]. Via a balanced interplay of protein kinases and phosphatases, more precisely of their cellular location, abundance, catalytic activity, specificity and affinity, protein phosphorylation is tightly controlled, which is crucial for this multilayered signal transmission process to maintain cellular integrity and functionality [3]. Aberrant kinase signalling has been found to play a major role in the evolution and progress of various human diseases such as oncological, immunological, neurological, metabolic, and infectious disorders [4]. Kinase inhibition is therefore a promising approach for 'molecularly targeted therapies' aiming at directly modulating the main disease drivers and deregulated cellular pathways. Consequently, small molecule kinase inhibitors have become important drugs over the past two decades. In 2001, imatinib (Gleevec) was the first kinase

*Maria Reinecke and Stephanie Heinzlmeir contributed equally.

Target Discovery and Validation: Methods and Strategies for Drug Discovery,
First Edition. Edited by Alleyn T. Plowright.

inhibitor to be approved by the Food and Drug Administration (FDA) for the targeted inhibition of BCR-ABL-positive chronic myeloid leukaemia (CML) [5] (Figure 4.1c). To date, about 50 approved kinase drugs are routinely used for (mainly cancer) patient healthcare, and a few hundred more molecules are evaluated in different phases of clinical trials.

Kinase Inhibitor Binding: The majority of these small molecules target the ATP binding pocket inside the kinase domain, which is highly conserved among protein kinases and other ATP binding proteins. Typically, protein kinase domains consist of two structurally and functionally different lobes: the N-terminal N-lobe and the C-terminal C-lobe, which are connected via a flexible hinge region [7]. The interface between the two lobes forms the catalytic centre of this enzyme class including the ATP binding pocket and the substrate binding site. Enzymatic action requires a structural make-up that is highly dynamic and allows the rapid interconversion between multiple conformations (so-called kinase breathing) [7, 8]. Depending on their molecular structure, kinase inhibitors interact to different degrees with pockets and amino acid residues within the ATP binding site. This interaction fingerprint determines those kinase conformations (e.g. active or inactive conformations) that are preferably bound over others, which is frequently used to classify ATP-competitive kinase inhibitors into type I, I½, and II inhibitors [9]. Besides these ATP-competitive binding modes, other small molecules target the neighbouring phospho-acceptor site of the kinase (type III) or an allosteric site remote from the catalytic centre (type IV). Bivalent inhibitors targeting both the ATP pocket and an allosteric binding site are categorized into type V, and covalent (reversible and irreversible) inhibitors into binding type VI [9].

(Poly)pharmacology of Kinase Inhibitors: Compound selectivity is a major consideration for drug discovery all the way from target validation through to clinical application, especially for ATP-competitive inhibitors. Due to the highly conserved nature of the ATP pocket, the design of selective ATP-competitive inhibitors remains challenging [10]. The requirement for selectivity is however highly dependent. On the one hand, high selectivity is a prerequisite for molecules that are used as tool compounds in basic research for studying the biology of particular proteins and has been defined as one of the key characteristics of chemical probes (chemicalprobes.org) (see Chapter 1 for more details). On the other hand, many approved and efficacious kinase inhibitors feature very promiscuous target profiles, resulting in multiple mode(s) of action. Polypharmacology might explain desired and undesired treatment effects and may in fact be valuable for successful therapy [11]. In any case and independent from its use as a therapeutic agent or a chemical probe, selectivity profiling remains crucial to understand a drug's mode of action and to anticipate its phenotypic effects [12].

Selectivity Metrics: Establishing a measure of compound selectivity is a challenging task because the value of the metric very much depends on its intended use, which greatly varies in different research areas [13]. Compound selectivity may be calculated, for instance, (i) to obtain a target-independent view on compound selectivity (e.g. identification of chemical probes in a large selectivity

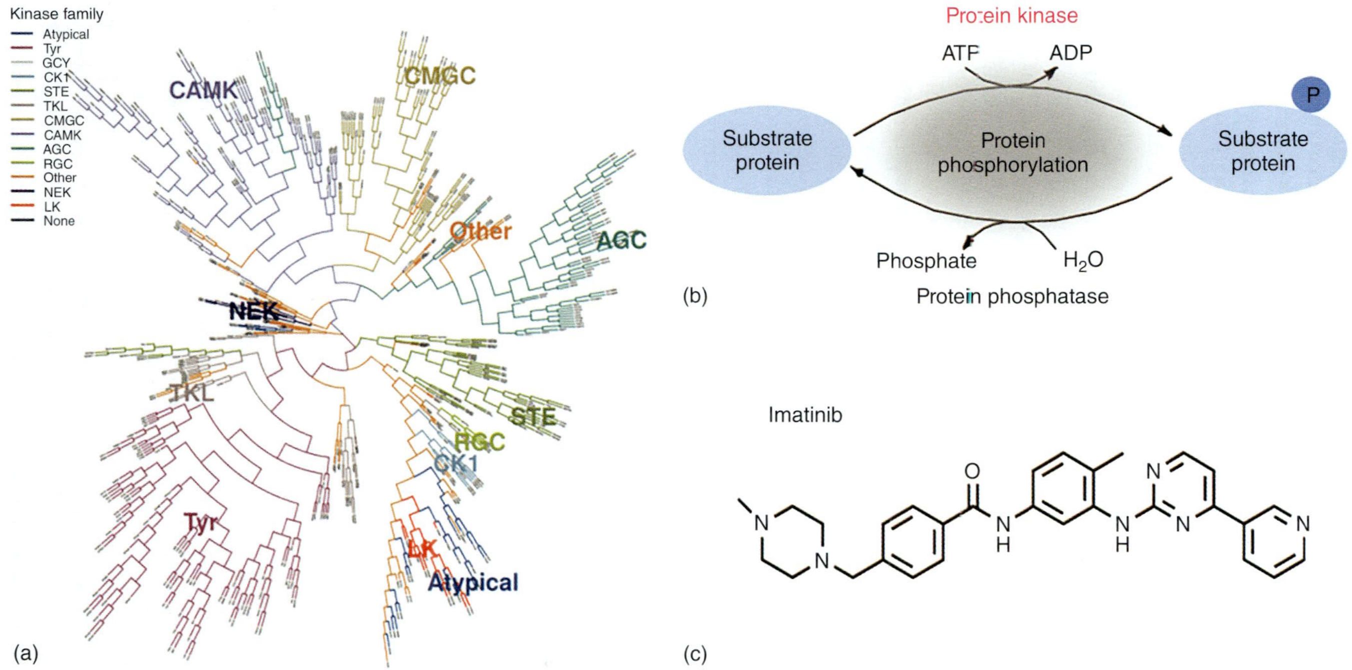

Figure 4.1 Human protein kinases. (a) Phylogenetic tree of human protein kinases. (b) Schematic representation of substrate protein phosphorylation by protein kinases under the consumption of the phosphate donor ATP and dephosphorylation by phosphatases along with the generation of free phosphate. (Source: modified from Heinzlmeir [6]). (c) Chemical structure of the clinical kinase inhibitor imatinib.

screen), (ii) to characterize the ability of compounds to selectively hit a particular target (e.g. in medicinal chemistry), or (iii) to quantify the preference of a compound to affect a particular mode of action or phenotype defined by a certain set of proteins (e.g. adverse and advantageous effects of clinical drug treatment) [13]. Technically, the quantification of compound selectivity is also dependent on the properties of assay technologies (activity or binding assay), experimental design (single dose or dose response), or input material (lysate or recombinant proteins). Several different metrics have been developed to compute compound selectivity, namely selectivity entropy [14, 15], selectivity score [16, 17], Gini coefficient [18], partition index [19], and concentration- and target-dependent selectivity (CATDS [20]). Selectivity entropy is a measure for the distribution of an inhibitor among all target proteins. It gives an idea about the quality of a compound to serve as chemical probe for any of these target proteins, but does not allow quantifying selectivity for a particular target or a particular concentration. The selectivity score divides the number of targets at a certain threshold concentration by the number of total screened proteins. Similarly, the Gini coefficient calculates the cumulative inhibition of all target proteins at a certain threshold concentration in relation to all tested proteins. These scoring systems account for the concentration dependency of compound selectivity and are well suited also for single-dose assay data, but cannot be used for a target-dependent view on selectivity. In contrary, the partition index describes the fraction of an inhibitor bound by a particular target protein in a pool of target proteins and thus facilitates target-dependent (but concentration-independent) determination of compound selectivity. The recently developed CATDS score calculates the fraction of compound binding to a certain target protein in relation to the sum of all binding events at a certain concentration. The CATDS scoring scheme provides more versatility for the calculation of selectivity in a concentration- and target-dependent manner, even when the size of the panel is variable. With the same data, different CATDS can be calculated such as $CATDS_{target}$, which describes the selectivity of a compound towards a particular target; $CATDS_{multi\text{-}target}$, which can be calculated if the selectivity of a compound against a group of proteins is of interest; or $CATDS_{MoA}$, which is designed to distinguish the selectivity of a compound for certain modes of action [20].

4.1.2 Chemoproteomic Profiling of Kinase Inhibitors

Kinobeads Technology: Despite their often remarkable success in the clinic, the mode(s) of action of many kinase inhibitors is often insufficiently understood, which hampers the adequate use and full exploitation of these very advanced molecules. To address this need, many technology platforms have been developed, offering the possibility to screen small molecules against large numbers of kinases and obtain a global view on inhibitor target profiles. In 2007, Bantscheff and co-workers introduced the concept of Kinobeads for profiling ATP-competitive small molecule kinase inhibitors [21] (Figure 4.2). The Kinobeads technology is a chemical proteomic approach that makes use of the structurally conserved ATP binding protein pockets and broad selectivity kinase inhibitors for the affinity enrichment of kinases and other ATP binding proteins.

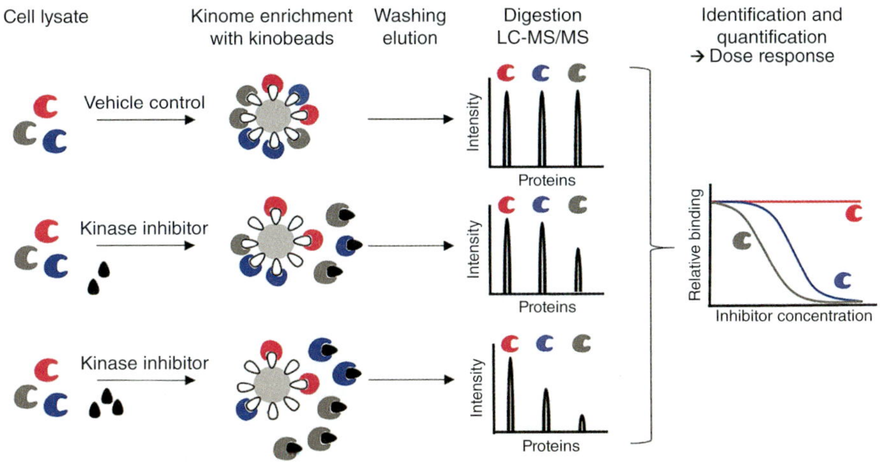

Figure 4.2 Schematic representation of the Kinobeads workflow. Cell lysates are pre-incubated with increasing drug concentrations or vehicle control. Kinobeads enrich kinases from native cell or tissue lysates. The free compound and Kinobeads compete for the same binding site of the kinase, which leads to reduced enrichment of the targets by Kinobeads. Both interactions occur in a reversible manner, establishing a three-membered thermodynamic binding equilibrium. Proteins are eluted from beads, digested, and measured via LC-MS/MS. Residual binding curves are generated based on the relative intensity values at each drug concentration and non-linear regression analysis.

Kinobeads consist of promiscuous kinase inhibitors immobilized on a solid matrix and enrich hundreds of these proteins from complex native cell or tissue lysates. When coupled to a quantitative mass spectrometry (MS) read-out, this technology enables the simultaneous identification and quantification of kinases and other ATP binding proteins in a native background. Target deconvolution of kinase inhibitors is accomplished by a competitive set-up where the lysate is treated with increasing concentrations of an inhibitor of interest. Both the compound and the Kinobeads compete for the same binding sites, leading to reduced enrichment of the targets by the Kinobeads and a dose-dependent loss of signal intensity for each protein target in the subsequent MS read-out (Figure 4.2) [20–22]. Resulting dose-response curves can be used for calculating EC_{50} values, which can then be converted into a dissociation constant by multiplying with a correction factor (see Section 4.1.3 for further explanation). When performing competitive pulldown experiments, only those inhibitors can be profiled that bind or alter the binding site that is also addressed by the affinity resin. ATP-competitive inhibitors can be examined, whereas most allosteric inhibitors do not score in the assay unless they alter the ATP pocket conformation in a way that makes it inaccessible for the affinity resin (e.g. the type IV inhibitor MK-2206 [20]). The number of native proteins constituting the 'screening panel' depends on the nature of the immobilized chemical probes and of the input biological material and only for some kinases on their conformation or activity. In most of the cases, Kinobeads bind kinases independently of their activation status, and, thus, assaying kinase activity using affinity matrices such as Kinobeads is restricted to a limited number of kinases and affinity probes [23–25]. Extension of assay coverage can be achieved by combining complementary affinity probes and complementary lysates (see Section 4.1.3). Such optimization steps as well as miniaturization/parallelization to 96-well plate format have culminated in the current Kinobeads protocol, allowing to profile any compound against ~350 native protein kinases [22].

Comparison to Similar Approaches: In contrast to Kinobeads that systematically address large parts of the human kinome, the classical chemical proteomic experiment uses an immobilized version of the compound of interest to enrich and identify solely its particular targets in an affinity pulldown [26–28] (see Chapter 2 for more details). Therefore, an analogue of the small molecule of interest usually needs to be synthesized to allow for covalent linkage to the solid support. This modification should ideally not affect the binding to the target proteins, which is in parts accomplished by prior analysis of the underlying structure–affinity relationships and adjusting linker lengths and coupling density. While it is possible to optimize the probe for binding to its main target (if known), binding to unknown but genuine off-targets cannot be accounted for and potentially introduces blind spots in the 'panel'. Throughput is a further major issue of this approach because each profiling requires chemical synthesis. To alleviate this limitation, wide-scope affinity matrices, such as Kinobeads or multiplexed inhibitor beads (MIBs) [29], can be used. They allow for specific enrichment (and competition) of large sub-proteomes and usually yield a more comprehensive view on a compound's target space than specific single-probe resins [21, 22, 30]. The KiNativ technology is such a relatively unbiased approach using desthiobiotinylated ATP to covalently link ATP binding proteins and subsequently enrich them via streptavidin [31]. Similarly to the Kinobeads approach, this lysate-based technology also enables broad assessment of target proteins beyond the protein kinase family (heat shock proteins or ABC transporters) and could also be used for tissues or other organisms [32]. Yet, determination of dissociation constants is complicated by the irreversible nature of the chemical probe. In comparison, the traditionally used screening panels that mainly consist of recombinantly expressed kinase domains do not offer the possibility of screening tissues or even other organisms. The usage of isolated protein kinase domains facilitates high throughput and yields robust and reproducible results, but does not accomplish close-to-physiological conditions as lysate-based technologies do. Complex native cell lysates contain endogenously expressed full-length proteins that have been functionalized in a cellular context and carry all the required post-translational modifications, cofactors, and binding partners. This often leads to differences in results between recombinant screens and lysate-based assays [33]. One recently developed technology, the NanoBRET assay [34], measures intracellular target engagement and binding affinities of ATP-competitive molecules in living cells. This approach is based on a kinase/luciferase fusion protein releasing a bioluminescence resonance energy transfer (BRET) signal upon binding of an ATP-competitive energy transfer probe. Compound affinity is determined by competitive displacement of this NanoBRET probe by a compound of interest. Upon binding, a dose-dependent decrease in NanoBRET energy transfer occurs, which can then be used for apparent intracellular affinity determination. This new technology is limited by the requirement of an expressed fusion protein and by the fact that just one kinase can be examined per experiment. However, it is so far the only method to determine whether a compound is able to permeate the cell membrane and to bind to a protein of interest in the presence of intracellular ATP concentrations.

4.1.3 Tips and Tricks Regarding Chemoproteomic Assay Development

Increasing Kinome Coverage: The overall number and type of kinases amenable to Kinobeads profiling depend on the composition of both the employed cell lysates and chemical probes [22]. Each cell comprises its individual kinome fingerprint in terms of expression of different kinases at different concentrations and activation states and engagement in protein–protein complexes. Recombinant assays excel by providing very high kinome coverage that is usually not obtained by chemical proteomic technologies such as Kinobeads because these rely on the cellular protein content. Proteins that are not inherently expressed by the cells are not accessible for affinity enrichment. This particular issue can be at least partially overcome by mixing lysates of different cell lines. This experimental set-up enables relatively broad kinome coverage for comprehensive selectivity profiling in a single chemoproteomic experiment [22]. Similar aspects need to be considered when designing the affinity resin and choosing the set of chemical probes for the affinity enrichment. The physicochemical and steric properties of a chemical probe determine its binding pose and affinity, and its adequate positioning within its target proteins may be optimized by the usage of different linkers in order to balance efficient enrichment and promiscuity of the affinity matrix. It is particularly important to consider the unspecific binding of proteins to the affinity matrix that can lead to high background, thus hampering the identification of target proteins. Unspecific binding mainly results from protein precipitation on the beads as well as the overall hydrophobicity of the affinity resin. The latter can be reduced by carefully evaluating the density of immobilized probes (adjusted when immobilizing the chemical probe to the solid support). Typically, lower coupling densities achieve better results. Bead washing conditions can also be optimized, but care has to be taken as the non-covalent nature of the enrichment will lead to loss of bound proteins over time. Hence, weak interactions may not be recovered. Importantly, in order to be able to distinguish genuine from background binding, competition pulldown experiments have to be performed.

Designing a Binding Assay: The Kinobeads technology is a typical *in vitro* binding assay, and setting up such an assay requires the consideration of several thermodynamic principles, such as binding equilibrium, association and dissociation kinetics, and enthalpic/entropic contributions to Gibbs free energy. These principles govern the various binding events between ligands, probes, and proteins and build the basis for how binding affinities and residence times of ligand–protein interactions are affected in chemical proteomic assays. Overall, the Kinobeads technology allows for the determination of thermodynamic parameters such as binding affinities (as derived from K_d^{app} values), but not of kinetic properties such as association (k_{on}) and dissociation (k_{off}) rates. Yet, the dissociation rate between affinity resin and protein strongly influences the success of a pulldown experiment. Short residence times on the beads may lead to loss of bead-bound proteins during the washing procedure and eventually to an overall signal decrease. Enthalpy and entropy also impact the experimental outcome. By immobilizing a compound onto a solid matrix, its degrees of freedom are reduced compared to the free compound. This increases the entropic contribution to Gibbs free energy and accordingly the binding affinity of the resin compared to the non-immobilized compound. Therefore, the Kinobeads technology is mainly suitable for profiling rather strong binding affinities in the nanomolar to low micromolar range, which feature longer residence times than weak interactions. The entropic change most likely affects binding kinetics in a way that proteins have a longer residence time on the beads. Hence, it is imperative to pre-incubate the lysate with the free compound for at least threefold of the longest residence time (if known) before affinity enrichment with the Kinobeads or other affinity matrices [35]. Slower association and dissociation rates can distort the binding affinities by preventing the establishment of a binding equilibrium in the experimental time frame.

Determining Binding Affinity: The determination of how strongly proteins bind their ligands is an essential step. Common measures include the assay-dependent half maximal inhibitory concentration (IC_{50}) and half maximal effective concentration (EC_{50}) or the assay-independent inhibition constant (K_i) and dissociation constant (K_d). The K_d describes the propensity of an inhibitor–protein complex to dissociate into its individual components at equilibrium. In a simple case of a two-membered equilibrium, the K_d can be described as the concentration of ligand that is necessary to occupy half of the binding sites of a target protein. In this case, K_d has molar units and is reciprocal to the affinity of the protein–ligand interaction. Several assay-specific aspects need to be considered to enable the determination of absolute and assay-independent binding affinities. Firstly, at fixed protein concentration and variable ligand concentrations, experimental K_d determination can only be accomplished if the protein concentration is lower than the K_d of the measured interaction. Since kinases are mostly considered low abundant signalling molecules, we assume that the target protein concentration is below the K_d concentration in a Kinobeads assay. However, that assumption may not always be justified, e.g. in case of overexpression of certain kinases or if another more abundant protein class can bind to the beads. Secondly, the affinity matrix should ideally not influence the binding equilibrium of a compound to its target protein. This is not the case for Kinobeads, where an assay-dependent EC_{50} value of a three-member interaction (Kinobeads–protein–free compound) is measured instead of the desired K_d of a two-state equilibrium (Figure 4.3a).

During the pre-incubation step, an equilibrium is established between protein, compound and protein–compound complex (Figure 4.3a, right). By adding Kinobeads, a certain portion of the 'free' proteins are bound by the Kinobeads (Figure 4.3a, left) and are consequently depleted from the binding equilibrium with the compound. Ideally, chemical probes should deplete less than 10% of the total protein amount, which is not achievable for all proteins in a highly complex chemoproteomic assay set-up. If protein depletion by the affinity matrix

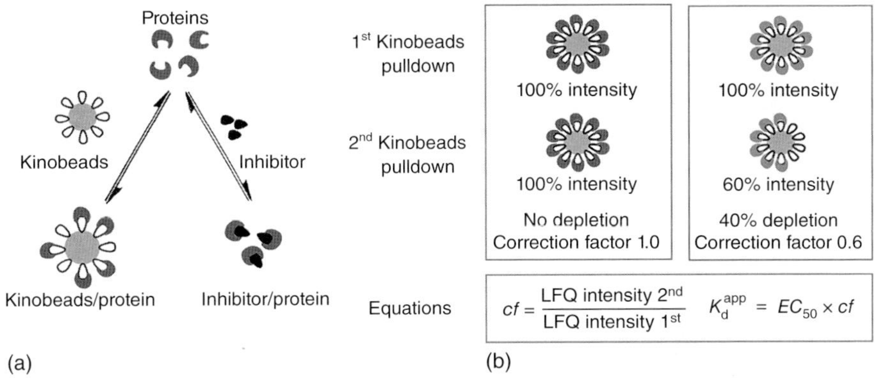

Figure 4.3 Determination of dissociation constants using Kinobeads. (Source: modified from Heinzlmeir [6]). (a) In a competitive Kinobeads pulldown experiment, a three-membered thermodynamic equilibrium is established between the affinity matrix, the target proteins and the kinase inhibitor. (b) Depending on the abundance and affinity of a particular protein to the beads, it will be (partially) depleted from the lysate. To account for this effect, a correction factor (*cf*) can be calculated by performing an additional pulldown using the depleted vehicle-treated lysate of the first pulldown and then dividing the LFQ intensity of the second pulldown by the LFQ intensity of the first pulldown. The determined ratio for a given kinase can be used to convert assay-dependent EC_{50} to assay-independent K_d^{app} values [32].

is not negligible, the compound–protein equilibrium is directed towards more dissociated species. The readjustment of the binding interaction between the protein and the free kinase inhibitor results in a shift of the measured EC_{50} values towards higher concentrations. The degree of depletion in a Kinobeads assay is dependent on protein abundance in the lysate, affinity to the affinity matrix and the effective Kinobeads probe concentration. Since none of these parameters are known beforehand, protein depletion needs to be examined experimentally. In order to do so, the correction factor concept introduced by Sharma et al. [36] was slightly modified for the Kinobeads assay [22]. Experimentally, two consecutive pulldowns of the vehicle-treated lysate are performed (Figure 4.3b). For each protein, the correction factor is calculated by determining the ratio of the intensity obtained in the second pulldown divided by the intensity measured in the first pulldown. Values close to 1 mean no or low protein depletion and values close to 0 indicate a high degree of protein depletion by the affinity matrix. Multiplying the correction factor with the EC_{50} values obtained from competitive pulldowns results in an apparent binding constant K_d^{app}, which describes the overall assay-independent affinity of a compound towards the different kinase species present in a particular lysate [20, 32].

4.2 Detailed Kinobeads Protocol

The following section will describe how a Kinobeads pulldown assay is performed and explain critical methodological steps in more detail. An overview of the workflow is shown in Figure 4.4. Briefly, native lysates are pre-incubated with

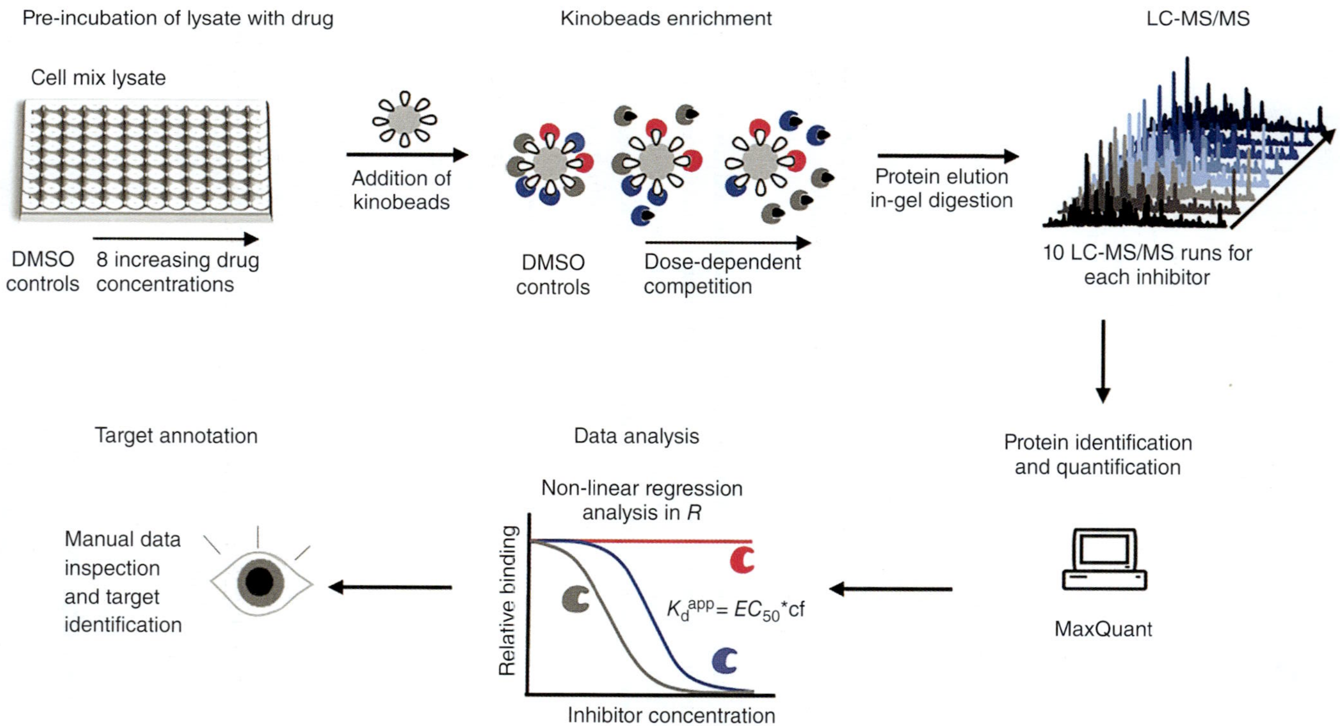

Figure 4.4 Detailed workflow of a competitive Kinobeads pulldown experiment. Kinobeads pulldowns are performed in 96-well format. Eight inhibitor doses are pre-incubated with the cell lysate. Subsequent enrichment of kinases and ATP binding proteins with Kinobeads leads to a competition between the free drug and Kinobeads for the active site of drug targets. Proteins are eluted from beads and digested, and the peptides are analysed via LC-MS/MS. Proteins and peptides are identified and quantified using MaxQuant/Andromeda. Dose-response curves are generated using a four-parameter log-logistic regression model, and target proteins are manually annotated.

compounds to establish binding equilibrium between the free compounds and their target proteins. Subsequently, Kinobeads are added to the lysates to enrich kinases from the lysates. Competition with the free drug leads to decreased binding of its target proteins to the Kinobeads as a function of increasing compound concentration. Bead-bound proteins are eluted, digested and subjected to a mass spectrometric measurement. Identification and label-free quantification (LFQ) of proteins are accomplished by state-of-the-art software such as MaxQuant [37]. Binding curves are generated by non-linear regression analysis.

4.2.1 Cell or Tissue Lysate

In principle, Kinobeads pulldown experiments can be performed using any kind of cell or tissue lysate as input material. For profiling purposes, it is favourable to achieve a high kinome coverage and thus choose a mix of cell or tissue lysates that covers as many kinases as possible. Alternatively, pulldowns can also be performed from lysates in which a particular compound effect was observed to deconvolute the target profile of a particular compound in a certain biological setting. In our laboratory, Kinobeads selectivity profiling is typically performed using a mixed lysate of four different cancer cell lines, namely, K-562, MV-4-11, SK-N-BE(2), and Colo205, which were selected to provide high kinome coverage [22]. To generate such lysates, cells are harvested at a cell confluency of approximately 80–90%. Native cell lysis is performed using a lysis buffer that preserves protein structures and complexes and also (partially) extracts membrane-bound proteins (0.8% IGEPAL CA-630, 50 mM Tris-HCl pH 7.5, 5% glycerol, 1.5 mM $MgCl_2$, 150 mM NaCl, 1 mM Na_3VO_4, 25 mM NaF, 1 mM DTT, protease inhibitor (SigmaFast, Sigma), and phosphatase inhibitor cocktails). Lysates are ultracentrifuged to remove all cell debris, and protein concentration is determined by colorimetric protein quantification assays, such as the Bradford assay. Cell lysates can be stored at −80 °C for several years before further use.

4.2.2 Affinity Matrices

The ε-version of Kinobeads [22, 38] is a mixture of seven broad-spectrum small molecule kinase inhibitors immobilized on sepharose beads (Figure 4.5): compound 1 (linkable PD173955), compound 5 (linkable vandetanib), compound 7 (purvalanol B), and BGT-226 are commercially sourced. Compound 13 (AKT probe), compound 19, and an analogue of omipalisib are synthesized in-house as reported previously [22, 38]. This mixture of affinity matrices is optimized towards the highest coverage of kinases within one experiment [22]. Compounds 1, 4, 13, 19 and BGT-226 are immobilized on *N*-hydroxysuccinimide (NHS)-activated Sepharose 4 Fast Flow beads (GE Healthcare, Germany) by covalent linkage via their primary amine, whereas compound 7 and linkable omipalisib are immobilized on 'reverse' NHS-activated sepharose beads through covalent linkage via carboxylic acid functional groups [22]. Here, we explain step by step how to immobilize a compound comprising either a primary or

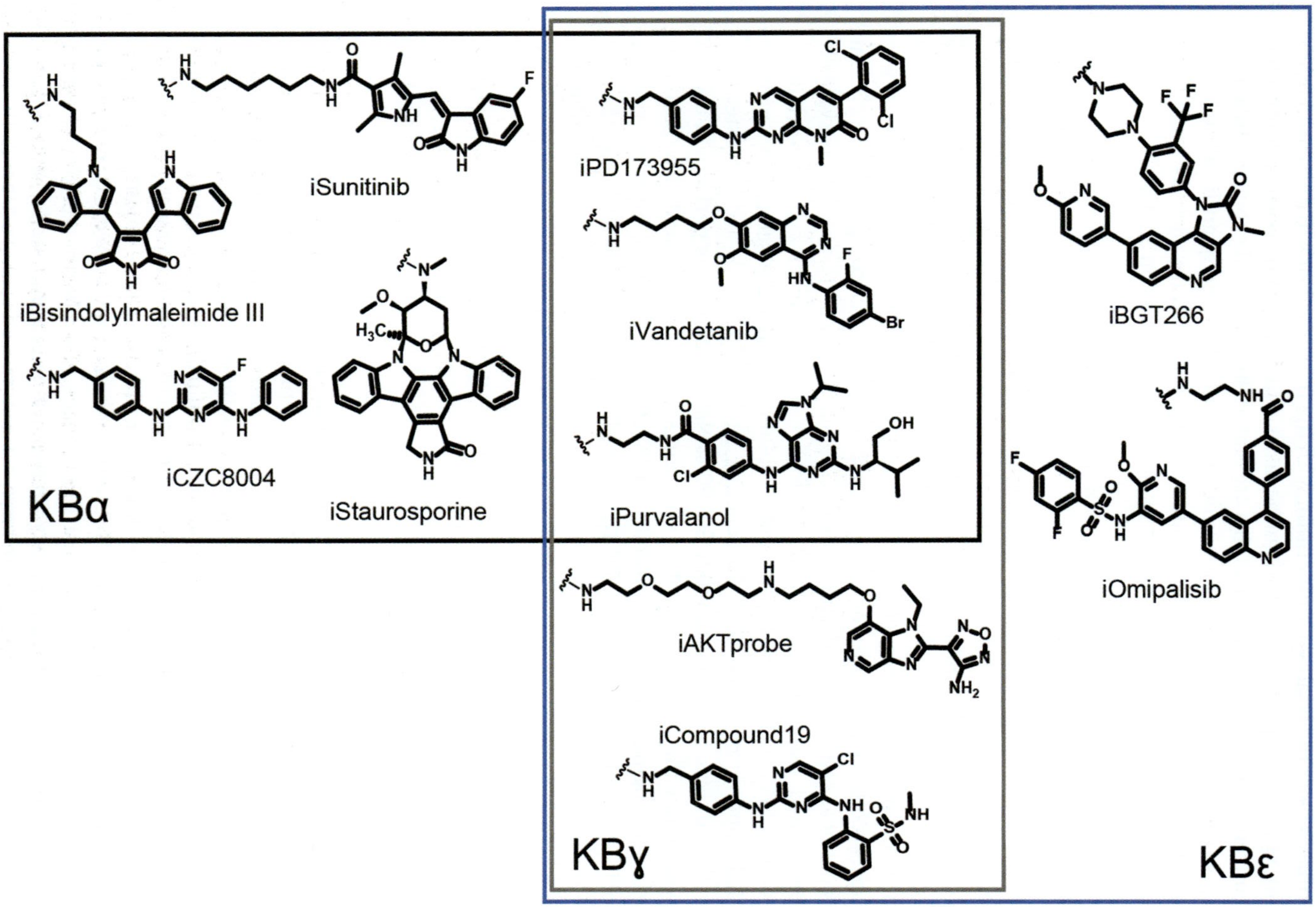

Figure 4.5 Milestones in the development of the Kinobeads affinity matrix. Chemical structures of the compounds that are included in three historical versions of Kinobeads (i: immobilized). The first version (KBα [21]) is marked in black, the version that allowed to establish the target landscape of clinical kinase drugs [20] (KBγ [22]) in grey, and the latest version including an extension to the PIK(K)s family of proteins (KBε [38]) in blue.

secondary amine or a carboxylic acid moiety onto NHS-activated sepharose beads (approximate capacity is 20 μmol/ml beads).

For coupling of compounds containing an amino group to NHS-activated sepharose beads, 1 ml of settled beads is washed four times with 10 ml dimethyl sulfoxide (DMSO) (centrifugation two minutes at 1200 rpm; supernatant is discarded). After washing, 1 ml settled beads are resuspended in 1 ml DMSO to yield a 1 : 1 slurry. The compound is added to the beads and mixed gently before beads are centrifuged (two minutes, 1200 rpm) and 20 μl of supernatant is taken for coupling control. Typically, coupling density is adjusted to 1 or 2 μmol compound/ml of beads, which was found to be useful for most kinase inhibitors. The coupling reaction is initiated by adding triethylamine (15 μl/ml of beads) and takes place for 20 hours on an end-over-end shaker at room temperature in the dark. On the next day beads are centrifuged, and 20 μl of supernatant is taken for coupling control. To block free remaining NHS groups on the beads, aminoethanol (50 μl/ml of beads) is added and incubated for another 20 hours at room temperature in the dark on an end-over-end shaker. Subsequently, beads are washed two times with 10 ml DMSO and five times with 10 ml ethanol (centrifugation two minutes, 1200 rpm) and stored as a 1 : 1 slurry in ethanol at 4 °C in the dark. To remove the *o*-nitrobenzenesulfonyl (*o*NBS) protecting group of compound 13, the beads are first washed five times with 15 ml dimethylformamide (DMF). Beads are resuspended in 1 ml DMF, and subsequently *N*-methyl-2-pyrrolidone (2 ml), 1,8-diazabicyclo(5.4.0)undec-7-ene (1.5 ml), and β-mercaptoethanol (1.5 ml) are added and incubated for 15 minutes in an end-over-end shaker in the dark. The supernatant is discarded and the procedure is repeated twice. Subsequently, beads are washed five times with 10 ml ethanol and stored as a 1 : 1 slurry in ethanol at 4 °C in the dark. Aliquots of the supernatant before and after coupling are collected as described to monitor for conversion by liquid chromatography-mass spectrometry (LC-MS).

For chemical probes containing a carboxylic acid functional group, 1 ml of NHS-sepharose beads is washed four times with 10 ml DMSO as described for amino compound coupling. In order to functionally 'reverse' the beads, an ethylenediamine spacer is introduced on NHS-sepharose beads to yield amino-sepharose beads with approximatively 4 μmol per ml beads available primary amines: a mixture of ethylenediamine (2.68 μl per ml of beads), aminoethanol (9.66 μl per ml of beads), and triethylamine (15 μl per ml of beads) is prepared, vortexed thoroughly, and added to the beads. After shaking for 20 hours on an end-over-end shaker at room temperature in the dark, beads are washed three times with 10 ml DMSO and twice with 10 ml DMF. These washing steps are crucial in order to remove remaining aminoethanol and ethylenediamine, which could react with the probe and thus reduce coupling efficiency. Washed beads are resuspended in 1 ml DMF (1 : 1 slurry), and the following is added sequentially: (i) the appropriate amount of COOH compound stock dissolved in DMF, (ii) 100 μl of *N*,*N*-diisopropylethylamine (DIEA) (prepared by dissolving 35 μl DIEA in 1 ml dry DMF), and (iii) 20 μl triethylamine. Beads are mixed and centrifuged (one minute, 1200 rpm), and 20 μl supernatant is taken for coupling control. The coupling reaction is initiated by adding the amino coupling reagent PyBrOP (4.7 mg/ml beads) or HATU (3.8 mg/ml beads) and incubated for 20 hours at room temperature in the dark on an end-over-end shaker. To acetylate the remaining free amines, a blocking reagent (NHS-acetate) is prepared by mixing equal volumes of 200 mM dicyclohexylcarbodiimide (DCC) and 200 mM NHS in a glass vial. Per 1 ml total volume of NHS/DCC mix, 11.4 µl acetic acid is added, and the reaction mixture is incubated at room temperature overnight. On the next day, beads are centrifuged, and 20 µl of supernatant are taken for coupling control. After washing three times with 10 ml DMSO, the remaining free coupling sites on the beads (1 : 1 slurry in DMSO) are reacted with NHS-acetate (10 µmol/ml beads) by addition of triethylamine (20 µl/ml beads) and incubation overnight at room temperature. Afterwards, beads are washed once with 10 ml DMSO and three times with 10 ml ethanol and stored at 4 °C in the dark. Aliquots of the supernatant before and after coupling were collected to control the coupling efficiency by LC-MS.

To determine the best loading density for a specific compound, beads with different densities (around 0.5–4 µmol compound/ml beads) are prepared. An affinity pulldown experiment is performed as described below, and the pulldown eluate is analysed by sodium dodecyl sulfate-polyacrylamide gel electrophoresis (SDS-PAGE) with silver staining read-out. If the density is too high, the bead surface might become excessively hydrophobic, and increasing unspecific binding can be observed by a rather overloaded SDS-PAGE. If the coupling density is too low, not all proteins that could theoretically bind will be enriched by the beads. Therefore, it is necessary to evaluate the best coupling density for each compound (clear and intense bands in an SDS-PAGE analysis) that is used for immobilization on sepharose beads. An optimal coupling density of 1 µmol/ml beads was determined for compound 1, BGT-226, and the omipalisib analogue. Compounds 5, 7, 13, and 19 are typically prepared with a coupling density of 2 µmol/ml beads. The γ-version of Kinobeads (5 compounds) is prepared by mixing the functionalized beads in a 1 : 1 : 1 : 1 : 1 mixture of probes 1, 5, 7, 15, and 19. The ε-version of Kinobeads (7 compounds) is prepared by mixing Kinobeads-γ, immobilized omipalisib analogue, and immobilized BGT-226 in a ratio of 2 : 1 : 1.

4.2.3 Kinobeads Competition Assay

For inhibitor selectivity profiling experiments as well as for affinity enrichment of kinases, the cell lysates of Colo205, SK-N-BE(2), MV-4-11, and K-562 are mixed in a ratio of 1 : 1 : 1 : 1 regarding to the total amount of proteins as determined by Bradford assay. If necessary the lysate mixture is diluted with lysis buffer (0.8% IGEPAL CA-630, 50 mM Tris-HCl pH 7.5, 5% glycerol, 1.5 mM $MgCl_2$, 150 mM NaCl, 1mM Na_3VO_4, 25 mM NaF, 1 mM DTT, protease inhibitor (SigmaFast, Sigma), and phosphatase inhibitor) to reach a protein concentration of 10 mg/ml. To reduce the NP-40 concentration, the lysate is diluted 1 : 1 with 1× compound pulldown (CP) buffer (50 mM Tris-HCl pH 7.5, 5% glycerol, 1.5 mM $MgCl_2$, 150 mM NaCl, 20 mM NaF, 1 mM sodium orthovanadate, 1 mM DTT, supplemented with protease inhibitor and phosphatase inhibitor). The mixed and diluted lysate is cleared by ultracentrifugation at 52 000 rpm for 20 minutes at 4 °C, and the supernatant is stored on ice.

For competition pulldowns, the mixed lysate (5 mg of total proteins per well) is pre-incubated with increasing inhibitor concentrations (e.g. final concentrations of 3 nM, 10 nM, 30 nM, 100 nM, 300 nM, 1 μM, 3 μM, or 30 μM) or with DMSO as vehicle control in a 96-deep-well plate. To do so, 5 μl of 200× compound stock solution (in DMSO) or DMSO alone is added to 1 ml of cell mix lysate in a 2 ml 96-deep-well plate (final DMSO concentration of 0.5%). Pre-incubation of lysate with compound takes place at 4 °C in an end-over-end shaker for 45 minutes. In the meantime, 70 μl slurry Kinobeads in ethanol per pulldown experiment are centrifuged (one minute, 1200 rpm, supernatant is discarded), and beads are resuspended with four bead volumes of 50% glycerol to prevent rapid settling of beads and ensure even and reproducible pipetting. 175 μl of the beads/glycerol mixture is pipetted to a 96-well filter plate (Porvair Combinatorial Microlute plate, unpacked with bottom frits, pore size 36 μm, polyethylene), washed twice with 1 ml CP buffer to remove the glycerol, and equilibrated once with 1 ml CP-0.4 buffer (1× CP buffer, 0.4% IGEPAL CA-630). The filter plate with beads is centrifuged (one minute, 1200 rpm) to remove residual buffer and the bottom is closed with a bottom mat. The pre-incubated lysate is transferred to cover the beads and the plate is closed with a top mat. After incubation for 30 minutes at 4 °C in an end-over-end shaker, the plate is centrifuged again for two minutes at 4 °C and 1200 rpm to collect the beads on the bottom of the filter plate. Afterwards, the bottom mat is removed first, and the filter plate is placed on a 2 ml 96-deep-well plate before removing the top mat to collect the lysate of the DMSO control. A second Kinobeads pulldown (pulldown of pulldown) is performed by incubating the DMSO lysate a second time with fresh beads in order to calculate the depletion factor for each protein. Subsequently, beads are washed three times with 1 ml CP-0.4 buffer, twice with 1 ml CP supplemented with 0.2% IGEPAL CA-630 (CP-0.2), and residual buffer is removed by centrifugation (one minute, 1200 rpm). To elute the proteins from the beads by denaturation and reduction of disulphide bridges, 40 μl 2× NuPAGE Lithium dodecyl sulfate (LDS) sample buffer supplemented with 50 mM DTT is added to the beads and incubated for 30 minutes at 50 °C and 700 rpm on a thermoshaker. The top mat is removed before the bottom mat, the filter plate is quickly placed on a 96-well plate, and proteins are eluted by centrifugation (three minutes, 1200 rpm). Samples are cooled down to room temperature or stored at −20 °C until further use. Proteins are alkylated with chloroacetamide by adding 4 μl of a 550 mM stock solution (final concentration of 55 mM) and incubated for 30 minutes in the dark. Afterwards, 20 μl Kinobeads pulldown eluate is loaded onto a 4–12% Sodium dodecyl sulfate (SDS) gel (NuPAGE, Invitrogen) and run for five minutes to concentrate and desalt the proteins. Proteins are then trypsin-digested by standard procedure and dried peptides are stored at −20 °C until MS analysis.

4.2.4 Mass Spectrometry

NanoLC-ESI-MS measurements of Kinobeads pulldown samples are performed using a Dionex UltiMate 3000 nano high performance liquid chromatography (HPLC) coupled online to an Orbitrap HF (Thermo Scientific) mass spectrometer. Peptides are dissolved in 20 μl 0.1% formic acid (FA) and half of the sample is injected. Peptides are delivered to a trap column (100 μm × 2 cm, packed in-house with Reprosil-Gold C18 ODS-3 5 μm resin, Dr Maisch, Ammerbuch) and washed at a flow rate of 5 μl/min in solvent A0 (0.1% FA in water). Subsequently, peptides are transferred to an analytical column (75 μm × 40 cm, self-packed with Reprosil-Gold C18, 3 μm resin, Dr Maisch, Ammerbuch) at a flow rate of 300 nl/min and separated using a 52 minutes gradient ranging from 5% to 33% solvent B (0.1% FA, 5% DMSO [39] in acetonitrile) in solvent A1 (0.1% FA, 5% DMSO in HPLC-grade water). The Orbitrap HF is operated in data-dependent acquisition (DDA) and positive ionization mode. Full MS spectra are acquired in the orbitrap over a mass-to-charge (m/z) range of 360–1300 m/z at a resolution of 60K using an automatic gain control (AGC) target value of 3e6 or a maximum injection time of 10 ms. Up to 12 peptide precursors are selected for fragmentation by higher-energy collision-induced dissociation (HCD) using 25% normalized collision energy (NCE), an isolation width of 1.7 m/z, a maximum injection time of 75 ms, and an AGC value of 2e5. Resulting fragment ions are recorded in the orbitrap. An inclusion list containing approximately 3700 kinase peptides m/z and their corresponding retention time values is enabled in the data acquisition regime. Dynamic exclusion is set to 30 seconds and singly charged precursors are excluded.

4.2.5 Peptide and Protein Identification and Quantification

Peptide and protein identification and label-free quantification (LFQ) of the MS raw data are performed using MaxQuant [37] with its built-in search engine Andromeda [40]. MS2 spectra are searched against all canonical protein sequences as annotated in the SwissProt reference database (human proteins only, 20 193 entries, downloaded 22 March 2016, internally annotated with PFAM domains). Carbamidomethylated cysteine is considered as fixed modification. Phosphorylation of serine, threonine, and tyrosine, oxidation of methionine, and N-terminal protein acetylation are typically set as variable modifications. Trypsin/P is specified as the proteolytic enzyme and up to two missed cleavage sites are allowed. LFQ and 'match between runs' options are enabled in MaxQuant. Search results are filtered for 1% peptide and protein false discovery rate (FDR) employing a target–decoy approach using reversed protein sequences.

4.2.6 Data Analysis

MS raw files of Kinobeads pulldowns from one particular drug are processed together as a self-contained experiment. The resulting file (proteinGroups.txt) is used for further filtering, normalization and curve fitting. Reverse hits, potential contaminants and proteins without intensity values are removed. Subsequently, protein raw and LFQ intensities are normalized to the corresponding DMSO control intensity to obtain the relative residual binding intensities (I_{rel}) for each protein group at every concentration. Dose–response curves for each protein group are then generated by a four-parameter log-logistic regression model (4.1) using an internally developed R-script that utilizes the 'drc' package:

$$I_{\mathrm{rel}}(c) = b + \frac{t-b}{1 + e^{s*(\log(c)-\log(i))}} \tag{4.1}$$

where c is the compound concentration and the four free parameters are the plateau of the fit b (bottom), the maximal residual binding t (top), and the hill slope s of the curve at the inflection point I (EC_{50}). I_{rel} values derived from LFQ intensities are preferably used. The apparent binding constant $K_{\mathrm{d}}^{\mathrm{app}}$ is calculated by multiplying the estimated EC_{50} with the protein-dependent correction factor (depletion factor). As already described, the correction factor of a protein is defined as the ratio of protein intensities in two consecutive pulldowns of the same DMSO-treated lysate.

Targets of the inhibitor of interest are annotated manually. A protein is considered a target if the binding curve shows a sigmoidal shape with a dose-dependent intensity reduction. The number of unique peptides and MSMS spectra are also taken into account and should ideally show the same behaviour as the binding curve with increasing inhibitor concentrations. Additionally, the protein intensity in the DMSO control sample is considered. Proteins with low peptide counts, MSMS spectra counts, or MS1 intensity are annotated as low confidence targets. Targets are considered direct Kinobeads binders if annotated in UniProt.org as protein or lipid kinase, nucleotide binders (e.g. helicases, ATPases, and GTPases), FAD cofactor containing proteins (e.g. NQO2) and heme-containing proteins (e.g. ferrochelatase [FECH]). Other proteins showing a dose response are often indirect Kinobeads binders (interaction partners/adaptor proteins), co-enriched as constituents of protein complexes captured by the Kinobeads.

4.3 Application Examples for Kinobeads

4.3.1 Expanding the Target Space of Kinobeads

Affinity Probes: The utopic goal when designing target class-specific affinity probes consists in achieving coverage and high affinity for all members – exclusively – of the particular target class. Alas, the ideal molecule able to enrich the whole human kinome has not yet been identified, and instead, sets of complementary probes are used to cover a large portion of the kinome. When the Kinobeads technology was first described in 2007 by Bantscheff et al. [21], the mixture of seven immobilized broad selective kinase inhibitors (Kinobeads-α; Figure 4.5) was able to enrich 269 human kinases from different tissues and cell lysates. In order to extend the target space of the Kinobeads, i.e. the 'panel' available for drug profiling, regular preparation and evaluation of novel affinity probes are performed. This continuous effort led to the development of several kinase family-specific probes, targeting, for example, the FGFR [41], VEGFR [42], JAK [43], PIKK [38], or AKT [44] family, all of which are important drug targets in pharmaceutical research. In order to better profile AKT kinase inhibitors, Pachl and co-workers [44] developed a chemical affinity

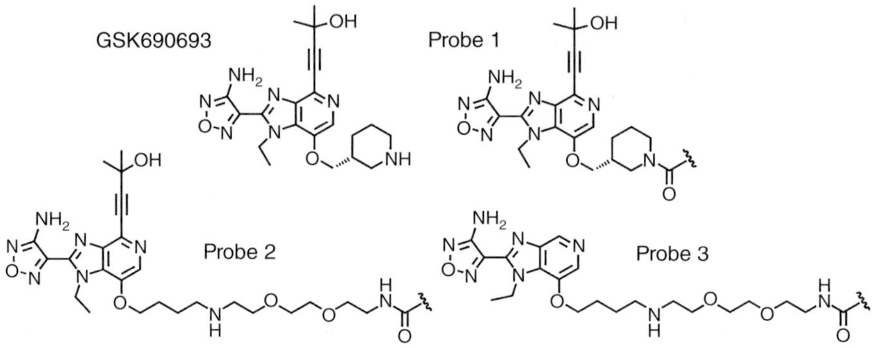

Figure 4.6 Chemical structures of the potent ATP-competitive AKT inhibitor GSK690693 and of three different affinity probes derived from that parent structure.

probe targeting AKT and related kinases based on the structure of the potent ATP-competitive AKT inhibitor GSK690693. The structure-activity relationship (SAR) study and the X-ray co-crystal structure with AKT2 provided by the inventors of GSK690693 [45] allowed to identify the best attachment point as well as a moiety that was described to provide selectivity. Hence, three probes were designed and prepared building on this information (Figure 4.6). The first matrix was made by simple immobilization of the compound via amidation of its secondary amine. The second probe kept the selectivity-providing moiety, but a spacer was introduced that allowed a basic amine to be maintained while allowing a better insertion in the pocket. The third used the same spacer, but the selectivity-providing moiety was omitted. Comparative pulldown experiments using the three probes were performed, revealing that the best promiscuity was obtained for the matrix featuring the spacer but without the selectivity-providing moiety (50 kinases). It was capable of capturing all three AKT isoforms (AKT1, AKT2, and AKT3) and, additionally, a considerable number of AGC kinases as well as members of the CMGC and CAMK family. Adding the new AKT affinity probe to the Kinobeads-α matrix extended kinome coverage to the AKT family.

Proceeding with the same retro-engineering strategy, probes were developed by Ku and co-workers to make VEGFR [42] and FGFR [41] family kinases accessible for the Kinobeads technology. FGFR-specific affinity probes were designed based on the chemical scaffold of the small molecule FGFR inhibitor PD-173074. The published co-crystal structure of PD-173074 and FGFR1 allowed insights into the binding mode of the inhibitor and facilitated the identification of appropriate linkage positions. In order to generate a VEGFR-specific affinity matrix, nine VEGFR inhibitors representing eight different scaffolds were selected based on a search of the literature. Analysis of the available co-crystal structures and SAR of the inhibitors leads to the prioritization of nintedanib as the lead structure for further probe design. For stable enrichment of the JAK family, Höfener et al. [43] identified three scaffolds. Analysis of X-ray structures allowed them to design linkable analogues, which were first docked and then synthesized. The probe based on the momelotinib series proved the most efficient, enriching 98 kinases in a triplicate experiment using a mixture of cell lysates, including JAK1, JAK2, and TYK2. Another example of the Kinobeads extension yielded Kinobeads-ε by addition of two probes targeting the PIKK and PIK families to the five probes constituting Kinobeads-γ. Here Reinecke et al. immobilized BGT-226 and an analogue of omipalisib allowing for subsequent profiling of ATM, ATR, mTOR, and PI3K inhibitors, whose primary targets were so far inaccessible to Kinobeads profiling [38]. These examples show how Kinobeads can be further fine-tuned to increase kinome coverage through the careful design of complementary affinity probes using the structural studies and SAR tables that medicinal chemistry provide to both seek for promiscuity and linkability. More generally, the combined probes should preferably have a complementary target profile so that each protein is enriched ideally only by one probe to prevent increased protein depletion. Additionally, the number of probes that are mixed should be kept to a minimum to avoid dilution effects.

Cell or Tissue Lysate: Chemical proteomic techniques such as Kinobeads are mostly lysate-based approaches providing several advantages over more classical recombinant activity or binding assays. Most other *in vitro* assays require genetic modification (e.g. fusion proteins), recombinant expression, and purification of individual target proteins, rendering the development of such assays tedious and cost intensive. The independence of genetic manipulation of biological systems to receive the required input material for the binding assay is one major advantage of the Kinobeads technology over recombinant assays. Using complex native lysates also provides the opportunity to examine the interaction of compounds and their target proteins in a close-to-physiological environment ensuring the presence of necessary cofactors, protein complex partners, and post-translational modifications defining the activity and conformation of most target proteins within the cell. Obviously, the used lysates differ in their protein composition depending on the biology of the underlying cell. This comes as a major advantage of the technology, which allows performing selectivity profiling of drugs in the biological or pathological model relevant to the intended use of the molecules. Indeed, the lysates can be produced from all types of biological input material constituting proteomes or sub-proteomes of cellular compartments, cell lines, primary cells or tissues. Selecting the appropriate lysate for a certain research question will not only reveal the (enrichable) kinome composition of the cell type or tissue of interest but will also (and most importantly) facilitate the identification of drug targets specifically inhibited in the disease-relevant cell type or tissue. The target space of the same drug may vary significantly depending on the differential expression and activity of protein kinases in different tissues, not only revealing tissue-specific modes of action but also explaining tissue-specific toxic side effects. For example, Kinobeads are capable of enriching 209 kinases from human placenta and 141 kinases from human liver tissue, showing both overlapping and exclusive sets of kinases (Figure 4.7a). Developing this thought further, lysates derived from all kinds of organisms can be utilized in a Kinobeads profiling assay, provided that their genomes have been sequenced. This unique feature of the approach greatly expands the potential of this technology to investigate inhibitors and protein targets of other origin than human (Figure 4.7b). As an example, we performed Kinobeads pulldowns in murine retina (122 kinases), bone marrow-derived dendritic cells (174 kinases), and liver mitochondria (50

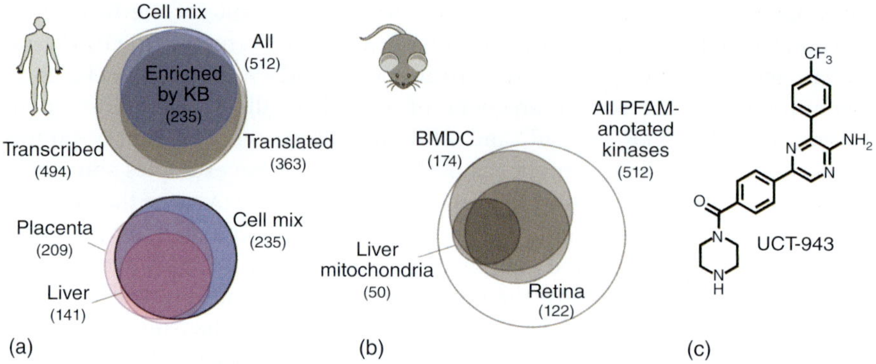

Figure 4.7 Kinase enrichment from lysates of different cellular origin using Kinobeads. (a) Kinobeads enrich 253 kinases from a mix of four different human cell lines (upper Venn diagram). Human tissues, including placenta and liver, comprise different kinase compositions and extend the space of enrichable kinases. (b) Kinobeads can also be used to profile tissues from other organisms such as mouse. (c) Kinase selectivity profiling of inhibitors in *Plasmodium falciparum* led to the discovery of UCT-943, a preclinical candidate for the treatment of Malaria.

kinases), identifying a total of 195 out of 512 PFAM-annotated murine protein kinases. Other model organisms used for Kinobeads profiling (unpublished data) included a zebrafish cell line or even non-mammalian model systems such as *Arabidopsis thaliana*, demonstrating the striking versatility of this technology. Kinobeads can also be used to investigate pathogens such as *Schistosoma mansoni* (115 out of 252 protein kinases detected [46]) and have already facilitated the discovery of kinase inhibitors targeting pathogens, such as *Trypanosoma brucei* [47] *or Plasmodium falciparum* [48] (UCT-943 [49]; Figure 4.7c). These organisms are usually insufficiently or not at all accessible by standard *in vitro* assays, opening completely new possibilities for lysate-based chemoproteomic technologies to perform drug discovery for infectious diseases.

When more comprehensive selectivity profiling of kinase inhibitors independent of a precise biological background is desired, different cancer cell lines with varying overexpressed signalling pathways can be mixed. Akin to the combination of affinity probes to cover the kinome, this concatenation of complementary kinomes creates a broad range of protein kinases (and other proteins) for selectivity profiling. Accordingly, our typically used combination of four different cell lines (COLO205, SK-N-BE(2), MV-4-11, and K-562) contains a total of 494 transcribed kinases (by RNA-Seq) and 363 translated kinases (by deep proteome profiling; Figure 4.7a), and Kinobeads are capable of enriching 253 of these [20].

4.3.2 Target Space Deconvolution of Small Molecule Kinase Inhibitors

Target Deconvolution for Mode of Action Analysis: Kinase inhibitors are usually rather promiscuous compounds, such that their biological impact must be considered as a complex interplay of many inhibitory effects rather than simplifying it to the inhibition of a single kinase and desired or undesired mode(s) of action must be carefully evaluated. Accordingly, a systematic and comprehensive evaluation of compound selectivity is required for a better understanding of drug perturbation and an informed targeted application, also of promiscuous inhibitors. From a clinical standpoint, off-target inhibition could be considered beneficial if proteins are affected that could potentially overcome the inhibition of a particular kinase (for instance, other family members) or that are known molecular resistance drivers (as known for MET or EPHA2 in the case of epidermal growth factor receptor [EGFR] inhibitor-resistant tumours [50, 51]). Multi-target drugs could also provide the opportunity of several modes of action that function in a concerted manner in defeating the disease [52–54]. As an example, the inhibition of pro-inflammatory immune responses could be beneficial during cancer therapy. However, off-target inhibition mediating toxic or adverse side effects could be detrimental for therapy outcome and will most probably lead to failure during clinical evaluation [11]. Besides protein kinases, the Kinobeads technology allows for the identification of additional non-protein kinase targets [55], including several metabolic kinases, other nucleotide binding proteins (e.g. helicases or GTPases), and a few FAD-containing proteins and heme-containing proteins. Examples for such unexpected non-kinase off-targets include glycogen phosphorylase (PYGL, PYGM, PYGB) [56], ribosyldihydronicotinamide dehydrogenase (NQO2) [21], or ferrochelatase (FECH) [20, 57]. This is of special interest since these proteins are not part of conventional screening panels, but may impact a drug's mode of action or explain adverse side effects. For example, it was found that about 15% of clinical kinase inhibitors bind to FECH [57], which may lead to the toxic side effect of photosensitivity as observed for the BRAF inhibitor vemurafenib. Another interesting aspect addresses the mode of action of prodrugs and their active metabolites. Kinobeads selectivity profiling showed that the target spectra and potencies of such pairs can vary considerably. Prodrugs may have more targets than their active metabolites (e.g. fasudil) or less (e.g. TG-100572 and the prodrug TG-100801) and might bind completely different proteins (e.g. barasertib, fostamatinib). Thus, careful target profiling of an inhibitor, the formulation and metabolites thereof, should be performed to comprehensively understand the mechanisms by which a clinical drug might exert its effects *in vivo*. In general, the data on 243 clinical kinase inhibitors profiled by the Kinobeads technology revealed that chemical proteomics holds the potential to substantially increase our understanding of the 'druggable kinome' and non-kinase off-target inhibition [20]. Comparison to publically available data from other kinase inhibitor screens [58, 59] or commonly used databases such as ChEMBL or Library of Integrated Network-based Cellular Signatures (LINCS) showed that many identified drug–protein interactions had not been reported before – rendering this technology a highly valuable tool for kinase inhibitor target deconvolution.

Example: Target Deconvolution of CHEK1 Inhibitors: CHEK1 plays a major role in coordinating the DNA damage response and overexpression was found

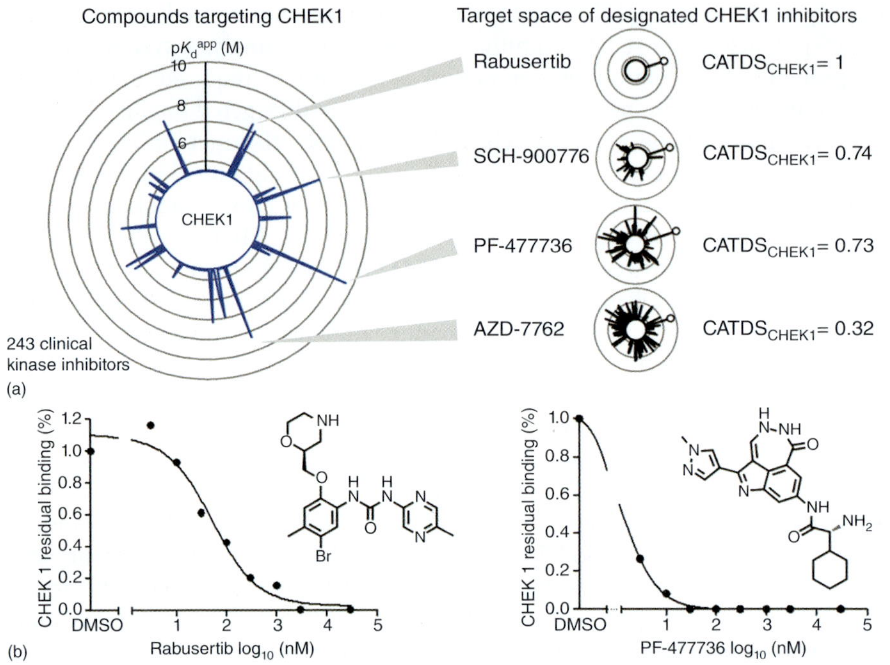

Figure 4.8 Target deconvolution of CHEK1 inhibitors (Source: Modified from Klaeger et al. 2017 [20]). (a) The radar plot on the left shows 19 identified CHEK1 binders and their affinities (protein-centric view). Each spike represents an individual clinical inhibitor and the length depicts inhibitor binding affinities as a pK_d^{app} value. The small radar plots on the right illustrate the target space of individual CHEK1 inhibitors (compound-centric view), each spike representing the binding affinity of an individual target protein to this particular inhibitor. The $CATDS_{CHEK1}$ scores at the corresponding K_d^{app} values are shown. (b) Target proteins are competed from Kinobeads, resulting in a dose-dependent decrease of MS signal intensity, as exemplified for rabusertib and PF-477736.

in numerous tumour entities including breast, colon, and liver [60]. Accordingly, CHEK1 is an important drug target in pharmaceutical research, and several inhibitors have been developed to target this serine/threonine-specific protein kinase. Studying the target space of 243 clinical kinase drugs revealed that 19 clinically relevant inhibitors bind to CHEK1 [20], 15 of which are not designated CHEK1 inhibitors (Figure 4.8a). The identified inhibitors bound CHEK1 with different affinities and hence reduced binding to Kinobeads in a dose-dependent manner, as exemplified in Figure 4.8b for rabusertib and PF-477736. Although the designated CHEK1 inhibitors AZD-7762, PF-477736, and SCH-900776 featured high affinity binding towards their intended target (K_d^{app}: 5, 0.2, 11 nM respectively), they also bound many other proteins, leading to rather low selectivity for CHEK1 (Figure 4.8a). In contrast, rabusertib exhibited high affinity (K_d^{app} = 43 nM) and was by far the most selective CHEK1 inhibitor in this screen ($CATDS_{CHEK1}$ = 1), qualifying it as a highly valuable chemical probe for CHEK1.

This application example demonstrates how the Kinobeads technology can be used for the thorough evaluation of binding affinities and selectivity of kinase inhibitors and how a protein- or compound-centric view of the screening results can inform different research aspects, for example, identifying chemical probes for a protein of interest or explaining mode(s) of action of kinase inhibitors.

Target Deconvolution of Irreversible Inhibitors: In the past decade, several kinase inhibitors have been developed to inhibit their kinase targets in a covalent, irreversible manner [61] (referred to as type VI inhibitors [9]). Prominent examples are afatinib and neratinib inhibiting EGFR or acalabrutinib and ibrutinib targeting BTK. These inhibitors contain a low reactive electrophile that reacts with a cysteine residue within or close to the binding site of the small molecule to the kinase [62], e.g. via a Michael addition. This strategy allows for long-lasting inhibition of the protein that is dependent on target protein turnover (e.g. degradation and synthesis rates) rather than on pharmacokinetic properties of the inhibitor (e.g. effective concentration and residence time). This type of inhibitor has to be evaluated even more carefully because specific or unspecific irreversible reactions probably lead to strong and long-lasting side effects. Kinobeads selectivity profiling is most often performed with ATP-competitive small molecule kinase inhibitors binding their target proteins in a reversible manner; in order to use it for profiling irreversible inhibitors, certain aspects need to be considered. For example, the reaction of the electrophilic compound and the cysteine depends on the redox environment and the local pH within the cell, which may vary strongly from the environment in lysates. Also, binding of such inhibitors usually follows two steps, the reversible binding of the compound to its binding pocket and subsequent reaction to form the covalent bond. Accordingly, these inhibitors can also reversibly bind and inhibit other kinases lacking a reactive cysteine in the appropriate position. Dittus and co-workers [63] introduced an approach for target identification of irreversible inhibitors using Kinobeads. They performed cell-based and lysate-based experiments in parallel in order to distinguish covalent and reversible binding of type VI inhibitors to kinase targets. To do so, either live cells or cell lysates were incubated with the compound prior to affinity enrichment of unbound kinases by Kinobeads. Non-covalent drug–protein interactions should undergo re-equilibration of the binding equilibrium after cell lysis and yield higher EC_{50} values in the lysate-based pulldowns as compared with the cell-based experiments. In contrast, EC_{50} values of covalent interactions should not be affected by cell lysis and dilution of the target protein. Potency of covalent targets might be even higher *in cellulo* because target engagement in cells might be more efficient than in lysate. In this study [63], the target space of the covalent BTK kinase inhibitors CC-292 and acalabrutinib were determined exemplarily. The covalently bound cellular target space of CC-292 consisted of the three kinases TEC, BTK, and BLK, whereas acalabrutinib solely bound BTK and TEC. Additionally, the kinases LIMK1, RIPK2, and RIPK3 were identified as reversibly bound inhibitor targets. This study [63] describes an elegant extension to the classical Kinobeads approach, revealing its technological potential towards profiling of inhibitors with unusual binding behaviour.

4.3.3 Opportunities Arising from Inhibitor Polypharmacology: Drug Repositioning

Drug Repositioning: A drug's mode of action needs to be considered within the biological background of the disease. Depending on protein expression levels and activities, a drug might affect different proteins in different tissues or disease backgrounds. Accordingly, target space deconvolution can open up new opportunities, such as the possibility of drug repositioning in other biological contexts. For instance, kinase inhibitors designed for treating oncogenic diseases could also be useful in inflammatory disorders, immune disorders, or neurodegenerative diseases. Indications outside oncology have very high safety hurdles, such that detailed insight into the target profile of kinase inhibitors can be helpful in order to estimate the drug's therapeutic index. So far, clinical kinase inhibitors have been designed for roughly 10% of all protein kinases validated as *bona fide* targets [64], but more and more protein kinases are found to be involved in diverse human diseases. This will lead to an increased demand of targeted inhibitors in the near future [64]. An improved characterization of a drug's target space may fill this gap by enabling the use of a compound for the targeted inhibition of formerly unknown off-target proteins. The prime example for drug repositioning is the BCR-ABL inhibitor imatinib, which was originally developed for the treatment of CML and is nowadays also used as a KIT inhibitor in gastrointestinal stromal tumours (GISTs) [65]. This approach becomes particularly attractive in light of the increasing application of precision medicine approaches, where patient tumours are molecularly profiled in order to inform individual treatment decisions (see Chapter 6 for more details). Off-label or compassionate use of available kinase drugs in other entities than the approved indication constitutes a valuable option to fully exploit the potential of these highly optimized molecules. Hence, comprehensive target profiling can foster drug repositioning, complement the search for novel compounds, and help to reduce the economic burden that arises from the development of new drugs.

Repositioning of Cabozantinib for FLT3-ITD-Positive AML: Cabozantinib is a MET and VEGFR inhibitor approved for the treatment of medullary thyroid cancer and advanced renal cell carcinoma [66, 67]. Kinobeads selectivity profiling revealed that cabozantinib binds several other proteins in addition to its designated targets, among them the kinase FLT3 (K_d^{app} = 53 nM; Figure 4.9a,b) [20]. A total of 30% of AML patients carry the FLT3-ITD (internal tandem duplication) mutation, resulting in a constitutively active receptor [68] and rendering FLT3 one of the most frequently mutated genes in AML. Since cabozantinib is already approved and safe for clinical use, it is of great interest as a potential candidate for repositioning in FLT3-ITD-driven AML. The effect of cabozantinib was examined in a preclinical study both *in vitro* and *in vivo*. Drug treatment of a panel of AML cell lines revealed that only FLT3-ITD cell lines were sensitive towards cabozantinib treatment, whereas FLT3 wild-type cell lines did not show reduced viability and proliferation. In addition, a xenograft mouse model using MOLM-13 (FLT3-ITD) and OCI-AML3 (FLT3 wild-type (FLT3-WT)) cells and bioluminescence read-out revealed a significant decrease of the tumour burden in MOLM-13 grafted mice upon drug treatment and a statistically significant

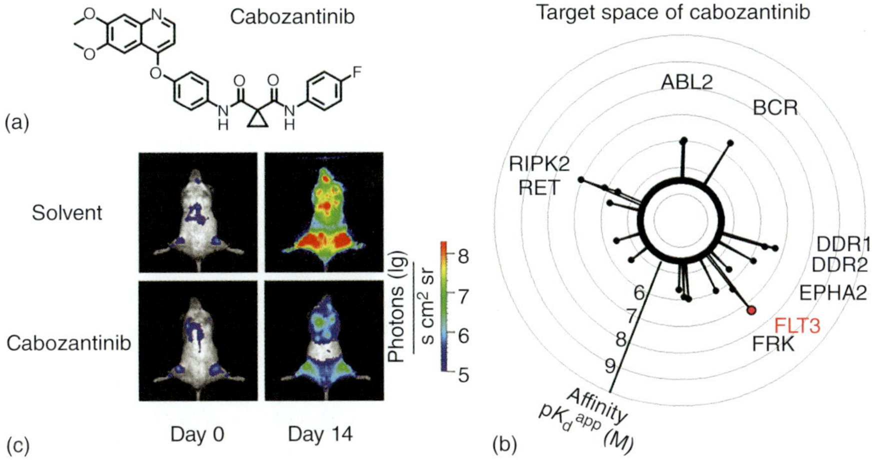

Figure 4.9 Repositioning of cabozantinib for FLT3-positive AML. (a) Chemical structure of cabozantinib. (b) Radar plot representing kinase targets with the corresponding affinities towards cabozantinib, each spike representing the binding affinity (pK_d^{app}) of an individual target protein to cabozantinib. (c) Whole-animal bioluminescence imaging of MOLM-13 (FLT3-ITD) xenografts on days 0 and 14 after treatment with cabozantinib or a vehicle control showing that the tumour burden is reduced after drug treatment (Source: Modified from Klaeger et al. 2017 [20]) AAAS.

positive effect on survival (Figure 4.9c). FLT3-WT xenografts were not affected by cabozantinib treatment and showed no differences in tumour burden compared with the vehicle control. This successful preclinical study [20, 69] illustrates the power of chemical proteomics to identify novel drug repurposing options and to support the initiation of new clinical trials.

4.3.4 Chemoproteomic-Guided Medicinal Chemistry

Chemoproteomic-Guided Drug Discovery: Drug discovery is often performed by traditional structure-based design relying on co-crystal structures of the target protein and the designed inhibitor candidates [70]. Hits identified in high-throughput screening (HTS) campaigns are optimized towards higher target affinity and improved pharmacokinetic properties. Yet, the impact of the desired drug–protein interaction on the selectivity of the novel ligands is often not considered in the early stages. In the past, the selectivity of inhibitor candidates was often only tested for very mature compounds and was not necessarily part of the lead optimization process. Many drugs fail during clinical evaluation, mainly due to insufficient efficacy or toxic side effects, both of which could be prevented by more thorough preclinical evaluation including early selectivity profiling of inhibitor candidates. Using selectivity profiling by chemical proteomics as guidance for the discovery of more selective inhibitors is a novel concept bearing several advantages as compared with the classical drug discovery approach [47, 71, 72]. Chemical proteomics can inform multiple steps of drug discovery including lead discovery, inhibitor design, and lead optimization as well as phenotypic model selection.

Lead Discovery: Recently, we published a comprehensive screen of 243 clinical kinase inhibitors that can facilitate the lead discovery process by identifying novel compound–protein pairs [20, 73]. The wealth of selectivity data generated in this screening effort allows for choosing appropriate lead structures comprising both favourable affinity towards a protein of interest and a favourable selectivity profile. The examined compound set included mature clinical fully developed kinase inhibitors, thus excluding typical drawbacks observed for leads derived from HTS, as, for instance, the detection of pan-assay interference compounds (PAINS [74]) or structures comprising unfavourable ADMET (absorption, distribution, metabolism, excretion, and toxicology) properties.

Lead Optimization: Chemical proteomics can further guide inhibitor design and lead optimization. Early selectivity profiling at the phase of lead optimization facilitates rationalized decisions towards more selective compounds and also allows for the early exclusion of inhibitor candidates that target unfavourable off-targets (e.g. FECH [57], ZAK [75]). At the same time, favourable co-targets (e.g. known resistance drivers) can be identified, ultimately allowing for the development of safe and highly specialized polypharmacological medicines. The coalescence of chemical proteomics and classical structural biology-guided medicinal chemistry can be very powerful and efficient in creating novel inhibitor candidates. One such methodology is a combined approach of selectivity profiling, protein crystallography, and kinase sequence alignment that was used to categorize 'druggable' amino acids according to their potential impact on affinity and selectivity of novel ligands [73]. Interactions with 'key residues' were proven to modulate the target spectra of a drug towards a certain target class, interactions with 'potency residues' were expected to increase affinity only, whereas engagement of 'selectivity residues' could enhance both affinity and selectivity. 'Scaffold residues' may build up hydrophobic pockets that could harbour hydrophobic moieties but do not allow for direct interactions. We have already used this classification to characterize important residues of MELK [20], ABL1, and EPHA2 [73]. In particular, using this approach, we evolved dasatinib into more selective EPHA2 inhibitors by specifically targeting selectivity residues, showing that this novel Kinobeads-bolstered analysis can help medicinal chemists to evaluate and prioritize potential drug–protein interactions in their ligand design.

Phenotypic Model Selection: Evaluation of the phenotypic effect of drug candidates is indispensable during preclinical evaluation. If the drug is not already designed for a particular phenotypic model, information gained from chemical proteomic experiments such as kinome expression profiling data of cell lines [76] and selectivity profiling of drug candidates [20] can help to select an appropriate phenotypic model according to the requirements of the presented inhibitor set. Combining this information enables the selection of a cell line for drug treatment experiments that comprises a kinase profile favourable for the evaluation of the inhibitor candidates – the protein of interest is highly expressed and ideally drives the cell growth, whereas other prominent targets of the inhibitors are rather low abundant, which, owing to the theory of kinase addiction, increases the possibility that the observed cellular effect might be more dependent on inhibition of the protein of interest rather than on other off-targets [71]. On the basis of this rationale, we selected the glioblastoma cell line SF-268 among the NCI60 panel to evaluate our novel EPHA2 inhibitors, since the expression of EPHA2 was high while many off-targets of this inhibitor series were comparatively lowly expressed, such as ABL and most other EPH receptors and SRC family proteins [71].

4.4 Kinobeads, Inhibitors, and Drug Discovery: Where Are We Heading?

4.4.1 What Is a Good Drug?

A change of perspective is required when using small molecule kinase inhibitors: scientists and clinicians need to accept and be fully aware of the fact that most kinase inhibitors are inhibiting more than only one target or target family and that biological systems and drug mode(s) of action interact as a complex interplay of many inhibitory effects [6, 52, 53]. The progress from a single-protein view to a system-wide evaluation could pave the way for better understanding of drug mode of action and an informed targeted application also of promiscuous inhibitors. Facing the reality of multicomponent phenotypes and the hurdles to create selective compounds, the question arises whether we really need single-target compounds [52]. The merit of highly selective compounds is under debate in the scientific community and needs to be discussed from several angles. Looking at clinical inhibitors that are already used in humans for targeted therapy, polypharmacology does not seem to be a major issue [53]. Many approved kinase drugs for oncology indications (e.g. dasatinib, midostaurin, brigatinib) have a very broad target profile inhibiting numerous kinases across the whole kinome. Modern clinical research is more and more evolving the idea of precision medicine [77, 78]. The basis for this approach is the understanding that a tumour is rather characterized by its molecular composition than by the cellular entity it emerged from. In precision medicine, the disease-driving molecular background of each patient is characterized to enable molecular tumour boards to suggest appropriate treatment options. This approach could indeed profit from highly selective compounds or combinations thereof that specifically target the pathogenic condition the individual patient suffers from [10] and allow for fine-tuned individualized therapy [53]. It is still a long way until precision medicine may evolve to be the standard of care; but if we succeed in providing adequate diagnostic tools and therapies, the usage of selective targeted therapies could be the future of clinical healthcare. From a scientific point of view, highly selective compounds provide the great opportunity to be used as chemical probes in target validation studies [10, 79] (see Chapter 1 for more details), thus offering a complementary approach to genetic methods such as RNAi or CRISPR/Cas [53] (see Chapter 9 for more details). Pharmaceutical inhibition has the advantage of being reversible and temporally controllable and interfering less with the overall cellular protein expression than the typically used genetic approaches. The choice and appropriate application of a chemical probe is difficult as it requires a thorough understanding of the molecule, its selectivity, and its mode of action [79, 80]. Unfortunately, many compounds are used as chemical probes in the scientific literature that are not suitable *per se* or not applied in an appropriate concentration, which could lead to false hypotheses. Highly selective molecules are valuable, but the development of truly selective inhibitors for each and every kinase is tedious. Considering the efforts that have been undertaken by experienced scientists in the past decades [81, 82], the question remains whether it is even feasible to reach this goal.

4.4.2 How Can We Discover New Drugs in the Future?

Traditional drug discovery efforts often follow a reverse pharmacology approach, where a protein of interest is selected and lead structures for targeting this protein are identified in a screen and further optimized during drug development [5–7]. Another even more historical approach, forward pharmacology, relies on phenotypic screening where compounds are tested for a particular biological response without prior knowledge of the molecular target. Nowadays, this approach is gaining significant interest again [83], mainly because many drugs generated in the reverse approach fail in clinical trials due to insufficient efficacy and because better target deconvolution strategies have been developed [84] along with significant advances in more complex and human-relevant assay systems, bioinformatics platforms, and associated technology (see Chapters 7, 10, and 11 for details). Combining phenotypic screening, chemical proteomics, and bioinformatics has the potential to revolutionize the way of designing new ligands in the future. A possible scenario could be to start from a cellular phenotype of interest and screen compounds for their phenotypic effect [85]. Optimally, these inhibitors are well profiled by chemical proteomics, such as the Kinobeads technology, and comprise target profiles that cover different target families with slight overlaps. A computational approach can then be envisaged to attribute the observed effect size of the inhibitor treatment to their target profiles and identify which protein targets are responsible for the observed effect. This analysis allows for characterization of the molecular contributors to the observed phenotype but also enables the rational selection of appropriate molecules to interrogate a certain phenotype instead of single proteins. It could even be useful to predict the phenotypic effect a compound may have according to its target profile. One such combination approach was developed by Gujral et al. [85] and was already tested successfully in-house in order to evaluate the anti-inflammatory effect of SIK2 inhibitors (identified by a Kinobeads drug screen) in an inflammatory background [20].

4.4.3 The Yin and Yang of Chemoproteomic-Guided Drug Discovery

The combination of multidisciplinary chemical biology and traditional medicinal chemistry is emerging and provides the opportunity to trigger advances in both disciplines, biology and chemistry [86]. Breaking down the boundaries between these traditional disciplines will generate new tools to interrogate biological function and to investigate the influence of drug treatment on the cellular level. Optimally, the interplay between chemical proteomics and medicinal chemistry functions as a yin and yang mechanism, where chemical biology facilitates the identification of novel molecular targets and lead structures and medicinal chemistry helps to create better compounds for further investigation or treatment.

Acknowledgments

The authors want to thank colleagues that contributed to the development and characterization of the Kinobeads technology, especially F. Pachl, D. Helm, X. Ku, B. Ruprecht, and J. Zecha, as well as A. Hubauer, M. Krötz-Fahning, and A. Klaus for technical assistance.

References

1 Manning, G., Whyte, D.B., Martinez, R. et al. (2002). The protein kinase complement of the human genome. *Science (New York, N.Y.)* 298: 1912–1934.
2 Hunter, T. (2012). Why nature chose phosphate to modify proteins. *Philos. Trans. R. Soc. London, Ser. B* 367: 2513–2516.
3 Fischer, E.H. (2013). Cellular regulation by protein phosphorylation. *Biochem. Biophys. Res. Commun.* 430: 865–867.
4 Blume-Jensen, P. and Hunter, T. (2001). Oncogenic kinase signalling. *Nature* 411: 355–365.
5 Radford, I.R. (2002). Imatinib. Novartis. *Curr. Opin. Investig. Drugs (London, England)* 3: 492–499.
6 Heinzlmeir, S. (2017). When chemical proteomics meets medicinal chemistry: Guided drug discovery towards EPHA2 inhibitors. Ph.D. Thesis, *Retrieved from mediaTUM Universitätsbibliothek Technische Universität München (urn:nbn:de:bvb:91-diss-20171215-1380642-1-5).*
7 Kornev, A.P., Haste, N.M., Taylor, S.S., and Eyck, L.F. (2006). Surface comparison of active and inactive protein kinases identifies a conserved activation mechanism. *Proc. Natl. Acad. Sci. U.S.A.* 103: 17783–17788.
8 Taylor, S.S. and Kornev, A.P. (2011). Protein kinases: evolution of dynamic regulatory proteins. *Trends Biochem. Sci* 36: 65–77.
9 Roskoski, R. Jr., (2016). Classification of small molecule protein kinase inhibitors based upon the structures of their drug-enzyme complexes. *Pharmacol. Res.* 103: 26–48.
10 Muller, S., Chaikuad, A., Gray, N.S., and Knapp, S. (2015). The ins and outs of selective kinase inhibitor development. *Nat. Chem. Biol.* 11: 818–821.
11 Reddy, A.S. and Zhang, S. (2013). Polypharmacology: drug discovery for the future. *Exp. Rev. Clin. Pharmacol.* 6: 41–47.
12 Wentsch, H.K., Walter, N.M., Buhrmann, M. et al. (2017). Optimized target residence time: type I1/2 inhibitors for p38alpha MAP kinase with improved binding kinetics through direct interaction with the R-spine. *Angew. Chem.* (International ed. in English) 56: 5363–5367.

13 Sutherland, J.J., Gao, C., Cahya, S., and Vieth, M. (2013). What general conclusions can we draw from kinase profiling data sets? *Biochim. Biophys. Acta* 1834: 1425–1433.
14 Uitdehaag, J.C. and Zaman, G.J. (2011). A theoretical entropy score as a single value to express inhibitor selectivity. *BMC Bioinf.* 12: 94.
15 Uitdehaag, J.C., Verkaar, F., Alwan, H. et al. (2012). A guide to picking the most selective kinase inhibitor tool compounds for pharmacological validation of drug targets. *Br. J. Pharmacol.* 166: 858–876.
16 Davis, M.I., Hunt, J.P., Herrgard, S. et al. (2011). Comprehensive analysis of kinase inhibitor selectivity. *Nat. Biotechnol.* 29: 1046–1051.
17 Karaman, M.W., Herrgard, S., Treiber, D.K. et al. (2008). A quantitative analysis of kinase inhibitor selectivity. *Nat. Biotechnol.* 26: 127–132.
18 Graczyk, P.P. (2007). Gini coefficient: a new way to express selectivity of kinase inhibitors against a family of kinases. *J. Med. Chem.* 50: 5773–5779.
19 Cheng, A.C., Eksterowicz, J., Geuns-Meyer, S., and Sun, Y. (2010). Analysis of kinase inhibitor selectivity using a thermodynamics-based partition index. *J. Med. Chem.* 53: 4502–4510.
20 Klaeger, S., Heinzlmeir, S., Wilhelm, M. et al. (2017). *The target landscape of clinical kinase drugs. Science*, 358. New York: N.Y.
21 Bantscheff, M., Eberhard, D., Abraham, Y. et al. (2007). Quantitative chemical proteomics reveals mechanisms of action of clinical ABL kinase inhibitors. *Nat. Biotechnol.* 25: 1035–1044.
22 Médard, G., Pachl, F., Ruprecht, B. et al. (2015). Optimized chemical proteomics assay for kinase inhibitor profiling. *J. Proteome Res.* 14: 1574–1586.
23 Ruprecht, B., Zecha, J., Heinzlmeir, S. et al. (2015). Evaluation of kinase activity profiling using chemical proteomics. *ACS Chem. Biol.* 10: 2743–2752.
24 Stuhlmiller, T.J., Miller, S.M., Zawistowski, J.S. et al. (2015). Inhibition of lapatinib-induced kinome reprogramming in ERBB2-positive breast cancer by targeting BET family bromodomains. *Cell Rep.* 11: 390–404.
25 Stuhlmiller, T.J., Earp, H.S., and Johnson, G.L. (2014). Adaptive reprogramming of the breast cancer kinome. *Clin. Pharmacol. Therap.* 95: 413–415.
26 Daub, H. (2015). Quantitative proteomics of kinase inhibitor targets and mechanisms. *ACS Chem. Biol.* 10: 201–212.
27 Rix, U. and Superti-Furga, G. (2008). Target profiling of small molecules by chemical proteomics. *Nat. Chem. Biol.* 5: 616.
28 Bantscheff, M., Scholten, A., and Heck, A.J. (2009). Revealing promiscuous drug-target interactions by chemical proteomics. *Drug Discovery Today* 14: 1021–1029.
29 Duncan, J.S., Whittle, M.C., Nakamura, K. et al. (2012). Dynamic reprogramming of the kinome in response to targeted MEK inhibition in triple-negative breast cancer. *Cell* 149: 307–321.
30 Schirle, M., Bantscheff, M., and Kuster, B. (2012). Mass spectrometry-based proteomics in preclinical drug discovery. *Chem. Biol.* 19: 72–84.
31 Patricelli, M.P., Szardenings, A.K., Liyanage, M. et al. (2007). Functional interrogation of the kinome using nucleotide acyl phosphates. *Biochemistry* 46: 350–358.

32 Lemeer, S., Zorgiebel, C., Ruprecht, B. et al. (2013). Comparing immobilized kinase inhibitors and covalent ATP probes for proteomic profiling of kinase expression and drug selectivity. *J. Proteome Res.* 12: 1723–1731.

33 Rudolf, A.F., Skovgaard, T., Knapp, S. et al. (2014). A comparison of protein kinases inhibitor screening methods using both enzymatic activity and binding affinity determination. *PLoS One* 9: e98800.

34 Vasta, J.D., Corona, C.R., Wilkinson, J. et al. (2018). Quantitative, wide-spectrum kinase profiling in live cells for assessing the effect of cellular ATP on target engagement. *Cell Chem. Biol.* 25: 206–214.e11.

35 Becher, I., Dittmann, A., Savitski, M.M. et al. (2014). Chemoproteomics reveals time-dependent binding of histone deacetylase inhibitors to endogenous repressor complexes. *ACS Chem. Biol.* 9: 1736–1746.

36 Sharma, K., Weber, C., Bairlein, M. et al. (2009). Proteomics strategy for quantitative protein interaction profiling in cell extracts. *Nat. Methods* 6: 741–744.

37 Cox, J. and Mann, M. (2008). MaxQuant enables high peptide identification rates, individualized p.p.b.-range mass accuracies and proteome-wide protein quantification. *Nat. Biotechnol.* 26: 1367–1372.

38 Reinecke, M., Ruprecht, B., Poser, S. et al. (2019). Chemoproteomic selectivity profiling of PIKK and PI3K kinase inhibitors. *ACS Chemical Biology* 14: 655–664.

39 Hahne, H., Pachl, F., Ruprecht, B. et al. (2013). DMSO enhances electrospray response, boosting sensitivity of proteomic experiments. *Nat. Methods* 10: 989–991.

40 Cox, J., Neuhauser, N., Michalski, A. et al. (2011). Andromeda: a peptide search engine integrated into the MaxQuant environment. *J. Proteome Res.* 10: 1794–1805.

41 Ku, X., Heinzlmeir, S., Liu, X. et al. (2014). A new chemical probe for quantitative proteomic profiling of fibroblast growth factor receptor and its inhibitors. *J. Proteomics* 96: 44–55.

42 Ku, X., Heinzlmeir, S., Helm, D. et al. (2014). New affinity probe targeting VEGF receptors for kinase inhibitor selectivity profiling by chemical proteomics. *J. Proteome Res.* 13: 2445–2452.

43 Hofener, M., Pachl, F., Kuster, B., and Sewald, N. (2015). Inhibitor-based affinity probes for the investigation of JAK signaling pathways. *Proteomics* 15: 3066–3074.

44 Pachl, F., Plattner, P., Ruprecht, B. et al. (2013). Characterization of a chemical affinity probe targeting Akt kinases. *J. Proteome Res.* 12: 3792–3800.

45 Heerding, D.A., Rhodes, N., Leber, J.D. et al. (2008). Identification of 4-(2-(4-amino-1,2,5-oxadiazol-3-yl)-1-ethyl-7-{[(3S)-3-piperidinylmethyl]oxy}-1H-imidazo[4,5-c]pyridin-4-yl)-2-methyl-3-butyn-2-ol (GSK690693), a novel inhibitor of AKT kinase. *J. Med. Chem.* 51: 5663–5679.

46 Andrade, L.F., Nahum, L.A., Avelar, L.G. et al. (2011). Eukaryotic protein kinases (ePKs) of the helminth parasite Schistosoma mansoni. *BMC Genom.* 12: 215.

47 Golkowski, M., Perera, G.K., Vidadala, V.N. et al. (2018). Kinome chemoproteomics characterization of pyrrolo[3,4-c]pyrazoles as potent and selective inhibitors of glycogen synthase kinase 3. *Mol. Omics* 14: 26–36.

48 Paquet, T., Le Manach, C., Cabrera, D.G. et al. (2017). Antimalarial efficacy of MMV390048, an inhibitor of Plasmodium phosphatidylinositol 4-kinase. *Sci. Transl. Med.* 9: eaad9735.

49 Brunschwig, C., Lawrence, N., Taylor, D. et al. (2018). UCT943, a next-generation plasmodium falciparum PI4K inhibitor preclinical candidate for the treatment of malaria. *Antimicrob. Agents Chemother.* 62 (9): e00012–e00018.

50 Koch, H., Busto, M.E., Kramer, K. et al. (2015). Chemical proteomics uncovers EPHA2 as a mechanism of acquired resistance to small molecule EGFR kinase inhibition. *J. Proteome Res.* 14: 2617–2625.

51 Amato, K.R., Wang, S., Tan, L. et al. (2016). EPHA2 blockade overcomes acquired resistance to EGFR kinase inhibitors in lung cancer. *Cancer Res.* 76 (2): 305–318.

52 Metz, J.T. and Hajduk, P.J. (2010). Rational approaches to targeted polypharmacology: creating and navigating protein-ligand interaction networks. *Curr. Opin. Chem. Biol.* 14: 498–504.

53 Knight, Z.A., Lin, H., and Shokat, K.M. (2010). Targeting the cancer kinome through polypharmacology. *Nat. Rev. Cancer* 10: 130–137.

54 Anighoro, A., Bajorath, J., and Rastelli, G. (2014). Polypharmacology: challenges and opportunities in drug discovery. *J. Med. Chem.* 57: 7874–7887.

55 Munoz, L. (2017). Non-kinase targets of protein kinase inhibitors. *Nat. Rev. Drug Discovery* 16: 424–440.

56 Kaiser, A., Nishi, K., Gorin, F.A. et al. (2001). The cyclin-dependent kinase (CDK) inhibitor flavopiridol inhibits glycogen phosphorylase. *Arch. Biochem. Biophys.* 386: 179–187.

57 Klaeger, S., Gohlke, B., Perrin, J. et al. (2016). Chemical proteomics reveals ferrochelatase as a common off-target of kinase inhibitors. *ACS Chem. Biol.* 11: 1245–1254.

58 Metz, J.T., Johnson, E.F., Soni, N.B. et al. (2011). Navigating the kinome. *Nat. Chem. Biol.* 7: 200–202.

59 Anastassiadis, T., Deacon, S.W., Devarajan, K. et al. (2011). Comprehensive assay of kinase catalytic activity reveals features of kinase inhibitor selectivity. *Nat. Biotechnol.* 29: 1039–1045.

60 Goto, H., Izawa, I., Li, P., and Inagaki, M. (2012). Novel regulation of checkpoint kinase 1: Is checkpoint kinase 1 a good candidate for anti-cancer therapy? *Cancer Sci.* 103: 1195–1200.

61 Singh, J., Petter, R.C., Baillie, T.A., and Whitty, A. (2011). The resurgence of covalent drugs. *Nat. Rev. Drug Discovery* 10: 307.

62 Liu, Q., Sabnis, Y., Zhao, Z. et al. (2013). Developing irreversible inhibitors of the protein kinase cysteinome. *Chem. Biol.* 20: 146–159.

63 Dittus, L., Werner, T., Muelbaier, M., and Bantscheff, M. (2017). Differential kinobeads profiling for target identification of irreversible kinase inhibitors. *ACS Chem. Biol.* 12: 2515–2521.

64 Edwards, A.M., Isserlin, R., Bader, G.D. et al. (2011). Too many roads not taken. *Nature* 470: 163.
65 Buchdunger, E., Cioffi, C.L., Law, N. et al. (2000). Abl protein-tyrosine kinase inhibitor STI571 inhibits in vitro signal transduction mediated by c-kit and platelet-derived growth factor receptors. *J. Pharmacol. Exp. Therap.* 295: 139–145.
66 Yakes, F.M., Chen, J., Tan, J. et al. (2011). Cabozantinib (XL184), a novel MET and VEGFR2 inhibitor, simultaneously suppresses metastasis, angiogenesis, and tumor growth. *Mol. Cancer Therap.* 10: 2298–2308.
67 Kurzrock, R., Sherman, S.I., Ball, D.W. et al. (2011). Activity of XL184 (Cabozantinib), an oral tyrosine kinase inhibitor, in patients with medullary thyroid cancer. *J. Clin. Oncol.* 29: 2660–2666.
68 Levis, M. and Small, D. (2003). FLT3: ITDoes matter in leukemia. *Leukemia* 17: 1738–1752.
69 Lu, J.W., Wang, A.N., Liao, H.A. et al. (2016). Cabozantinib is selectively cytotoxic in acute myeloid leukemia cells with FLT3-internal tandem duplication (FLT3-ITD). *Cancer Lett.* 376: 218–225.
70 Kuhn, P., Wilson, K., Patch, M.G., and Stevens, R.C. (2002). The genesis of high-throughput structure-based drug discovery using protein crystallography. *Curr. Opin. Chem. Biol.* 6: 704–710.
71 Heinzlmeir, S., Lohse, J., Treiber, T. et al. (2017). Chemoproteomics-aided medicinal chemistry for the discovery of EPHA2 inhibitors. *ChemMedChem* 12: 999–1011.
72 Golkowski, M., Vidadala, R.S., Lombard, C.K. et al. (2017). Kinobead and single-shot LC-MS profiling identifies selective PKD inhibitors. *J. Proteome Res.* 16: 1216–1227.
73 Heinzlmeir, S., Kudlinzki, D., Sreeramulu, S. et al. (2016). Chemical proteomics and structural biology define EPHA2 inhibition by clinical kinase drugs. *ACS Chem. Biol.* 11: 3400–3411.
74 Pouliot, M. and Jeanmart, S. (2016). Pan assay interference compounds (PAINS) and other promiscuous compounds in antifungal research. *J. Med. Chem.* 59: 497–503.
75 Vin, H., Ching, G., Ojeda, S.S. et al. (2014). Sorafenib suppresses JNK-dependent apoptosis through inhibition of ZAK. *Mol. Cancer Therap.* 13: 221–229.
76 Frejno, M., Zenezini Chiozzi, R., Wilhelm, M. et al. (2017). Pharmacoproteomic characterisation of human colon and rectal cancer. *Mol. Syst. Biol.* 13: 951.
77 Jameson, J.L. and Longo, D.L. (2015). Precision medicine – personalized, problematic, and promising. *New Engl. J. Med.* 372: 2229–2234.
78 Hollingsworth, S.J. (2015). Precision medicine in oncology drug development: a pharma perspective. *Drug Discovery Today* 20: 1455–1463.
79 Arrowsmith, C.H., Audia, J.E., Austin, C. et al. (2015). The promise and peril of chemical probes. *Nat. Chem. Biol.* 11: 536–541.
80 Blagg, J. and Workman, P. (2017). Choose and use your chemical probe wisely to explore cancer biology. *Cancer Cell* 32: 9–25.

81 Li, B., Liu, Y., Uno, T., and Gray, N. (2004). Creating chemical diversity to target protein kinases. *Comb. Chem. High Throughput Screening* 7: 453–472.

82 Fedorov, O., Sundstrom, M., Marsden, B., and Knapp, S. (2007). Insights for the development of specific kinase inhibitors by targeted structural genomics. *Drug Discovery Today* 12: 365–372.

83 Zheng, W., Thorne, N., and McKew, J.C. (2013). Phenotypic screens as a renewed approach for drug discovery. *Drug Discovery Today* 18: 1067–1073.

84 Lee, J. and Bogyo, M. (2013). Target deconvolution techniques in modern phenotypic profiling. *Curr. Opin. Chem. Biol.* 17: 118–126.

85 Gujral, T.S., Peshkin, L., and Kirschner, M.W. (2014). Exploiting polypharmacology for drug target deconvolution. *Proc. Natl. Acad. Sci. U.S.A.* 111: 5048–5053.

86 Plowright, A.T., Ottmann, C., Arkin, M. et al. (2017). Joining forces: the chemical biology-medicinal chemistry continuum. *Cell Chem. Biol.* 24: 1058.

5

Label-Free Techniques for Target Discovery and Validation

Daniel Martinez Molina and Michael Dabrowski

Pelago Bioscience AB, Banvaktsvägen 20, Solna, 17148, Sweden

5.1 Introduction

To validate a therapeutic hypothesis, it is necessary for the intended drug to reach the intended site of action in the patient and deliver the intended outcome. This proof of concept is normally reached in phase II clinical trials. However, recent studies show a decreasing trend in success rates, with the predominant cause of failure being a lack of efficacy [1]. It is generally accepted that a majority of efficacy failures are attributable to insufficient target engagement (TE). As a consequence, considerable efforts are being made to identify and validate therapeutic targets in terms of disease relevance and to quantify TE of the hits, leads, and candidate drugs.

In this chapter, we limit the discussion of label-free techniques to methods that do not require modification or addition of the analyte, substrate, or binding partner, i.e. methods that do not require a reporter or externally added 'marker' to monitor the system. Examples of such markers are tags or probes on the protein studied (His, biotin, nonnatural amino acids) or labelling of the molecule studied (radioactive, heavy atoms [mass], fluorophores [optics]). The term label-free is, however, most frequently associated with biophysical methods that utilize biophysical characteristics such as charge, size, structure, and denaturation temperature to monitor the system studied. The advantage of label-free methods is that they yield detailed data on the molecular interactions between binding partners or molecules studied in drug discovery and development.

It is this characteristic of accurate reporting on the molecular interactions in a native, unperturbed system that makes label-free techniques particularly attractive and useful in drug discovery. In recent decades, label-free techniques have replaced an increasing number of traditional labelled formats throughout the drug discovery value chain, from target identification to clinical development. In this chapter, we will focus on the use and utility of such assays in the preclinical target discovery and validation phases, with an emphasis on a technique called the cellular thermal shift assay (CETSA). Due to the versatility and multiple readout formats of label-free methods in general and the platform of CETSA

Target Discovery and Validation: Methods and Strategies for Drug Discovery,
First Edition. Edited by Alleyn T. Plowright.

in particular, we will also investigate the scope of applications beyond the first target validation experiments.

In our definition of label-free methods, surface plasmon resonance (SPR) and CETSA using tagged proteins are not true label-free techniques. However, because of the widespread use of SPR in drug discovery and the similarity of phenomena studied in CETSA and its versions using tagged proteins, we include these techniques in the comparison.

5.2 CETSA: How It All Began

The CETSA method was invented in the academic group of Professor Pär Nordlund at Karolinska Institutet in Sweden. Prior to CETSA, the Nordlund group was among the international leaders in X-ray crystallographic structural studies of proteins. The group placed a heavy focus on proteins involved in nucleotide metabolism, but they were also early adopters of high-throughput (HT) target cloning and developers of techniques for screening protein expression levels and solubility. The cloning and screening pipeline contained very diverse protein families with little in common with regard to natural ligands. Therefore, the Nordlund laboratory recognized early the need for biophysical measurements that proved the binding of specific compounds or ligands to the studied protein, rather than setting up protein-specific functional assays for each cloned target. Such methods did not just prove the binding of a compound to the target protein; they also helped reveal, for example, which buffers and additives would have a favourable effect on the crystal-forming properties of the proteins [2, 3]. One of the key factors to understanding crystallizability was attributed to protein solubility, which can be rapidly assessed by monitoring the thermostability of a protein.

The laboratory had access to instrumentation for high-throughput dynamic light scattering (StarGazer), which allowed rapid stability measures. Together with the Thermofluor technique, a purified protein could be screened against libraries of potential ligands as well as put through large two-dimensional screens of buffers, pH, salts, and additives to understand which parameters affected protein stability the most. In both StarGazer and Thermofluor, heat is applied to the purified protein solution, causing the protein to denature and subsequently precipitate in a protein-specific manner. In Thermofluor, the unfolding process can be monitored using a hydrophobic probe. This probe is quenched by water, and only when the protein unfolds, revealing its hydrophobic surfaces, does it fluoresce. StarGazer, based on dynamic light scattering, monitors how the sample is occluded as a function of increasing heat and subsequent precipitation.

In parallel, the group worked with method development with the aim of screening large construct libraries for solubility. The employed screens were performed by means of filtering out insoluble protein aggregates such as inclusion bodies, where the soluble protein fraction could be captured and quantitated directly from the overexpression cellular system. It was during this time, while observing both how small molecules could shift the stability of a particular isolated protein and how the solubility of a tailored protein construct could also be monitored while overexpressed in a complex environment such as the cell, that Professor Nordlund connected these observations and suggested the first experiments that laid the ground for CETSA. The hypothesis was that proteins inside the cell would denature and precipitate in a protein-specific manner as a consequence to an applied heat pulse. The experimental outline was simple: heat a cell slurry or lysate to a range of temperatures and then separate precipitated proteins from soluble proteins by centrifugation (or filtration). The precipitated proteins could be recovered from the pellet and the soluble proteins from the supernatant. With increasing temperature, the amount of protein in the pellet would increase, and the amount of protein in the supernatant would decrease. Using specific antibodies, it would be possible to study specific proteins without the need of any tags. With the addition of a compound that bound the protein of interest, the melting temperature would shift, resulting in more soluble protein being present at higher temperatures than in the control sample.

The first experiments were conducted on overexpressed proteins in *Escherichia coli*, but as soon as the proof-of-principle experiments had been completed, the work turned to mammalian cells grown as cell lines in flasks or extracted from tissues. In the process of developing the method, the inventor also recognized the impact of being able to quantify interactions in live cells in a label-free manner, both to study cellular events and to be applied in drug discovery to prove and quantify TE. This realization and the fact that the method was novel lead to a patent application [4], which was first granted in the United Kingdom in 2013.

In the subsequent pioneering proof-of-concept paper, which was published in *Science* [5], we set out to explain the principle behind the method. The use of western blots was perfect to illustrate the method. Specific antibodies showed that the correct molecular weight was identified, and the disappearance of the protein band as a function of increasing temperature was very illustrative. The paper showed how the addition of certain ligands could shift the stability of the studied proteins, all clinically relevant targets, in a dose-dependent manner in both the intact cell and the lysate. The ligands were chosen to highlight specific events in the cell (such as drug transport and activation), how certain molecules could be selective and bind to one class of proteins but not the other, and how drugs at different stages of development had different abilities to engage with the target protein. With this publication, the CETSA method was introduced as a label-free method to study TE in the physiologically relevant environment of an intact cell (Figure 5.1).

The general outline of a CETSA experiment can be summarized in four key steps, namely, treat, heat, separate, and detect, and this combination is the backbone of the CETSA formats covered below. This chapter is not intended to give a detailed outline of the CETSA protocol, which has been covered elsewhere [6, 7]. However, it is important to understand that the combination and possible variations of the key steps of the method allow it to be carried out in many different ways. For example, either the sample can be treated at a fixed dose to give a qualitative TE indication, or the concentration of the compound can be altered to yield quantitative concentration–response curves, the so-called isothermal dose–response fingerprints (ITDRFs).

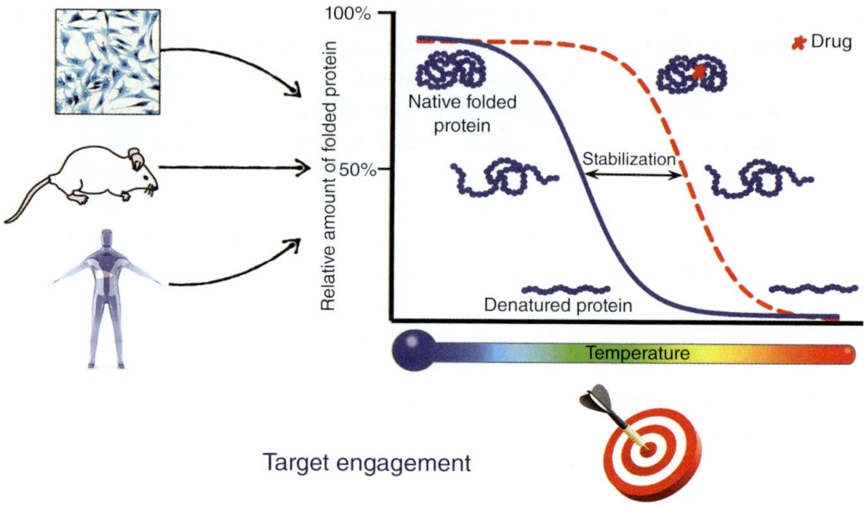

Figure 5.1 The cellular thermal shift assay (CETSA) principle. As in traditional TSAs, the amount of soluble protein in a solution decreases when heated to increasing temperatures. This melting behaviour can be shifted by addition of a protein ligand. With CETSA, the protein solution can be made up of unpurified protein from all protein containing sample sources without the need for any protein labels or modification to the ligand.

The sample matrix should comprise cells from any species that best represents the biology of interest or offers the best model system. It can be derived from cell cultures, plants, or tissues from any source. One important, sometimes limiting, factor is that the cells used in the experiment need to be aliquoted to carry out the experiment. With solid tissue, this either involves physical separation of the cells by enzymatic treatment, lysate preparation, or the cutting of tissue into equally sized pieces, with the latter being the most challenging in practice.

The heating device and the technique used to separate soluble from precipitated protein can be adjusted to fit the experimental needs and instrumentation of the laboratory.

The heating step is the first and only perturbation to the system in the CETSA protocol and is carried out just prior to the final detection step. Hence, the heating step needs to be highly controlled and, preferably, as brief as possible, to allow a distinction between the stability of protein in the treated and control samples.

It is worth noting that quantitative results from concentration–response curves (ITDRF) generated at fixed temperatures are apparent and will be dependent on a number of factors, for example, the cell line used (biological context of the target), the buffer, or heating time. It is therefore also important to be consistent when handling the samples after the heating step. The absolute temperature also affects the obtained values, where a higher temperature typically requires more compound to saturate and stabilize the target protein fully, giving a lower apparent TE potency.

Finally, the protein detection setup will be of major importance. Because the CETSA method is protein centric, in principle, any method that enables the quantification of a soluble (or aggregated) protein can be used.

To date, three main formats have been established and will be explained in greater detail in the next section. Apart from the classical CETSA experiment, using a western blot readout, more advanced formats based on mass spectrometric analysis have become highly valuable since it gives information on key events in the cell at the proteome level in an unbiased manner. The third format, known as CETSA HT, allows high-throughput generation of many data points, enabling, for example, the screening of compound libraries for cellular TE. In CETSA HT, dual antibody detection (preferably with antibodies that recognize only the native folded protein) simplifies and reduces the protocol since the separation step often does not require centrifugation or filtration – this distinction between soluble and precipitated protein is made by the antibodies.

Regardless of the instrumentation and detection setup, an experiment can be carried out in intact cells or lysates. If the cells are lysed prior to the heating step, the method is more similar to a traditional thermal shift assay (TSA), albeit a lysate-based CETSA still takes place in a much more complex solution containing the native proteins and ligands.

There are several important differences between conducting an experiment in an intact cell or lysate format. In short, in the intact cell setting, biology is still 'switched on', and a lipid membrane shields the cellular content. If a stability shift is observed in targeted CETSA, it is because the compound has passed the lipid bilayer, resisted cellular breakdown, been activated (if necessary), and finally found its way to the target protein at a high enough concentration to affect the melt curve of that protein population. In the lysate experiment, only very few biological pathways are likely to be active, target-protein complexes and chaperones may not be intact in such a diluted environment, and importantly, there is no cell membrane to shield the cellular contents from the surroundings.

In the early days of CETSA development, the difference between intact cell and lysate experiments could be used to study, for example, active transport into or out of the cell. With western blots, such experiments were carried out in a target-by-target approach. The first indication we got that CETSA could also be used to monitor pathways and signalling events was while studying how the addition of cyclic AMP (cAMP) affected protein kinase A (PKA) (Figure 5.2).

PKA is present as a dimer of dimers (two regulatory subunits and two catalytic subunits) in the cell, and when this tetramer is intact, it also melts in unison, i.e. all subunits show the same melting behaviour. This was the first time we realized that complexes of different proteins are often denatured in a concerted manner. When cAMP levels rise in the cell, for example, by G-protein coupled receptor (GPCR)-triggered signalling, cAMP molecules bind to the regulatory subunits of PKA, leading to structural rearrangements that cause the tetramer to dissociate. The catalytic subunits are now free to phosphorylate target proteins in the cell. With targeted antibody-based CETSA, we could follow how cAMP binding stabilized the regulatory subunits, while the subsequent dissociation caused the catalytic subunits to become destabilized. Using mass spectrometry (MS)-based detection however, no prior knowledge is needed to design a similar experiment for other proteins and complexes, since the readout is unbiased and reports on actual events among thousands of proteins in the cell.

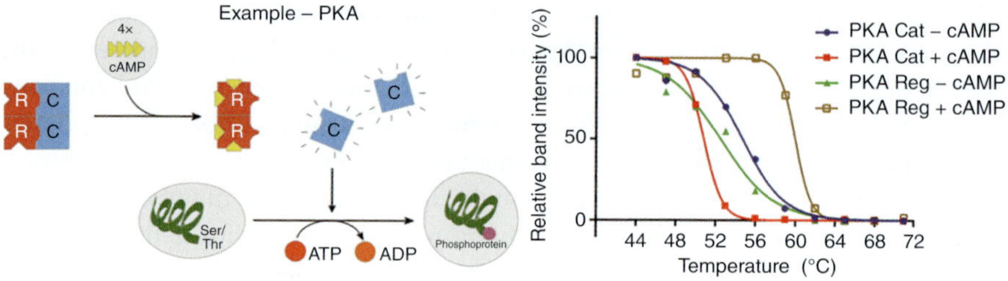

Figure 5.2 Protein kinase A activation occurs as a response to increased levels of cAMP in the cell. The holoenzyme is composed of two regulatory and two catalytic subunits. Each regulatory subunit (red) can bind two cAMP molecules. This causes a conformational change that results in a dissociation and activation of the catalytic subunits (light blue). The catalytic subunits have many substrates (green) for their kinase activity, leading to different cellular effects, depending on cell type and target availability. Right panel: in its inactive tetrameric form, the regulatory and catalytic subunits have similar melting profiles (triangles and dots, respectively); however cAMP addition causes a net stabilization of the regulatory subunit (open squares) and the catalytic subunits to become destabilized (squares).

We published the PKA finding together with several other important examples of how CETSA MS can be used [8], not only to look at the target of interest but also to understand pathway effects caused by the binding of a ligand to signalling proteins. The implications of these experiments also resulted in another patent application [9] on the use of CETSA to identify and validate biomarkers in the cell as well as more detailed reports on coprecipitation of cellular protein complexes [10].

5.3 The CETSA Formats

5.3.1 CETSA Classics

In the original CETSA format, also called a 'CETSA Classics' experiment, the final protein detection is accomplished using western blots (Figures 5.3 and 5.4).

Despite the simple detection setup, this format allows the analysis of very complex experiments and is readily performed in different sample matrices, allowing a seamless translation of results. Since the publication of the proof-of-concept paper in 2013, the number of yearly references has increased steadily, and at the time of this writing, approximately 200 reports have been published where CETSA data have been generated to prove TE. A large majority of these publications utilize the CETSA Classics approach, primarily in a quantitative setting, not looking at dose-dependent stabilization using ITDRFs.

Researchers have realized the general applicability of CETSA, although the proof-of-concept paper reported mainly on proteins targeted by anticancer drugs. The studies by these early adopters strengthens the notion that CETSA is a versatile method, as it has been applied to many different target families and cell matrices. In a vast majority of the reports, human immortalized cell lines have been used, but there are also examples of studies performed in plant cells, human brain tissue, bacterial cells, and yeasts.

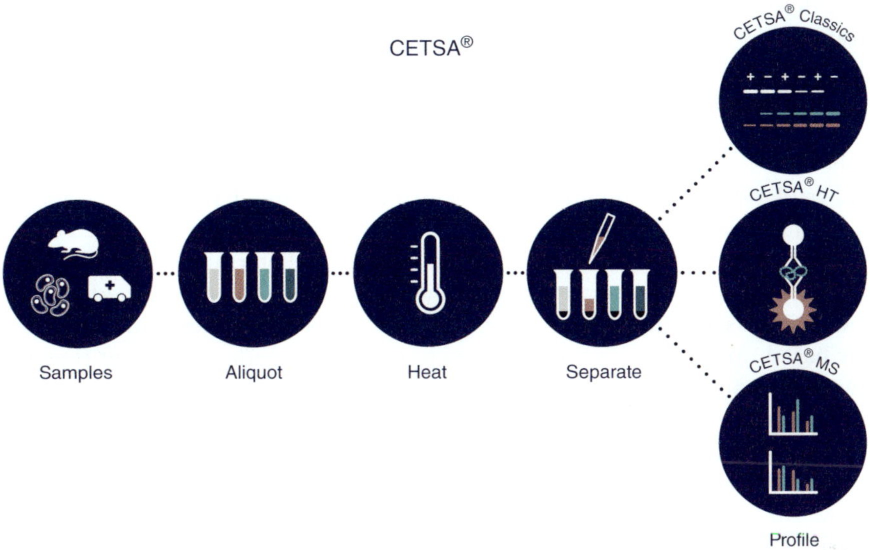

Figure 5.3 The CETSA workflow. The three main CETSA assay formats all share the same assay principle. The samples are treated (and aliquoted), heated to a specific temperature or range of temperatures followed by separation of the soluble from insoluble protein. In the final step, the remaining soluble protein amount is quantified. CETSA Classics and CETSA HT are based on antibody detection, either in western blot format or using (homogeneous) ELISA systems. The use of mass spectrometry-based detection allows proteome-wide studies of ligand effects.

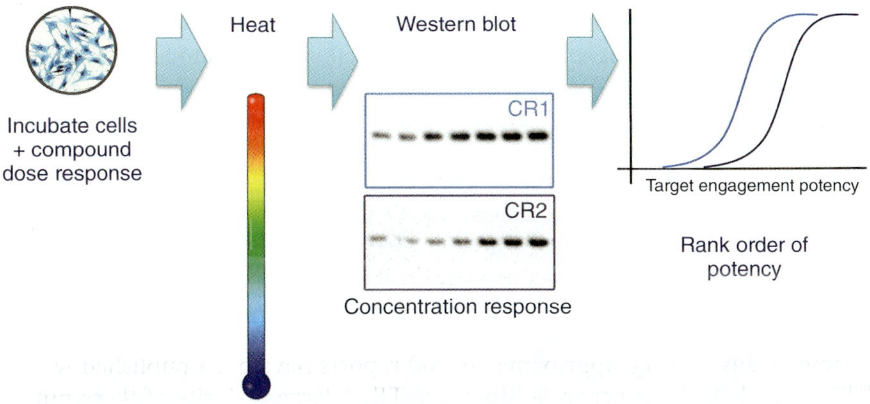

Figure 5.4 CETSA Classics is the method format first described. It uses western blot detection to quantify protein amounts. Despite limited sample throughput, it allows easy translation between cellular matrices and rapid evaluation of target engagement.

It should also be noted that since the Classics format is dependent on antibody detection, there will be limitations owing to antibody availability and performance. For example, in the crop science field, the availability of reliable antibodies has turned out to be a limiting factor for targeted CETSA studies. Similarly, when turning to tissue samples, the presence of host IgGs and the high abundance of certain plasma proteins may interfere with antibody detection and therefore limit its use.

The main advantage of the CETSA Classics format is the ease of setting up and validating the assay. While the western blot readout is low in throughput, it allows detailed identification and control of the selected proteins based on electrophoretic separation. Hence, the classics format is well suited as an early and rapid validation of how amenable a specific protein is to CETSA analysis and as a control of results obtained in other CETSA formats. Once the specific conditions for the classics assay on the selected protein are determined in one sample matrix, it can rapidly be transferred to different sample matrices. The fact that the CETSA assay reports on the same phenomenon of changes in thermal stability based on the drug–protein interaction together with the ease of transfer between sample matrices makes the classics format very well suited for translational assays. As such, the classics format allows detailed studies of drug TE of the native protein target in cells, animal tissues, and samples obtained from humans, without adding translational errors due to changes in the applied technology. The limited throughput of the classics format is also less of a challenge in translational studies since such studies are performed on a limited number of drug candidates. It is therefore likely that the main utility of the classics format in the future will be in translational studies using cellular systems, animal tissues, and samples obtained from healthy volunteers and patients.

5.3.2 CETSA HT

Shortly after the publication of the proof-of-principle CETSA paper, the use of homogeneous dual antibody detection was explored together with the team at the Chemical Biology Consortium Sweden at SciLifeLab in Stockholm. Such a format would allow CETSA to also be used as a screening assay in a plate format (Figure 5.5). In the first proof-of-concept paper [11], a small library consisting of approximately 12 000 compounds was screened. The target of choice, thymidylate synthase (TYMS), is central in the dividing cell; moreover, TYMS has a rich literature, and many tool compounds are available. The screened library consisted of both lead-like compounds and known drugs (the Prestwick Library, http://prestwickchemical.com/libraries-screening-lib-pcl.html) and nucleosides.

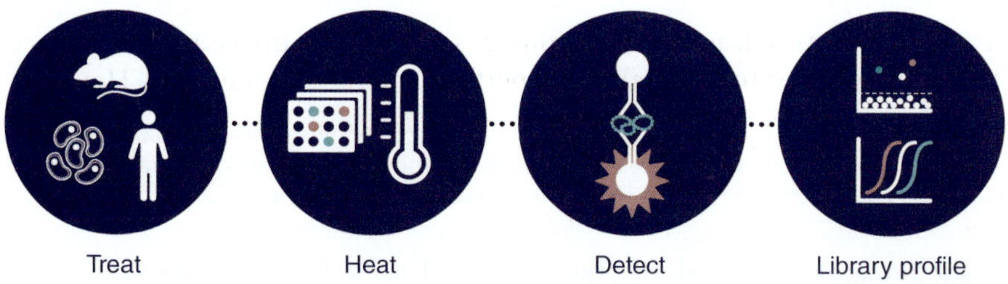

Figure 5.5 CETSA HT allows for fast generation of many data points by virtue of employing microtiter plates. The typical application is hit conformation and screening of compound libraries. The separation step normally carried out using centrifugation can be omitted if the assay antibodies are able to discriminate between native and denatured/precipitated protein.

Interestingly, the hits from the first screening campaign were not only nucleosides but also some existing drugs identified as binders. The latter were not known to bind TYMS, and a number of these compounds were also prodrugs, i.e. compounds that needed cellular activation in order to bind to the target protein. Since such compounds would have been missed in traditional biophysical screening assays, this again highlights the value of cellular assays early in the drug discovery value chain (also see Chapter 7 for a broader description of human-relevant assay systems).

In CETSA HT, it is possible and preferred to overcome the centrifugation step used in the other CETSA formats. The homogeneous format allows the use of antibodies that can distinguish between folded and denatured (and precipitated) protein; therefore the demands on the antibodies used are higher than those in western blots. Therefore, one limiting factor for the use of the format is the availability of antibodies, specifically in newly identified and less validated targets. Hence, variants of CETSA HT have emerged where tagged proteins are used. These tags may range from small His- or FLAG-tags, for which there are affinity tools available, to large constructs using entire protein molecules as reporters. Examples of the latter are the NanoLuc® luciferase technology from Promega, which requires the addition of organic compounds to produce light, or DiscoverX's InCELL Hunter™, which requires both the addition of an enzyme acceptor fragment and a chemiluminescent substrate. For these non-label-free methods, careful interpretation of the results will be needed due to the potential interference of the tag with the cellular phenotype in general and the cellular function of the proteins in particular.

Nevertheless, for the majority of targets for which the antibody availability allows the researchers to screen for CETSA HT compatible antibodies, the following requirements need to be fulfilled: the antibodies should work in pairs with the assumption that once the antibodies are bound in close enough proximity, they should either combine into a functional enzyme (so-called enzyme fragment complementation) or be able to excite each other by resonance energy transfer. For an exhaustive description of how to best screen antibody pairs that will be suitable for CETSA HT, please see Ref. [6].

We have now evaluated several dozen targets (ranging from small cytosolic targets to nuclear receptors and membrane proteins) using homogeneous assays primarily from PerkinElmer and Cisbio Bioassays. Similar to what is known for CETSA Classics, as well as other antibody-based methods, the assay performance will be directly linked to the quality and performance of the antibodies. However, there are also differences in, for example, the sensitivity of the different protein quantification methods, but no exhaustive analysis has been made to firmly say that one method is superior (in terms of sensitivity) to another.

One observation is that for large screens to be carried out, a typical CETSA HT assay often requires a large number of cells, which can preclude screens in scarce or expensive primary cells. Therefore, many of the activities in Pelago Bioscience's laboratories are focused on miniaturization of the assay system as well as multiplexing, both with regard to other CETSA targets and with alternative endpoint assays.

Recently, there have been two reports of developing formats that allow CETSA measures in a high-content, high-throughput single-cell immunofluorescent-based format [12, 13]. Both of these reports addressed the issue of high cell consumption per well in a typical CETSA HT assay, which was also a key motivation for further method development. Apart from this imaging format being more sensitive due to its fluorescent readout, these studies also highlighted the importance of being able to keep the assayed cells adherent to the wells of the plate during incubation with drug and subsequent detection steps. The latter is an important improvement. Previous protocols require adherent cells to be detached from their growth support, which may potentially hinder the cellular physiology because of shearing forces or enzymatic treatment during the detachment step. We expect future development reports to include multiple readouts of cellular response in combination with CETSA TE determination, as well as the wider applicability of this promising new format in larger compound screens.

The HT format allows the generation of thousands of data points per day, which enables studies of drug–target interactions on the physiologically relevant form of the target using entire compound libraries. However, throughput is currently limited by the plate–plate transfer step between the heating and detection steps and, to a certain extent, the use of immortalized cell lines. Once these limitations are overcome by increased automation of the workflow and optimization of detection sensitivity, the high-throughput format will allow full high-throughput screening (HTS) campaigns on entire large compound collections using millions of data points. Then, the screening campaigns can also be executed in more disease-relevant samples, such as primary cells, and in more mechanism-relevant 3D cultures or organoids (see Chapter 7 for more information on these types of cellular systems).

Several of the homogeneous formats validated in the detection step of CETSA HT allow multiplexing of proteins and cellular readouts. By developing multiplexed assays in the HT format, it will be possible to employ panels of targets to assess selectivity and safety by monitoring orthogonal pharmacology and liability targets in parallel. The development of such panels holds promise for large time and cost savings in the preclinical phases of drug discovery as well as maximizing the amount of relevant information from a single assay.

The microtiter plate-based HT format is well suited for a standardized setup and protocol and will therefore allow the development of kits combining the CETSA protocol with a validated homogeneous protein detection step. Such kits will not only facilitate the generation of large datasets with low variation, which is needed in larger screening campaigns, but also enable the monitoring of clinical markers of drug–target interactions.

5.3.3 CETSA MS

The implications of being able to multiplex the readout was understood early, and the first experiments with a mass spectrometric readout were performed by the Nordlund group in early 2011, almost in parallel with the first western blot experiments. The first CETSA paper describing the CETSA approach with

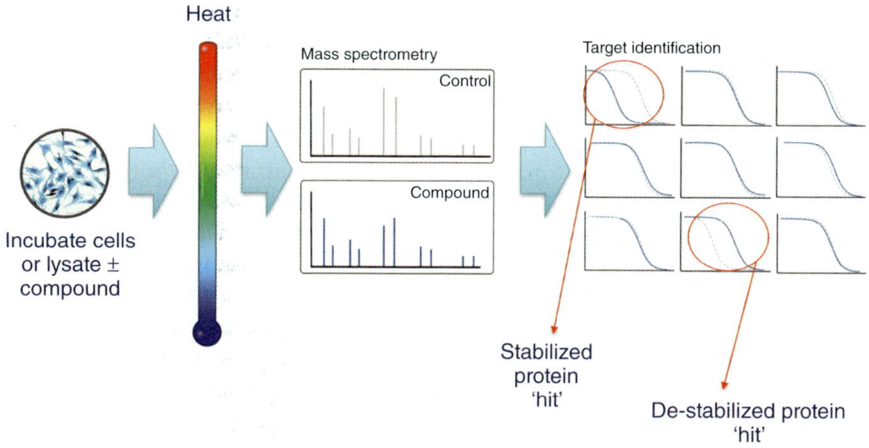

Figure 5.6 CETSA MS is the most demanding of the different CETSA assay formats, both regarding instrumentation and data analysis. The unbiased format allows proteome-wide drug profiling, making it ideal for biomarker investigation, target deconvolution, and evaluation of ligand selectivity and specificity profiles.

an MS endpoint was published in 2014 together with colleagues at Cellzome [8] (Figure 5.6).

Combining the CETSA hallmark of studying the effect of drug–target interactions in relevant physiological settings on thousands of proteins in parallel therefore proved to be a very powerful format. The advantages of the unbiased format were recognized early on as a vast improvement in selectivity and specificity profiling with the assessment of an unprecedented number of targets assessed (~6000 proteins) and without limitations to specific target classes. This led to selectivity profiling of several drugs and tool compounds and identification of a number of targets linked to clinically observed side effects. In this first CETSA MS report, a beautiful example of such was shown, where dasatinib, which is known to bind BCR-ABL, could be profiled. It was already known that the BCR-ABL fusion protein was not amenable to the CETSA method and no shifts could be observed in the fusion protein, while c-Abl alone showed distinct stabilization with both dasatinib and imatinib. However, in the CETSA MS study, several proteins showed dose-dependent dasatinib stabilization in intact cells but without any response in lysates. One of these was CRKL, a known downstream effector of BCR-ABL and a previously proposed treatment response biomarker. The comparison between intact cell and lysate experiments, especially when the primary target is believed to be a membrane protein, is thus very valuable for understanding the mode of action (MoA) of small molecule inhibition and for identifying TE biomarkers.

One year after the first CETSA MS paper, the Superti-Furga group presented a CETSA MS study on crizotinib, methotrexate, and diverse cellular metabolites [14]. Crizotinib, as expected, bound to MTH1, a subsequently de-validated target that has been shown not only to bind to a large number of compounds (a so-called frequent hit) but also to not be responsible for the effects previously described.

Also, methotrexate was shown to bind to dihydrofolate reductase (DHFR), neatly reproducing the results from the proof-of-principle western blot-based CETSA paper.

Shortly after the Superti-Furga paper, the Cellzome group extended the original assay format to use detergents and therefore also included membrane proteins in CETSA MS, which had until then been a limitation in target space [15]. The method was developed further when in 2016 Cellzome introduced the so-called 2D format [16], where multiple concentrations were tested at a dozen temperatures, giving a better understanding of the dose-dependent effects of small molecule inhibitors. This paper and several others [17, 18] have since shown that CETSA MS can be used to understand the MoA of compounds and discover targets of compounds that can explain adverse clinical side effects and even to identify prognostic and stratification biomarkers.

CETSA MS is different from other proteomics approaches in that it reports on functional changes rather than on the abundance of a protein and its modifications. The ability to resolve both the direct binding mode of a compound and the pathway effects is why CETSA MS lends itself very favourably to the deconvolution of the MoA of phenotypically characterized drugs as discussed below. This is true for compounds identified through phenotypic screening as well as repurposing of candidates in the clinical stages or even marketed drugs since CETSA MS can be performed on all sample matrices and species containing the biology of interest. The detailed reporting on signalling changes on the whole proteome level in physiologically relevant samples is also why CETSA MS is now employed to describe the time course of drug interactions in important cellular phenomena such as drug resistance as well as to understand fundamental aspects of cell cycle regulation [19, 20].

In conclusion, studies of the effects of preclinical development candidates in physiologically relevant sample matrices on the whole proteome level will allow the identification of liability target panels and potential biomarkers to facilitate the development of novel therapies. A number of therapies in use today are hampered by debilitating side effects; it is therefore tempting to speculate that the profiling of clinical samples will allow identification of safety, stratification, and dose-monitoring markers.

5.4 Target Discovery

5.4.1 Generation of Active Hit Molecules

The first step after validating and agreeing on prosecuting a target linked to a therapeutic hypothesis is to find active hit compounds. The large pharma companies and several established biotech companies have access to large diversity libraries, which are then tested by HTS campaigns. This process necessitates assays capable of generating 10–100 000 datasets per day in a highly automated fashion. Therefore, such screening is not always possible because of high resource needs and costs and access to large diversity libraries or the selected assay methodology is not HTS compatible. The latter is often true for label-free technologies, where these technologies lack throughput and the necessary automation or high costs per data point. This is true for most CETSA HT formats because of the limited automation developed to date. Recently, however, variants of CETSA (sometimes referred to as lazy or labelled CETSAs) using tagged proteins in combination with enzyme complement luminescence [21, 22] have been evaluated for high-throughput library screening. Although lazy CETSA is not a true label-free assay, as it employs a tagged overexpressed protein, such applications may enable full CETSA HT campaigns in the future. Today, label-free screening is often applied with good success in the early target discovery stages using smaller libraries either instead of a full HTS campaign, enabling HTS or following the primary screen. In the next section, we will discuss a number of applications of label-free technologies in early target discovery.

5.4.2 Tool Generation (Small Screens to Identify Tool Compounds)

To prosecute a target and generate novel leads, it is necessary to establish a toolbox of reagents and assays. This is always a daunting task, and many parameters need to be addressed while remaining true to the therapeutic hypothesis being probed. Considerations regarding the strategy for generating actives include throughput, cost, and physiological relevance. Establishing the toolbox can be particularly challenging for a target hypothesis that is novel and therefore has very little prior validation and availability of established reagents. Similarly, when prosecuting targets by a novel approach, such as new binding site(s) or modes of regulation (allosteric, protein–protein interaction [PPI], and structural interference/correctors), tools to validate and prosecute such mechanisms can be scarce. In other cases, the target may not have a specific substrate or may have multiple substrates, such as transcription factors. Assays generating actives on such targets may simply not be possible by traditional labelling methods. In such projects, a label-free screen can be set up to identify the initial library of tool compounds, which in turn can be used to validate the screening cascade towards identifying drug-like leads. A CETSA assay for such novel targets can then be established if affinity reagents can be generated or are available. For very novel targets, the availability of affinity reagents can be an issue. In such situations, validation of a limited number of tool compounds can be performed using the CETSA MS format.

5.4.3 Target Classes That Are In and Out of Scope and Difficult Targets

As discussed in the previous section, targets with no clear or specifically relevant substrate can be difficult to prosecute by labelled methods. Examples include transcription factors, proteases, and many epigenetic targets, as well as classic drug targets such as (orphan) GPCRs and ion channels. In many such cases, it may be difficult to set up a relevant efficacy assay since this process will occur downstream of TE and will often use nonnatural substrates. This gap is particularly well filled by traditional TSAs since TE can be quantified and hits filtered based on TE potency as a measure of affinity. Please see the comprehensive review by Renaud et al. of TSA utility in drug discovery [23]. Once hits are identified and ranked on TE potency, the efficacy can then be determined in a downstream substrate conversion format. When the TE structure–activity relationship (SAR) is established and correlated with the efficacy measure in such substrate conversion assays, one can then choose the more predictive assay of the two as the primary screening cascade assay because it is very unlikely that the SAR for an established lead series will shift to a new MoA.

GPCRs are often difficult to analyse with antibodies or affinity-based methods and therefore possibly better evaluated with TSAs using protein preparations reconstituted using detergents or vesicles than with CETSA. Ion channels as therapeutic targets can be prosecuted using cell lines and plate-based electrophysiology when screening large numbers of compounds. This method format allows a functional characterization of the small molecule effects and are therefore often a better choice than TSAs. Most remaining targets should be better served by TSAs, SPR, or a CETSA assay.

5.4.4 Focused or Iterative Library Screening

Instead of running full campaigns in HTS or uHTS on large diversity libraries, one can adopt strategies to generate actives from much smaller compound collections. Focused library screening based, for instance, on target class or stratified subsets from the full chemical library can yield results much faster and more cost effectively than a full HTS. Iterative screening, when the initial hits guide the subsequent selection of library compounds for screening, can also be applied to rapidly develop actives and hit series. When such strategies for the generation of actives are employed, label-free technologies are well suited as the primary assay to identify and filter hits for further development into lead series.

5.4.5 Fragment Library Screening

The use of smaller ~200 Da molecular weight fragment molecules as building blocks and starting points to generate leads is called fragment-based lead generation (FBLG) or fragment-based drug discovery (FBDD) [24]. The starting points for such campaigns are library collections of 1000–10 000 fragments. Such approaches can be very effective when good resolution structural data are available to guide the design of new molecules, providing a rationale for combining the fragments into full-size leads with high affinity and selectivity. The fragments have a generally low affinity for the target compared to a full-size lead molecule because of the limited number of interactions with the protein of interest. It is therefore necessary to test fragments at 10–100 times the concentrations typically applied in primary screens in other *in vitro* assays. Label-free biophysical screening of fragment libraries has therefore become the standard approach to generate starting points for FBLG since these assays generally tolerate high concentrations of test compounds. The most widespread label-free assay format in such campaigns is probably the TSA, which is carried out on isolated proteins. TSAs rely on and quantify the thermal denaturation shift upon, for example, ligand addition or buffer composition. Most frequently, the protein is overexpressed and purified, either in its full-length form or in a truncated version. There are numerous TSA screening formats available, each having different strengths and limitations in terms of protein properties, detection, and throughput of the format. For a more exhaustive evaluation of the available TSA formats used in preclinical drug discovery, please see Ref. [25]. CETSA HT offers an advantage over such TSAs as there is no need for recombinant protein production or purification. The actives will be identified by interaction with the native protein, and the screen can be carried out in both lysate and intact cells, which will then yield information on whether the target is available in the physiologically relevant setting.

5.4.6 Hit Confirmation

Whether the generation of active compounds against the target of interest is carried out by testing very large chemical diversity libraries or smaller focused campaigns, screening is performed at a single or very few concentrations and conditions. Such campaigns can yield from hundreds to a few thousand hits divided over several chemotypes in both clusters and single compound hits (singletons). To confirm the validity of such hits, they are usually tested in an orthogonal readout assay. It is particularly important to confirm the hits in a cellular assay if they are generated by an *in vitro* assay on the naked protein target. The CETSA HT format is particularly well suited to bridge this gap since it offers the opportunity to confirm cellular TE on the native form of the target in the physiologically relevant setting of a living cell. The added advantage of using CETSA HT for hit confirmation is that it can then serve as the affinity measure in a screening cascade post-hit confirmation.

5.4.7 Phenotypic Hit Deconvolution to Discover Targets

Before combinatorial chemistry, molecular biology, genomics, and pharmacology took centre stage in drug discovery during the 1980s and 1990s, the development of novel therapies was driven by phenotypic observations in either human or animal studies. However, it has been realized in the last decade that pure affinity-based targeted drug discovery for first-in-class and novel molecular MoA programmes may be less efficient than phenotypic approaches [26]. When benchmarking the efficiency by which new drugs are discovered, it seems at least for novel molecular MoA that the phenotypic approaches offer a relevant alternative [27]. This has led to a renewed focus on phenotypic testing in advanced or more disease-relevant cellular systems, which in turn increases the demand for deconvoluting the MoA of such phenotypically identified hits and leads. The primary target as well as liability targets can be identified, and the relevant target screens as well as counter screens can be established to more broadly profile hit molecules or rescreen against the identified target(s). Hence, while extremely challenging, deconvolution of the target interaction and MoA will de-risk, facilitate, and accelerate the development of phenotypic hits from the bench to human testing.

The traditional deconvolution strategies employed are the profiling of hits in cell panel tests by correlating multiple phenotypic readouts from annotated datasets (for example, BioMAP® from Eurofins) and binning them by typical features to narrow down the list of potential MoA. Such profiling is followed up by siRNA and CRISPR techniques to modulate the individual protein targets at the gene expression level to validate if target modulation phenocopies the effect of the hit molecule (see Chapter 09 for more details). However, such deconvolution strategies are often time consuming and dependent on the particular phenotype used for the MoA binning being well defined and annotated. Furthermore, the expression-based target confirmation has the obvious disadvantage of being based on modulating the gene and therefore the whole function or abundance of the protein rather than more specific target modulation at the protein level and hence differing effects on signalling pathways. An alternative to the gene-centric approach is offered by the protein-centric deconvolution approach based on affinity probes in chemical proteomics (see Chapter 2 for more details). In this case significant time and effort is often required to effectively develop the affinity probe as well as the bias that the probe will introduce in the target fishing. Finally, it may be difficult to assess the pathway effects when only fishing out direct binding partners and their complexes using elution after fishing in a lysed sample matrix.

CETSA MS may provide some alternatives since the assay can be carried out in the physiologically relevant sample matrix, reproducing the phenotypic test condition in the living cell or tissue, and can be performed directly using the intended drug without any need for affinity probes (Figure 5.7). The target identification is unbiased with regard to MoA, albeit certain target classes are less readily resolved for direct binding based on the thermodynamics of such targets (GPCRs and ion channels, as discussed previously). However, since the CETSA MS assay is performed in live cell incubation, it will also allow the identification of functional changes in the pathway downstream of the primary target binding event. The resolution of the potential efficacy driving pathways is unique to the CETSA MS method. In contrast to other proteomics formats, CETSA MS reports general changes in the functional status of the proteins involved in the signalling pathway. Normally, only the abundance of a protein species is measured, for instance, in phospho- or glycoproteomics. Due to the resolution of both direct

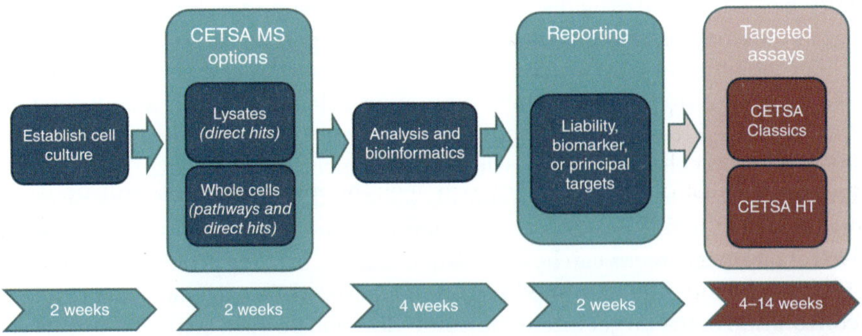

Figure 5.7 Deconvolution flow using CETSA. Comparison of the drugs profile in intact cells and lysate allows identification of both direct hits and shifts caused by downstream signalling events, leading to loss or gain of interactions, phosphorylations, or cellular relocalization. The identified targets can then be followed up in targeted CETSA assays.

binding and pathway effects, CETSA MS profiling also offers the opportunity for the early discovery of potential biomarkers. This combination of CETSA with an unbiased shotgun protein quantification approach for target identification and deconvolution of MoA has recently proven useful to identify the molecular mechanism of phenotypically identified compounds with antiproliferative effects and potential applications in oncology [17]. In this study, the authors profiled two similar acting compounds, a131 and a166, with the CETSA MS method using the same cells and incubation conditions as in the phenotypic assay. The CETSA MS melt curve profiling identified PIP4K2A and PIP4K2C as common molecular hits between the two compounds. These findings were functionally verified by the compounds' ability to potently inhibit the PIP4K2C enzyme activity *in vitro*. Subsequent knockdown experiments using multiple siRNAs against all PIP4K isoforms induced cell cycle arrest – a phenocopy of a131 and a166 treatment. Interestingly this study also identified ferrochelatase (FECH), a protein in the heme synthesis pathway as a target for a131. However, FECH has previously been identified as a promiscuous binder of multiple drugs [8]. The promiscuous drug binding of this protein was further substantiated by siRNA studies showing no effect on cell cycle by knockdown of FECH.

Since the CETSA MS format uses a significant amount of LC-MS/MS resources and comprehensive specialized data analysis, it can often be advantageous to set up targeted CETSA Classics or HT assays to further prosecute the identified efficacy or liability targets. An example of targeted CETSA Classics used to verify cellular TE was employed by AstraZeneca scientists to in fact *de-validate* a target hypothesis [28]. In this report, the authors showed that in spite of selective, specific, and potent inhibition of MTH1 with a series of tool compounds, no antiproliferative effect of the MTH1 inhibition was observed. Cellular TE on MTH1 was quantified with CETSA and correlated with SPR on the immobilized enzyme. Finally, siRNA and CRISPR techniques were employed to knock down MTH1 expression, similarly without effect on cell proliferation *in vitro*. Next, scientists from Bayer translated the findings to the *in vivo* setting showing no effect of tumour size after dosing with cellular active MTH1 inhibitors [29].

5.5 Target Validation

5.5.1 Binding Modes

Assessment of binding modes is an area where label-free methods are frequently employed because of the detailed reporting on the molecular interaction between compound and target. Label-free assays can be used to study the kinetics of the interaction or competition experiments. SPR is frequently employed to test large numbers of compounds for their kinetics of binding and unbinding the target to determine the true K_d of the interaction. However, in this format, the purified or recombinant protein target is immobilized on the matrix, which may affect the binding mode. Final confirmation of binding mode requires structural studies where, for example, nuclear magnetic resonance (NMR) can provide a detailed identification of the binding site and structural rearrangements occurring in a protein upon compound binding. Similarly, X-ray crystallographic studies can reveal high-resolution details of compound binding modes. However, neither NMR nor X-ray crystallography is compatible with large numbers of compounds.

5.5.2 Selectivity, Specificity, and Safety

As lead compounds proceed through optimization, they are tested in multiple selectivity and specificity assays of increasing complexity and cost. As the lead series mature towards the selection of prenomination and candidate drugs, increasing numbers of selectivity and specificity tests are introduced. Commonly used selectivity and safety testing are cardiac liability ion channels, kinase and enzyme panels, or broad diversity panels that can be selected based on the site of action, intended administration, and therapy area for which the drug will be used. In addition, alternative approaches, for example, the use of kinobeads for kinase selectivity, can also be used (see Chapter 4 for more details). All of these approaches will inform about potential liabilities and general specificity of the tested molecules. However, often the selection of which target panels to employ are, in the early discovery phases, either generic or determined by the individual project and available resources, the experience of the team, and the legacy knowledge of the target in focus. The target panels themselves contain a limited number of targets and often a range of readouts depending on the target. In general, labelled formats are used including radioactive ligand binding, substrate conversion or functional measures, for example, ion channel testing in plate-based electrophysiology screening. The variety of methods employed can often complicate a direct comparison of the results.

The CETSA MS format allows an unprecedented number of targets to be tested in parallel, which in turn allows a direct comparison between the data obtained on all targets in parallel. There is no preselection of targets, and the method is unbiased on target classes and can, like all CETSA assays, be employed on all sample matrices that contain the biology of interest. Such physiologically relevant profiling may in the future enable a very thorough de-risking and safety profiling of molecules possibly even before they are dosed in man. As an example, scientists at GlaxoSmithKline and EMBL profiled the histone deacetylase (HDAC) inhibitor panobinostat (trade name Farydak, marketed by Novartis) in 2D CETSA MS profiling experiments (varying both temperature and concentration) in the human HepG2 cell line and lysates thereof [16]. They identified the expected pan-HDAC interaction by dose-dependent stabilization of HDAC1, HDAC2, HDAC6, and HDAC10, but they also discovered a previous unknown binding partner of panobinostat: the phenylalanine hydroxylase (PAH). As a specificity control, vorinostat (another HDAC inhibitor) was also profiled and shown to stabilize several HDACs but not PAH. The functional effect of panobinostat was verified in an enzymatic assay in liver cells where panobinostat inhibited tyrosine synthesis with a half maximal inhibitory concentration (IC_{50}) value of 190 nM. In man, loss-of-function mutations in the PAH gene leads to impaired phenylalanine metabolism and causes phenylketonuria. Likewise, PAH inhibition can lead to decreased tyrosine levels, which can cause symptoms mimicking hypothyroidism, which is also known as a common panobinostat side effect. Taken together, these observations lead the authors to speculate that PAH is the molecular target responsible for some of the panobinostat side effects.

5.5.3 Translation Bench to Bedside (via Animals)

Traditionally, label-free assays have been used in the early phases of preclinical discovery to filter early active molecules. After the initial identification of hits and development of lead series, the focus is typically shifted from affinity to efficacy first in cellular assays and later *in vivo* models. Such efficacy assays tend to make use of phenotypic readouts and reporter labels with good success. However, the invention of label-free methods such as CETSA allows the label-free quantification of TE in all sample matrices, including living cells and tissues. It is therefore now possible to correlate the efficacy with TE determined by the CETSA method. The added advantage is that there is no translational error as a project moves between cellular assays and tissue, since the basic assay protocol is identical in all sample matrices [5].

Within the research area of oncology, project compounds are often assessed for their antiproliferative activity in immortalized cancer cell lines, which are then used for grafting into immunocompromised mice to provide the well-known xenograft models. Efficacy is assessed by measuring tumour shrinkage after dosing. In both experiments, CETSA Classics can be used to quantify the occupancy of the compound on the target and thus correlate TE with efficacy translating from the cellular system to tissue. Similarly, it is possible to assess TE in tissues from PK/PD studies using the same CETSA assay. Normally, the relationship between the incubation concentration (*in vitro*) from the cell studies and the effective dose (*in vivo*), together with the PK/PD data, is used to translate the efficacy of the drug from *in vitro* to *in vivo*. With the addition of occupancy or TE quantifications using CETSA in the setup described above, the strength of the correlation can be increased, and the certainty that efficacy is driven by occupancy of the selected target is substantially strengthened. This, in turn, will support the target hypothesis of the pharmacological effect. Similarly, the CETSA suite of assays can be used to measure and quantify occupancy in samples from healthy volunteers and patients. Since the assay can be performed by *ex vivo* incubation, it is possible to frontload and de-risk projects by assessing TE in human samples before any lead optimization work is carried out.

An example of this utility was done with a candidate drug from the Swedish biotech company Medivir inhibiting cathepsin S. The lead candidate molecule stabilized cathepsin S with a CETSA EC50 of 16 nM when incubated with live immortalized cells expressing cathepsin S. When the candidate drug was dosed directly in whole blood and the peripheral blood mononuclear cells (PBMCs) separated out in a Ficoll gradient, the CETSA EC50 of stabilization was 20 nM (Figure 5.8).

This utility in translational science is quite atypical compared with that of an unlabelled assay technology, and it is therefore difficult to benchmark CETSA against other label-free methods in this area. However, the use of CETSA certainly limits the necessity to develop radioactive labelled ligands for measuring

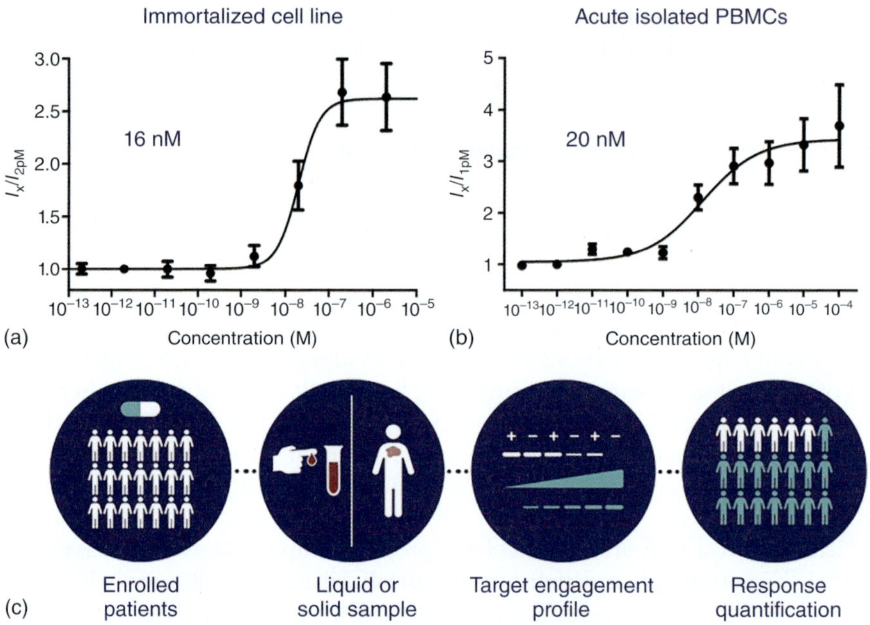

Figure 5.8 *In vitro*-to-*in vivo* translation. CETSA assays can be used to translate target engagement between sample matrices. The top panels show concentration–response curves to determine target engagement potency of a candidate drug incubated in live cultures of transformed B lymphocytes (9001) (a) and in acutely isolated PBMCs after incubation in whole blood (b). Panel (c) show the intended analysis flow using CETSA profiling to correlate the target engagement and efficacy endpoints in healthy volunteers and patients.

occupancy and distribution *in vivo* and provides an alternative method with promising broad utility in translational science.

5.6 Conclusion

Label-free techniques are well established and have proven their utility and value in targeted drug discovery. They deliver precise information on the interaction between the test molecule and the protein target, albeit this detailed information is often reported in the absence of other interaction partners or on somewhat perturbed systems of immobilized, recombinant, or purified protein. The invention of the CETSA method has presented a new dimension to the label-free arsenal of methods by adding the opportunity to monitor drug–target interactions on the native target in cells or tissue, thereby combining the strength of the label-free methods unperturbed reporting on molecular interactions with physiological relevance of the living cell. We expect that for proteins amenable to CETSA analysis, the method will greatly facilitate target discovery, validation, and translation in the years to come. The combination of an unperturbed physiologically relevant measure of affinity and a relevant efficacy measure in a disease-relevant human system has the potential we believe to significantly reduce the time from discovery to bedside for new medicines.

References

1 Arrowsmith and Miller (2013). Trial watch: phase II and phase III attrition rates 2011-2012. *Nat. Rev. Drug Discovery* 12: 569.
2 Ericsson, U.B., Hallberg, B.M., Detitta, G.T. et al. (2006). Thermofluor-based high-throughput stability optimization of proteins for structural studies. *Anal. Biochem.* 357 (2): 289–298.
3 Vedadi, M., Niesen, F.H., Allali-Hassani, A. et al. (2006). Chemical screening methods to identify ligands that promote protein stability, protein crystallization, and structure determination. *Proc. Natl. Acad. Sci. U.S.A.* 103 (43): 15835–15840.
4 Nordlund, P. (2011). Methods for determining ligand binding to a target protein using a thermal shift assay. WO2012143714A1, filed 18 April 2011, application 18 April 2012. PCT/GB2012/050853.
5 Martinez Molina, D., Jafari, R., Ignatushchenko, M. et al. (2013). Monitoring drug target engagement in cells and tissues using the cellular thermal shift assay. *Science* 341 (6141): 84–87.
6 Jafari, R., Almqvist, H., Axelsson, H. et al. (2014). The cellular thermal shift assay for evaluating drug target interactions in cells. *Nat. Protoc.* 9 (9): 2100–2122.
7 Franken, H., Mathieson, T., Childs, D. et al. (2015). Thermal proteome profiling for unbiased identification of direct and indirect drug targets using multiplexed quantitative mass spectrometry. *Nat. Protoc.* 10 (10): 1567–1593.
8 Savitski, M.M., Reinhard, F.B., Franken, H. et al. (2014). Tracking cancer drugs in living cells by thermal profiling of the proteome. *Science* 346 (6205): 1255784.
9 Martinez Molina, D. and Nordlund, P. (2014). Method for identifying a biomarker indicative of a reduced drug response using a thermal shift assay. WO2015145151A1, priority date 25 March 2014, application filed 25 March 2015, PCT/GB2015/050895.
10 CSH, T., Go, K.D., Bisteau, X. et al. (2018). Thermal proximity coaggregation for system-wide profiling of protein complex dynamics in cells. *Science* 359 (6380): 1170–1177.
11 Almqvist, H., Axelsson, H., Jafari, R. et al. (2016). CETSA screening identifies known and novel thymidylate synthase inhibitors and slow intracellular activation of 5-fluorouracil. *Nat. Commun.* 7: 11040.
12 Axelsson, H., Almqvist, H., Otrocka, M. et al. (2018). In situ target engagement studies in adherent cells. *ACS Chem. Biol.* 13 (4): 942–950.
13 Massey, A.J. (2018). A high content, high throughput cellular thermal stability assay for measuring drug-target engagement in living cells. *PLoS One* 13 (4): e0195050.

14 Huber, K.V., Olek, K.M., Müller, A.C. et al. (2015). Proteome-wide drug and metabolite interaction mapping by thermal-stability profiling. *Nat. Methods* 12 (11): 1055–1057.
15 Reinhard, F.B., Eberhard, D., Werner, T. et al. (2015). Thermal proteome profiling monitors ligand interactions with cellular membrane proteins. *Nat. Methods* 12 (12): 1129–1131.
16 Becher, I., Werner, T., Doce, C. et al. (2016 Nov). Thermal profiling reveals phenylalanine hydroxylase as an off-target of panobinostat. *Nat. Chem. Biol.* 12 (11): 908–910.
17 Kitagawa, M., Liao, P.J., Lee, K.H. et al. (2017). Dual blockade of the lipid kinase PIP4Ks and mitotic pathways leads to cancer-selective lethality. *Nat. Commun.* 8 (1): 2200.
18 Miettinen, T.P., Peltier, J., Härtlova, A. et al. (2018). Thermal proteome profiling of breast cancer cells reveals proteasomal activation by CDK4/6 inhibitor palbociclib. *EMBO J.* 37 (10). pii: e98359.
19 Dai, L., Zhao, T., Bisteau, X. et al. (2018). Modulation of protein-interaction states through the cell cycle. *Cell* 173 (6): 1481–1494.e13.
20 Becher, I., Andrés-Pons, A., Romanov, N. et al. (2018). Pervasive protein thermal stability variation during the cell cycle. *Cell* 173 (6): 1495–1507.e18.
21 Dart, M.L., Machleidt, T., Jost, E. et al. (2018). Homogeneous assay for target engagement utilizing bioluminescent thermal shift. *ACS Med. Chem. Lett.* 9 (6): 546–551.
22 McNulty, D.E., Bonnette, W.G., Qi, H. et al. (2018). A high-throughput dose-response cellular thermal shift assay for rapid screening of drug target engagement in living cells, exemplified using SMYD3 and IDO1. *SLAS Discovery* 23 (1): 34–46.
23 Renaud, J.-P., Chung, C.W., and Danielson, U.H. (2016). Biophysics in drug discovery: impact, challenges and opportunities. *Nat. Rev. Drug Discovery* 15: 679–698.
24 Jhoti, H., Williams, G., Rees, D.C., and Murray, C.W. (2013). The 'rule of three' for fragment-based drug discovery: where are we now? *Nat. Rev. Drug Discovery* 12: 644–645.
25 Silvestre, H.L., Blundell, T.L., Abell, C., and Ciulli, A. (2013). Integrated biophysical approach to fragment screening and validation for fragment-based lead discovery. *Proc. Natl. Acad. Sci. U.S.A.* 110: 12984–12989.
26 Swinney, D.C. and Anthony, J. (2011). How were new medicines discovered? *Nat. Rev. Drug Discovery* 10: 507–519.
27 Sedrani, R. and Wiesmann, C. (2014). The discovery of first-in-class drugs: origins and evolution. *Nat. Rev. Drug Discovery* 13: 577–587.
28 Kettle, J.G., Alwan, H., and Bista, M. (2016). Potent and selective inhibitors of MTH1 probe its role in cancer cell survival. *J. Med. Chem.* 59 (6): 2346–2361.
29 Ellermann, M., Eheim, A., and Rahm, F. (2017). Novel class of potent and cellularly active inhibitors devalidates MTH1 as broad-spectrum cancer target. *ACS Chem. Biol.* 12 (8): 1986–1992.

6

Reverse Translation to Support Efficient Drug Target Selection and Stratified Medicine

Lauren Drowley[1] *and Martin Armstrong*[2]

[1] *UCB Pharma, 701 W Main Street, Suite 200, Durham, NC, 27701, USA*
[2] *UCB Pharma, Chemin du Foriest, Braine-l'Alleud, B – 1420, Belgium*

6.1 Introduction: the Challenge

One of the major challenges faced in drug discovery is the decrease in R&D productivity, which is largely driven by the high attrition rate seen in the clinic. This has led to significantly increased costs for bringing new drugs to market, with a recent estimate being $2.5 billion per new drug approval [1]. When assessing the driving factors for this high attrition rate, it was reported that the majority of the failures are due to lack of efficacy and toxicity [1, 2]. The reduced R&D productivity can also be seen in the fact that many of the new drugs that are successful in gaining regulatory approval do not end up being successful on the market as they fail to significantly differentiate from the standard of care [2, 3]. This decline in productivity can be linked to reduced innovation, as there has been a decline in the proportion of late-stage targets in the pipeline that are classified as first in class, as well as in the percentage of approvals considered first in class [3]. Using annual peak sales as an estimate to assess this decline, there has been a decrease of almost 50% over recent years, though peak sales increased in 2017 [3, 4].

A focus in drug discovery going forward is to minimize this risk and to reduce attrition and cycle times in development. Of the many factors contributing to determining the efficacy of a drug, perhaps the biggest factor is ensuring that the right target has been selected early on in the drug discovery process. Although many factors go into selecting and prioritizing the 'right target', the most important is undoubtedly knowledge that your target is intrinsically linked to the disease that is being treated and that modulating it will favourably affect the disease phenotype [5]. It is considered that increasing use of genetics during research will alleviate some of the problems associated with the selection of drug targets and lead to optimized target selection.

Target Discovery and Validation: Methods and Strategies for Drug Discovery,
First Edition. Edited by Alleyn T. Plowright.

6.2 Genetics to Date in Drug Discovery

Until recently there has been anecdotal evidence that drug targets with a human genetic linkage to the disease are likely to be successful targets, with the oft quoted examples of CCR5, sclerostin, PCSK9, and others. However, beyond selected examples, it was uncertain as to how important this was and how much weight should be given to genetic evidence when selecting drug targets. Recently work has emerged that has helped to clarify and quantify this.

In a longitudinal review of AstraZeneca's small molecule drug projects between 2005 and 2010, Cook et al. [6] explored the most important determinants of project success. While recognizing that the reasons for project success and failure are complex and, usually, multifactorial, it was shown that those projects with a human genetic linkage between the target and the disease indication were successful (or still open at the time of the review) 73% of the time versus 43% of projects without this evidence.

This concept was further validated and quantified by Nelson et al. [7] who looked at historical drug trial information on drugs across all stages of development and the evidence of genetic linkage between the target and the primary disease indication. It was concluded that selecting genetically supported targets could double the success rate in clinical development (Table 6.1). Taking the analysis one stage further, the authors looked at whether that evidence came from genome-wide association studies (GWASs) (i.e. common genetic variation generally applied to larger cohorts of common diseases or phenotypic traits versus control populations) or from rare Mendelian (single-gene) traits, which were derived from Online Mendelian Inheritance in Man (OMIM). It was observed that those targets with supporting evidence from OMIM were more successful than those with evidence from GWASs. Furthermore, in 2004, 5 out of the top 10 individual drugs sold (Lipitor, Zocor, Procrit, Plavix, Zyprexa) had correlates with monogenic disorders [8].

Many companies are now leveraging genetics and genetic data to support not only their drug target selection but also selection of their target patient population. Until recently it is fair to say that the promise of genetics had not

Table 6.1 The relative value of genetic support for the probability that a target–indication pair progresses along the drug development pipeline (based on historical drug trial information).

	p(progress with genetic support)/ (progress with no genetic support)		
Progression	**GWASdb and OMIM**	**GWASdb**	**OMIM**
Phase I to phase II	1.2 (1.1–1.3)	1.2 (1.1–1.3)	1.2 (1.1–1.3)
Phase II to phase III	1.5 (1.3–1.7)	1.4 (1.2–1.7)	1.6 (1.3–1.9)
Phase III to approval	1.1 (1.0–1.2)	1.0 (0.8–1.2)	1.1 (0.9–1.3)
Phase I to phase III	1.8 (1.5–2.1)	1.8 (1.4–2.1)	1.9 (1.5–2.3)
Phase I to approval	2.0 (1.6–2.4)	1.8 (1.3–2.3)	2.2 (1.6–2.8)

Source: Nelson et al. 2015 [7]. Taken from Springer Nature.

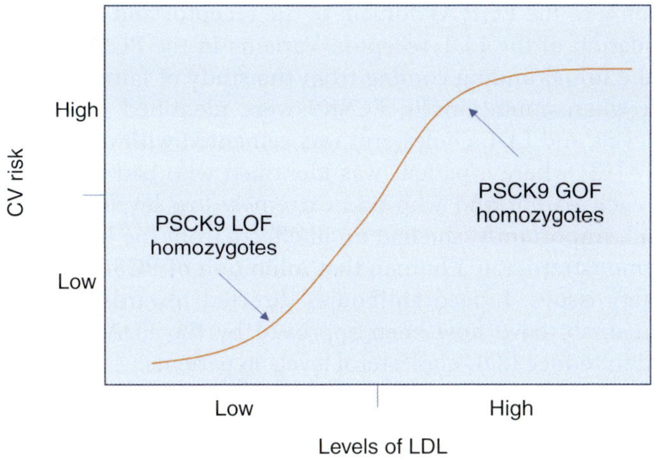

Figure 6.1 An 'experiment of nature' using the PCSK9 example. PCSK9 gain-of-function (GOF) mutations lead to high levels of LDL cholesterol and high cardiovascular (CV) risk, whereas people with loss of PCSK9 function have low levels of LDL cholesterol and low CV risk. Source: Plenge et al. 2013 [2]. Adapted from Springer Nature.

been fully realized in its impact on drug discovery and development. However, technological advances and our ability to cost effectively generate, analyse, and interpret whole genome sequence (WGS) data, as well as the emergence of more publicly available datasets and initiatives, are promoting the more routine use of genetics within the industry.

At a basic level, the aim is to identify gene variants that perturb gene function in a certain direction and that result in the disease phenotype to be treated. Aspirationally, the pharmaceutical industry would like to link a series of alleles (variant forms of a gene) for a target, including gain-of-function and loss-of-function (LOF) variants that together can mimic a dose–response curve of a drug affecting that target. If this can be linked to relevant clinical information, an estimation of the effect of perturbing this target can be seen in a relevant human system and would provide significant information in the efficacy and safety of that target, leading to high confidence in moving forward with drug discovery [1]. These 'experiments of nature', demonstrated in Figure 6.1, can bring value throughout the drug discovery process as they can aid in target identification, help to predict potential safety concerns, and identify target patient populations [9]. Despite the clear value, there are challenges in the process, including identification of the mutation/genetic locus that is believed to be driving a phenotype of interest, validation of the causality, and translating that biology into a drug discovery programme [10].

One of the most notable examples of the value of human genetics in drug discovery is the story of the proprotein convertase subtilisin/kexin type 9 (PCSK9) antibodies. *PCSK9* encodes the PCSK9 protein that regulates the number of low-density lipoprotein (LDL) receptors, which in turn regulate the levels of LDL cholesterol in the blood by binding to LDLs and removing them from the bloodstream [11]. With more LDL receptors present, LDL cholesterol gets removed more quickly from the blood. PCSK9 reduces the number of LDL receptors through binding to the EGF(A) domain of the receptor and initiating the intracellular degradation of the LDL receptor. Variants in the PCSK9 gene were identified, with the initial finding coming from the study of families with hypercholesterolaemia where mutations in PCSK9 were identified [12]. The link between PCSK9 levels and LDL cholesterol was cemented with data from the Dallas Heart Study [13] where a patient was identified who had inherited LOF mutations from each parent and who had extremely low levels of LDL cholesterol in the blood. Importantly, she had no ill effects from the low levels of LDL cholesterol, demonstrating in a human that inhibition of PCSK9 would not lead to severe safety issues. Indeed antibodies directed towards PCSK9, alirocumab and evolocumab, have now been approved by the FDA and are successfully being used to reduce LDL-cholesterol levels in patients.

PCSK9 is a clear example of how genetics can drive new target discovery, but it is oncology that is often regarded as the 'poster child' for the use of genetics to impact drug discovery and personalized therapy and where genetics has been used to great effect. One example is the epidermal growth factor receptor (EGFR) and the emergence of resistance to EGFR inhibitors. EGFR is a receptor protein that is located on the cell surface and is involved in cell growth and division. Overexpression of EGFR in lung cancer has been known for several decades, and mutations that result in this phenotype confer advantages to tumours, enhancing growth, survival, invasion, and metastasis [14]. Monoclonal antibodies, such as cetuximab, and small molecule tyrosine kinase inhibitors that target the receptor catalytic domain of EGFR, such as gefitinib and erlotinib, have been used clinically in the treatment of non-small-cell lung cancer patients. However, the emergence of mutations in the catalytic kinase domain of the receptor, including the T790M mutation, led to reduced effectiveness of the early targeted therapies in these patients and required new drug molecules to target this mutation [15]. This finding has led to the discovery of new therapies to target the EGFR T790M mutation including osimertinib for the treatment of advanced non-small-cell lung cancer harbouring the EGFR T790M mutation [16].

Table 6.2 highlights a small portion of the drugs that have reached the market across different disease areas with a level of supporting genetic evidence, both prospective and retrospective.

6.3 Genetic Strategies for Target Discovery

As is shown in the PCSK9 example described previously and the data presented by Cook et al. [6] and Nelson et al. [7], using human genetic variation to gain confidence in potential drug targets can be a highly successful approach to identify and provide supporting evidence for selection and prioritization of drug targets. There are different strategies that can be employed to achieve this, and these are evolving with the technologies, analytics, and knowledge within the field.

Table 6.2 Drugs that have reached the market that have some level of supporting genetic evidence.

Drug	Indication	Genetic evidence	Target	Type of evidence
Evolocumab/ alirocumab	Hyperlipidaemia	*PSCK9*	PSCK9	LOF *PCSK9* mutations result in lower LDL-C levels and protect against CHD, whereas GOF *PCSK9* mutations have elevated LDL-C plasma concentration and hypercholestero-lemia
Ustekinumab	Psoriasis	*IL23A, IL23R, IL12B*	IL23/IL12	SNPs in IL12B that encode for p40 subunit are associated with psoriasis susceptibility. IL12 and IL23 share the p40 subunit
Aripiprazole/ risperidone	Schizophrenia	*DRD2*	DRD2	Multiple SNPs in close proximity to dopamine receptor D2 are strongly associated with schizophrenia
Tezacaftor/ ivacaftor	Cystic fibrosis	*CFTR*	CFTR	A mutation in CFTR (deletion at position 508) causes CFTR protein to break down before it can reach the membrane and transport chloride
Secukinumab	Psoriasis	*TRAF31P2*	IL-17	TRAF3P2 encodes IL-17 receptor adapter, and SNPs in TRAF3P2 are associated with psoriasis
Burosumab	X-linked hypophos-phatemia	*PHEX*	FGF23	Patients with mutations in *PHEX* leading to a loss of activity have increased levels of FGF23 and low levels of phosphate
Pegvaliase	Phenylketonuria	*PAH*	PAL	Patients with mutations in PAH leading to loss of activity accumulate phenylalanine
Ruxolitinib	Myelofibrosis	*JAK2*	JAK1/2	GOF mutations in JAK2 underlie myeloproliferative disease

(*continued*)

Table 6.2 (Continued)

Drug	Indication	Genetic evidence	Target	Type of evidence
Avatrombopag/ eltrombopag/ romiplostim	Thrombo-cytopenia	*MPL*	MPL	GOF mutations in MPL lead to the overproduction of abnormal megakaryocytes and an increased number of platelets
Binimetinib/ vemurafenib/ encorafenib	Melanoma	*BRAF*	BRAF/MEK	Mutations in BRAF (V600E or V600K) lead to increased activation/activity towards MEK and increased cancer growth
Romosozumab	Osteoporosis	*SOST*	SOST	Mutations in SOST reduce the levels of functional proteins, leading to excessive bone formation
Belimumab	Systemic lupus erythematosus	*TNFSF13B*	BLyS	Mutation in TNFSF12B (insertion/deletion, GCTGT > A) results in a shorter transcript that escapes microRNA inhibition, increasing levels of soluble BAFF and increased risk for SLE

Note: At the time of writing romosozumab has only been approved in some regions.

6.3.1 GWAS

The sequencing of the human genome in 2003 and the subsequent mapping of relatively common genetic variation into haplotype maps across the genome, by the International HapMap Project, provided the basis for the application of GWASs to identify genes linked to diseases and phenotypic traits [17]. GWASs examine the genetic variation across individuals to determine if any of the variation is associated with a phenotype or a disease. These observational studies take advantage of the natural variation that occurs, with any two human genomes differing in millions of ways. These differences can range from small variations, such as single nucleotide polymorphisms (SNPs) where individual nucleotides are changed, to larger variations, such as deletions where portions of DNA have been lost, insertions where portions of DNA have been added, and copy number variations where sections of the genome have been repeated. Any of these naturally occurring variations can cause changes in a person's phenotype, which can be anything from physical properties such as hair colour to increased or decreased risk of getting a disease [17].

GWASs rely on linkage disequilibrium (LD) in the correlation structure that exists among DNA variants in the human genome as a result of evolution, including finite population size, mutation, recombination rate, and natural selection. The statistical power to detect these associations between genetic variants and a trait depends on the sample size, the distribution of effect sizes of causal genetic variants that are segregating in the population, the frequency of those variants, and the LD between genotyped variants and unknown causal variants [18]. GWASs have been traditionally performed using SNP arrays, which are technologies that query a large but discrete number of validated genetic variants that have proven to have a measurable population frequency, i.e. they are relatively common. These are genotyped in cohorts of cases and controls and statistical approaches used to identify SNPs that associate with the disease trait.

The set-up of GWASs can also influence the loci identified, as comparing cases to controls may be more likely to pull out genes active in early phases of disease, whereas to understand genes that affect prognosis or the course of the disease may require a within-case design, as has been shown with Crohn's disease [19].

It was thought that the application of GWASs to human disease would open the floodgates for the identification of novel drug targets for complex and common diseases. However, it can be considered that the impact of GWASs to inform novel target identification has been disappointing. The reasons for this are varied but include:

1. Lack of specificity: Many GWAS SNPs are located between genes and can be linked to a number of genes and SNPs in a region (via a concept called linkage disequilibrium). This means that in many cases it is difficult to identify not only the causative variant, but which gene(s) are affected by the SNP.
2. Lack of validation/replication: Given the number of SNPs that are queried and the statistical approaches used to analyse the data, large numbers of cases and controls are generally needed to provide the power to detect significant association. In this respect, GWAS has been used to explore common diseases/traits where (relatively) large case control cohorts are available. However, findings have been difficult to replicate, which can partially be explained by the developing understanding that common disease is not necessarily driven by a common variant(s) and that common diseases actually arise from multiple different interacting genes and mechanisms that present with a common phenotype [18]. This means that often there is a heterogeneity, or noise, within the cohorts with multiple genes and mechanisms involved, and GWAS fails to take into account the impact of multiple rare variants across multiple mechanisms. Attempts to address this issue include increasing the cohort size or performing meta-analysis, but both increase the noise within the study and suffer from the problem of lack of consistency and depth in the phenotypic end points studied.
3. Lack of causal relationship: GWASs frequently identify genes 'associated' with a disease or trait, rather than 'causative of'. When SNPs are located between genes, it is difficult to assign causality (as discussed in point 1 [20]).

These issues have been excellently reviewed by Loos [21], who cite the example of the FTO locus, where multiple SNPs in the introns of the FTO gene were shown to be associated with increased body mass. Despite replication in other studies, the actual role of FTO in obesity has yet to be established.

Despite some of the issues, recent advances have enhanced the GWAS approach, which will increase the utility of GWAS in drug discovery. The advent of WGS and associated advances in analytical approaches will likely allow a more accurate approach to GWASs. Being able to query rare and common variants across the genome and to assess the impact of multiple mutations across a gene and within a pathway and to be able to derive polygenic risk scores will allow a deeper understanding of the role of genetics in common and complex diseases.

Methods are improving for functional follow-up of risk variants identified in GWAS, which have allowed for improved filtering and prioritization of variants. The integration of genetic data, with tissue-level gene expression data will further strengthen the utility of this approach. The databases such as GTEx and ENCODE, among others, have provided the opportunity to examine variants and has also highlighted that tissue-specific resources will become increasingly useful [22].

Once the variants that may play a role in disease risk have been identified from GWASs, there still remains a large piece of work to validate these findings, trying to address the gap between the genetic sequence and the phenotypic consequence [18], which will be addressed in depth later in this chapter.

6.3.2 Rare Disease Genetics

With approximately 3 billion base pairs in the human genome, and every individual carrying approximately 35–40 *de novo* mutations, this means that in the 6.7 billion people in the world, every base pair compatible with human life has been knocked out in someone, somewhere in the world [23]. Where this leads to a phenotype of interest and the correct samples can be obtained, it is a relatively easy task to identify the causal gene.

Using rare disease genetics to inform drug discovery is an attractive approach as the gene function perturbations are often stronger and more penetrant than in GWAS, making it easier to assess the functional consequences of the identified rare variants (Figure 6.2). Similarly, rare variants are more likely to be disease specific as broad effects could lead to lethality. The hope is that this approach will open a lens into novel disease mechanisms that have a common disease correlate as well as providing more evidence to support pathways/genes implicated by more common variants identified in GWASs. The work of Nelson also highlighted that targets derived from rare, single-gene Mendelian disorders (OMIM) were likely to be more successful drug targets than those derived from GWAS. This can be explained by the fact these genes are actually causative in driving the disease, so by targeting the gene there is increased likelihood of directly impacting the disease. In UCB this has led to looking for drug targets where nature has done the key target identification and validation experiments for us, i.e. where a mutation in a gene directly leads to a disease.

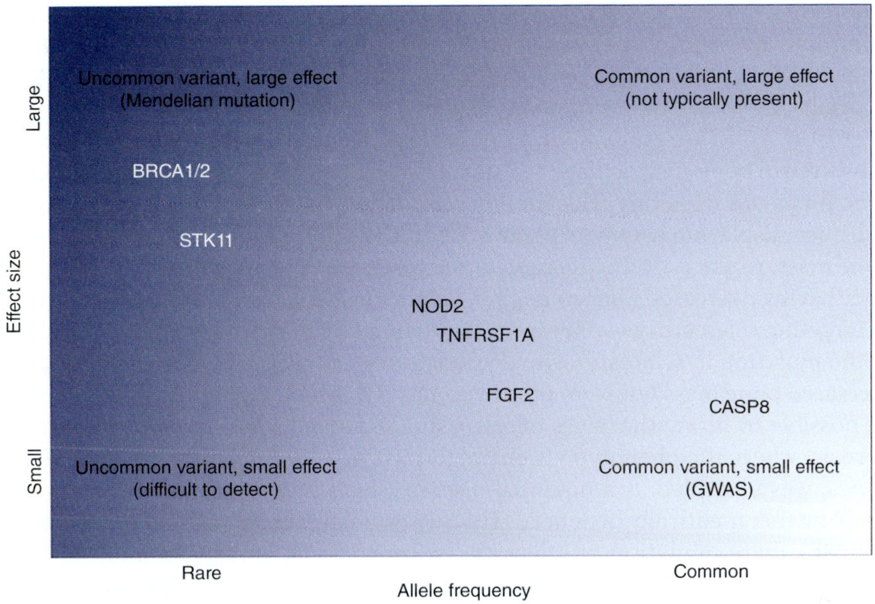

Figure 6.2 GWASs typically identify common variants with small effect sizes (located in lower right), whereas rare disease genetics discovers rare variants with large effect sizes (upper left). Source: Bush and Moore 2012 [24]. Adapted from PLOS.

6.3.2.1 Rare Mutation → Rare Disease Drug Discovery

In terms of drug development, the question arises as to the strategic direction of the company. An economic case can be difficult to make for extreme orphan indications where the costs of drug development could outweigh possible financial returns. However, some cases have been pursued and proven to be viable, such as phenylketonuria (PKU). PKU is a rare inherited disorder affecting approximately 1 in 10–15 000 people caused by mutations in the phenylalanine hydroxylase (PAH) gene, which results in low levels of the phenylalanine hydroxylase enzyme and build-up of phenylalanine in the body, leading over time to toxicity. The effects of the disease can be partially managed by reducing the amount of phenylalanine in the diet, but another treatment strategy was identified to more directly address the defect in PKU patients by replacing the function of the deficient enzyme [25]. Pegvaliase was approved by the FDA in 2018 for PKU patients and is a phenylalanine-degrading enzyme that acts as a substitute for the enzyme that is deficient in PKU.

6.3.2.2 Rare Mutation → Common Disease Drug Discovery

One of the concepts in pursuing rare/extreme phenotypes for target identification is that it will lead researchers into novel mechanisms that may then be translatable to common diseases with phenotypic correlates, opening up larger markets and making the endeavour economically viable. Although this translation from rare to common can prove challenging, many examples do exist. One well-known example of how rare disease genetics can inform drug discovery is the story of sclerostin. A rare autosomal recessive genetic disorder exists called van Buchem syndrome and is prevalent in a specific population in South Africa and is characterized by sclerosteosis, i.e. bone overgrowth and increased bone mass [26]. Crucially, the new bone is of good quality. The mutation in the gene coding for sclerostin, SOST1, results in an LOF of the sclerostin protein, which is mainly expressed in bone and cartilage and normally inhibits bone formation by blocking Wnt/β-catenin signalling. This finding was further validated in mice, with knockout mice displaying a similar phenotype to the sclerosteosis patients with high bone mass, whereas overexpression of sclerostin had the opposite effect, with the mice having decreased bone mass [27]. Further evidence supporting the potential of targeting sclerostin as a therapy was provided by the identification of carriers of the mutation in sclerostin who demonstrated reduced levels of sclerostin and increased bone mass but were otherwise healthy, which highlighted that it could be possible to titrate the levels of sclerostin and avoid safety issues [26]. Osteoporosis, where the phenotype is characterized by reduced bone mass and weak bones, was identified as a potential disease where reducing levels of sclerostin could be therapeutically beneficial. This was validated in animal models of osteoporosis, where inhibition of sclerostin by monoclonal antibodies induced new bone formation and improved bone strength. This has led to the development on an antibody, romosozumab, which at the time of printing is in phase III clinical trials [27].

6.3.3 Somatic Mutations

The ability to deep sequence the genome using WGS approaches, i.e. the ability to generate 100s–1000s of sequences covering the same base pairs, has opened up the ability to explore somatic variants of drivers of disease. Somatic mutations occur *de novo* in specific tissues, rather than germline mutations that are inherited and so are present in all cells in the body. Deep sequencing allows the identification of rare mutations in affected cells against the backdrop of the normal genome in unaffected cells. Although the concept of somatic variants is well established within the oncology space, its utility in other disease is beginning to become appreciated.

Focal cortical dysplasias are a set of highly intractable human epilepsies resulting from focal tissue overgrowth in the regions on the brain. Since many of these patients are referred for surgery as the only remaining treatment option, resected tissue has been available for study, and deep sequencing approaches have identified somatic mutations in a number of genes that are in, and result in overactivity of, the mTOR pathway [28]. This has opened the possibility of now treating epilepsy with inhibitors of the mTOR pathway, as opposed to resorting to more risky surgical approaches. mTOR inhibitors do exist, such as rapamycin and everolimus, but chronic treatment with these drugs presents potential issues [29]. The ability to explore other drivers of this pathway could lead to more efficacious and safer treatment options.

6.3.4 Analytical Approaches

As the costs of next-generation sequencing have dropped and the technology has become more widely accessible, generally the problems now lie not in the generation of data, but in the analysis and then the interpretation of that data. Although outside the scope of this chapter, it is relevant to mention at a high level the analytical approaches that are being developed to address this area.

Analysis techniques for GWAS are now well established and routinely applied. Associations are expected to meet a statistically defined genome-wide significance, corrected for multiple testing, that defines a positive association. Ideally replication should also be presented.

The analysis of rare diseases and extreme phenotypes from WGS data has been an active area of analytical development over the recent years. Many software packages are now publicly available to support these analyses, and there are no hard criteria or set analytical approaches to these areas. Generally individual institutions have their own preferred pipeline and criteria that they apply to the analysis. Within UCB we have developed an automated pipeline (Figure 6.3) that allows us to quantitatively assess a genetic variant against four criteria:

- Frequency/rarity: We do not expect to see the variant represented to any great extent in population reference databases. Similarly any inheritance patterns can be considered in the case of any family history.

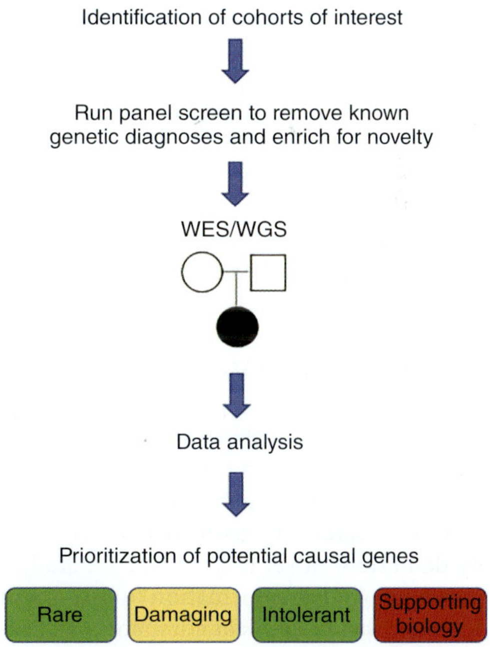

Figure 6.3 Pipeline for identifying and prioritizing mutations. WGS, whole genome sequencing; WES, whole exome sequencing.

- Predicted pathogenicity: Variants are scored for the predicted effect of the variant on gene function using a combination of software.
- Gene intolerance: In general we would expect that the gene is predicted to be intolerant to harbouring and retaining mutations, implying that it has an important biological role and that mutations in the gene would not be evolutionarily tolerated.
- Related biology: In the search for novelty, it is important to get as many pointers as possible to tell us if we are in the correct area with our predictions. To support this a tool was developed internally that provides the ability to look at the pathway and nearest neighbours to the starting gene, apply publicly available data on diseases related to these genes, and use sematic similarity approaches to provide a quantitative measure of phenotypic similarity [30]. An over-representation of genes that share traits with phenotypic similarity to the starting gene gives confidence that your gene is involved in the suspected biology.

Variants are quantitatively scored for each criterion and we apply a prioritization of variants based on an overall assessment of all criteria, as opposed to applying hard cut-offs. This allows us to fully assess the outputs and not dismiss potential candidates. The selection of the preferred genes is then driven through a multidisciplinary team review, with input from the clinicians who know the case, disease area experts, bioinformaticians, and geneticists.

WGS approaches are now being applied to 'common' diseases, complex phenotypes, and quantitative traits. This requires a different set of analytical approaches that support polygenic analysis, i.e. the effects of multiple genes on the phenotype as well as gene and pathway burden analysis, which is the overall mutational burden of rare variants at play within a gene and/or pathway in relation to the phenotype [31]. While the analytical approaches for gene-centric variants are becoming better established, the next challenge will be to develop approaches that support the same amount of rigour for intergenic regions available through WGS.

Finally it is pertinent to mention that this work is *in silico* and the outputs are predictions. The only true way to confirm that the correct gene has been identified is through functional validation (see Section 6.4).

6.4 Functional Validation

In the pharmaceutical industry, a desire to be first on the market is balanced with the desire to be best in class, which often creates a dichotomy in the desired profile for new targets, including those that come from genetics [32]. Furthermore there is a natural tension that exists in the desire to have novel drug targets. By definition, novel targets will generally come with a lack of additional supporting biological information to back them, i.e. an inherent level of uncertainty, whereas pharmaceutical companies want a degree of certainty about potential targets before committing to investments. This is also complicated by the fact that the first outputs from the genetic work are essentially bioinformatically and statistically led hypotheses. All of this together points to the fact that the genes emerging from the discovery phases are the starting point and not the end point and that functional validation is required to prove the hypothesis, establish the link between the gene and a disease mechanism, and then translate that knowledge into a druggable target.

6.4.1 Prioritization of Putative Mutations

The first challenge that exists is the prioritization and selection of emerging genes linked to the biology of interest that have the most promise for successful translation as drug targets. One of the approaches to move forward genetic targets is described by the Pfizer group in the area of schizophrenia where targets are prioritized by annotating a list of potential genes with additional data, including tissue-specific mRNA expression, known functional variation, disease-associated rare mutations, and prior literature knowledge [10]. This is a logical approach as it will prioritize targets with increased confirmation. These will then be further pursued by bringing together multidisciplinary teams with expertise in areas such as specific biology, animal models, partners from toxicology, drug safety, and chemistry, highlighting the benefit of bringing together different disciplines and sets of information to enhance target selection and speed up drug discovery. Starting from an initial 125 SNPs associated with schizophrenia, this process allowed the company to reduce this down to a list of 1–3 targets for potential follow-up.

Even in the situation where well-understood genes/mechanisms emerge from this workflow, the challenges of safety, druggability, and establishing a relevant set of preclinical end points to test the functional consequence and causality of the gene/mechanism in disease persist [10]. The process discussed below (Figure 6.4) is a general workflow of how many companies move from genetic findings to drug targets, though targets with existing validation can move through this process, particularly the validation stage, much more quickly.

6.4.2 Determining Functional Consequence of Mutation

6.4.2.1 Publicly Available Data

Establishing the directional effect that the variant has on the gene and the mechanistic impact are issues faced in the validation process. Access to relevant human patient tissue can provide one method to address this by providing direct data on the functional consequence of the mutation, as has been shown by looking at RNA expression in patient cells [33]. However, for many diseases, it is difficult to access relevant patient tissue (e.g. in the case of disorders of the central nervous system [CNS]), and the functional impact of the mutation may not be equivalent or present in more accessible tissue or fluids.

With the increasing amounts of publicly available datasets and information sharing platforms, examining databases with functional information should be a first port of call. Tools such as GeneMatcher allow the sharing of information that can allow the identification of additional patients with the same mutation and phenotype, which increases the confidence that the initial gene selection was correct. Other publicly accessible databases such as GeneCards, which provides information on human genes, and Kyoto Encyclopedia of Genes and Genomes

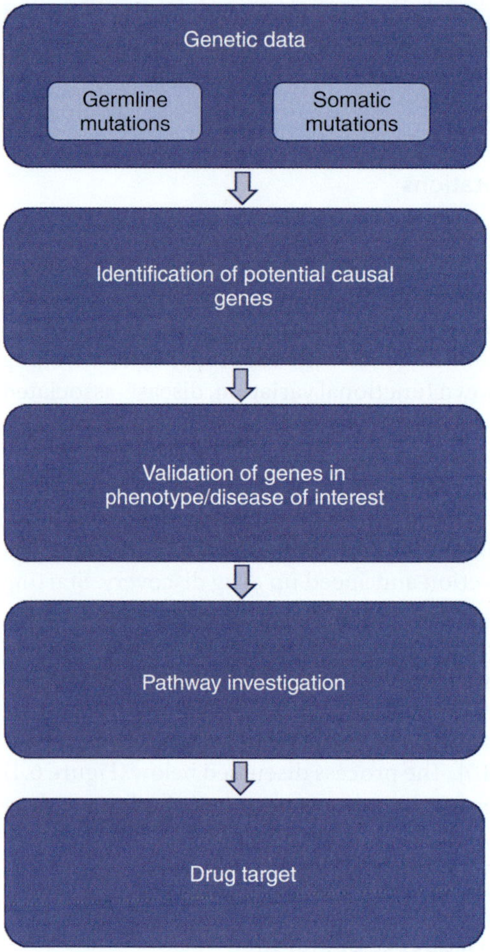

Figure 6.4 Path from generation of genetic data to a potential drug target.

(KEGG), which provides information on cellular functions of genes/proteins, are useful starting resources. Databases of systematic knockout and phenotyping in animal models are available, such as the International Mouse Phenotyping Consortium [34], which can also provide a resource to support gene to mechanism deconvolution.

6.4.2.2 Systems Biology

As the cost of genotyping has decreased, there has been a rapid increase in new genes being discovered that are linked with disease but whose biological function is not well understood, leading to challenges in translating those genes into actionable hypotheses without protein and pathway-level information. One way to move forward is to use systems biology to connect the genomic data to the biology of interest. This concept is exemplified in the psychiatric cell map initiative [35], which focuses on an approach using convergence (Figure 6.5). This framework is built from the concept that diverse biological perturbations that increase risk for a disease are likely to converge mechanistically. In order to facilitate the

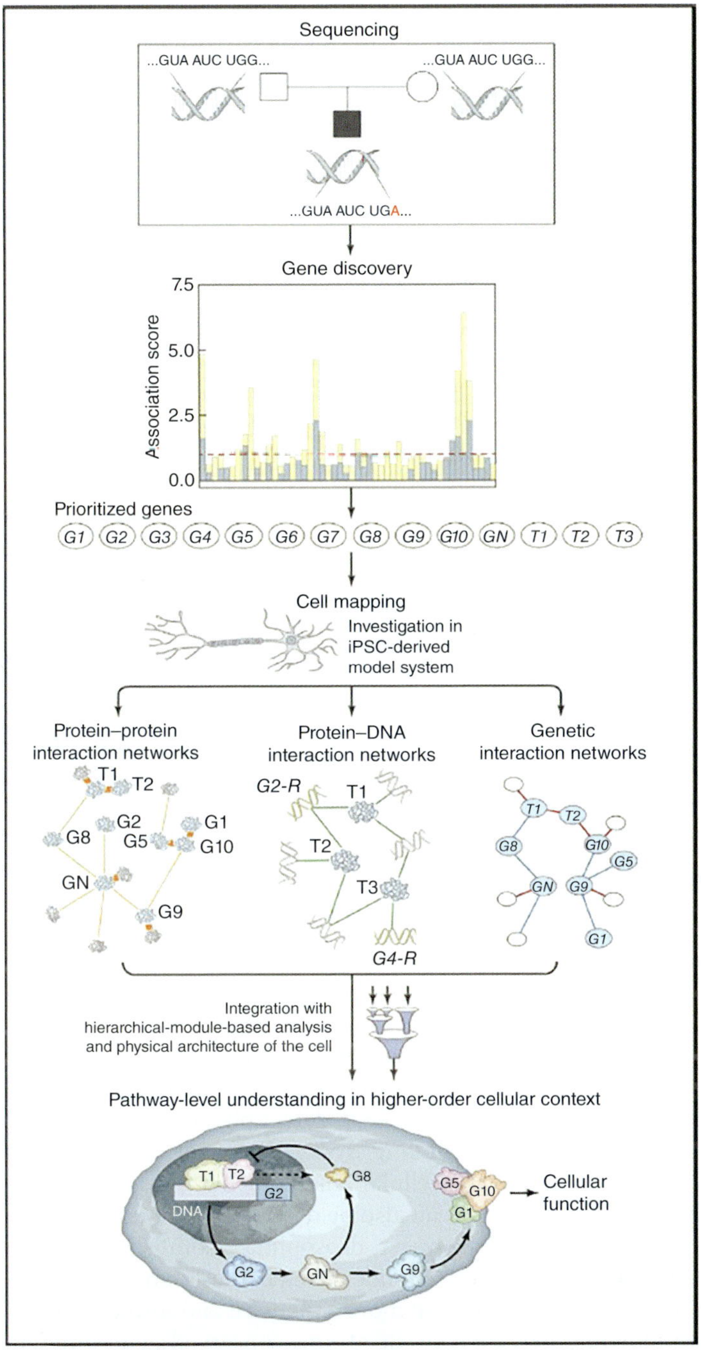

Figure 6.5 Using systems biology to connect genetic data to biology of interest. The first step is generating the data, which can then be prioritized and mapped onto interaction networks (protein/protein, protein/DNA, and genetic) that identify connections and can be integrated to generate pathway-level hypotheses for follow-up. Source: Willsey et al. 2018 [35]. Taken from Elsevier.

interpretation of genomic data, it would be highly useful to be able to put the data into context by placing the mutations into the biological pathways they affect [36, 37]. Another example that highlights the value of systems biology was recent work performed by Srivistava et al. [38], where they developed and validated a predictive framework for drug discovery that combines gene expression data with causal reasoning. Using this system, they were able to predict the tyrosine kinase receptor Csf1R as a potential therapeutic target in epilepsy, which was then validated in *in vivo* epilepsy models [38].

6.4.2.3 Model Systems: 'The Tissue Is the Issue'

While 'generic' databases and systems biology approaches can help to develop and/or strengthen a hypothesis, these do not always hold information on the tissue-specific effect of a specific mutation, which is a common issue when the strategy of pursuing rare/extreme phenotypes is employed. Oftentimes, this requires additional approaches, and there are many models that can be used to dissect the biology and increase confidence (highlighted in Table 6.3), including rescuing the phenotype and recapitulating the patient phenotype in model systems. Rescuing a phenotype is often done by using patient-derived cells with the genetic defect and reintroducing the wild-type version of the gene or overexpressing the gene variant and knocking it down/out. For this approach, there needs to be a phenotype that can be measured that is related to the disease, such as the levels of LDL cholesterol in the case of PCSK9 described earlier.

When patient tissue is difficult to access, as in CNS and cardiac diseases, induced pluripotent stem cell (iPSC) technology now offers an opportunity to create disease-specific models (see Chapter 7 for further details). Either a patient's cells can be taken from an accessible source, such as skin, and reprogrammed into iPSCs that can then be differentiated into the cell type of interest, or a genetically normal iPSC line can be modified to contain the mutant of interest [39]. There are numerous examples of how this has been used to understand the mechanisms underlying disease in disorders caused by single mutations. One area where it has been used with positive impact is in cardiovascular disease where beating cardiomyocytes can be differentiated from iPSCs. To better understand the functional consequence of a mutation underlying familial hypertrophic cardiomyopathy, Lan et al. [39] created patient-specific iPSC-derived cardiomyocytes with the missense mutation (Arg663His) in the MYH7 gene. They were able to detect phenotypes associated with hypertrophic cardiomyopathy, including dysregulation of calcium levels and cycling, contractile arrhythmia, and cellular enlargement.

The functional impact of the variants can also be determined by expression in other model systems, such as cell lines, yeast, drosophila, zebrafish, and mice. These models can provide the greatest confidence that the identified gene is causal in the phenotype of interest, but are more expensive and lower throughput, and a negative outcome may be a result of non-conserved gene function between humans and the model species. An example of how this validation can fit into the workflow was published by a consortium focused on atrial fibrillation [40]. Using GWAS datasets, they were able to identify a number of novel loci, including TBX5, GJA1, NEURL, CAND2, and CUX2 [41]. Both TBX5 and

Table 6.3 Model systems that are used to validate genetic findings, highlighting benefits, and drawbacks of each system.

Models	Benefits	Throughput	Drawbacks
Patients samples	High translatability	Very low	Can be difficult to access, small amounts available
Cell line	Cost effective, easy to use, easy to expand, greater reproducibility than primary cells	Medium to high	Potentially altered phenotype compared to patients/primary cells, reduced translatability
Primary/iPSC	More physiologically relevant, phenotype more similar to patient	Medium	Limited availability, maintenance of phenotype, donor variability
Yeast	Easy to use, simple to manipulate	High	Can be used for only the portion of human genes where orthologue/paralogue exists
Fly	Simple to manipulate, inexpensive for animal model	Medium	Not all human genes are present; some diseases not suitable
Zebrafish	Good for development model, simple manipulation	Low to medium	Not all human genes are present; some diseases not suitable
Mouse	More similar to humans (anatomy, physiology, and genetics), better model for more complex diseases	Low	Not completely translate to human

GJA1 are known to play a role in cardiovascular physiology, so only the three novel genes were taken forward into an embryonic zebrafish model where the candidate genes were knocked down using morpholino oligonucleotides and the fish examined for morphological and functional changes. In this case, of the three genes tested, they found that two of them (NEURL and CAND2) led to increased action potential durations in the zebrafish [41].

6.4.3 Druggability: From Validation of a Gene to a Druggable Target

Translating the prioritized candidates into a drug target and the strategy for drugging the mechanism is very highly context dependent. In its simplest form, once directionality of the effect has been established, direct inhibition of gain-of-function targets and activating, potentiating, or replacing LOF targets is the obvious strategy. Examples of these direct approaches can be found, with the enzyme replacement in the PKU example stated previously as one.

Gain-of-function mutations can be treated by direct inhibition of the protein or by targeting other members of the pathways. An example of how a genetic finding can lead to a therapy that directly targets the cause of the disease is the case of transthyretin-mediated amyloidosis, which is a rare autosomal dominant condition that leads to neurodegeneration. It is caused by a mutation in the TTR gene, which leads to aggregation of misfolded monomers, and affects approximately 50 000 people worldwide [42]. Alnylam developed a short interfering RNA (siRNA) therapeutic that directly interferes in the disease process by blocking production of the protein [43]. Targeting directly downstream of the mutation can also be effective, as seen in cryopyrin-associated periodic syndromes (CAPS). CAPS are three diseases that are caused by mutations in the same gene, *NLRP-3*. Mutations in this gene are gain of function and result in increased levels of activated IL-1B and inflammation. Treatments such as canakinumab, which neutralizes IL1B activity, and rilonacept, which blocks IL1B signalling, are effective [44]. In the case of canakinumab, Novartis took advantage of CAPS to test their lead antibody, as CAPS was a rare disease with a well-defined and understood genetic profile. After efficacy was shown in that system, they were able to move into other diseases that had dysregulation of the same inflammatory process, such as systemic juvenile idiopathic arthritis.

In many cases the identified gene itself may not be a tractable target. Functional genomics and validation approaches can be used to establish the perturbed pathway, and once this is understood, the pathway can be 'walked' to identify a more tractable entry point. Tuberous sclerosis is a rare genetic disorder that is caused by LOF mutations in the TSC1 and two genes. The resulting phenotype of benign tumour growth is driven by activation of the mTOR pathway. In this case Novartis has developed a rapamycin analogue, everolimus, to directly target the mTOR protein [29]. In this way the directly causative gene remains untouched, but the overgrowth is halted.

Even if a set of mutations are found that are clearly linked to disease, it may be considered 'undruggable' for traditional drug discovery. However, other advances in new modalities, such as targeted protein degradation, oligonucleotides, and gene editing, will allow for targets previously considered 'undruggable' to now be taken forward [45].

6.5 Forward-Looking Perspectives

The tools available now to researchers allow a great amount of data to be generated and analysed, yet the field is still in an accelerated rate of evolution. Considering genetics alone, then two highly interrelated approaches, molecular taxonomy and precision medicine, are emerging that warrant mention as those that are likely to have a great impact on the use of genetics in drug discovery and development, as well as advancements in data integration that support these approaches.

6.5.1 Molecular Taxonomy of Disease

As the understanding of the molecular and genomic variations in common disease progresses, incorporating this information into diagnosis and treatment could transform medicine [46]. As a by-product of the increased activity into the genetic basis of disease, there is an increasing ability to define the molecular taxonomy of diseases, i.e. to move away from a phenotypic/clinical descriptor of a disease to a more precise description based on the underlying molecular mechanism driving it. Again, oncology has led the way in this area, where tumours are no longer defined by their location, e.g. lung, breast, etc., but by the molecular mechanism driving it in an individual, e.g. EGFR+ and HER2+. Within the prostate cancer field, studies have been able to identify several recurrent genomic alterations that are involved in primary prostate cancer including mutations, copy number changes, and gene fusions [47]. To achieve this, tumour samples were analysed by pathologists for tumour grading and then characterized by DNA and RNA/miRNA sequencing, DNA methylation arrays, and SNP arrays. This study demonstrated that many genomically distinct subsets of prostate cancer exist and can be used to establish a molecular taxonomy of disease, with 74% of all primary prostate cancers falling into seven distinct molecular classes [36]. However, despite this success, 26% of the tumours were not able to be defined in these classes, implying that there are additional levels of information that may be necessary for full classification.

6.5.2 Precision Medicine

Precision medicine is a rapidly developing approach to treat diseases that aims to take into account the differences between individuals in a population, such as variations in genetics, environment, and lifestyle. The increasing understanding of the molecular taxonomy of disease helps to drive the ability to more precisely design medicines. Again, the cancer field has led the way. The EGFR example was discussed previously but is an excellent example of precision medicine [16, 48]. Another example from the oncology area is in melanomas, where BRAF mutations are present in more than 40% of patients [49]. Great clinical success has been seen with vemurafenib, which inhibits a mutated form of BRAF with a substitution of glutamic acid for valine at codon 600 [50]. Unfortunately, many patients are resistant, highlighting that there may be other drivers of the disease in those patients. As more information has emerged on the complex crosstalk between the RAS/RAF/MEK/ERK signalling pathways, it has been shown that a combination therapy that inhibits both BRAF and MEK is more effective [51].

An example outside of oncology that focuses on the genetic variation between individuals is the new therapies for cystic fibrosis (CF). CF is caused by mutations in the cystic fibrosis transmembrane conductance regulator (CFTR) gene. Over two thousand different mutations have been reported in CFTR, with the result being defects in ion transport that lead to decreased clearance of mucus, increased bacterial colonization, and inflammation [52]. The mutations in CF have been separated into different classes depending on the functional impact of the mutations. Mutations of the CFTR gene in class III produce protein that is trafficked to the cell membrane but do not respond normally. One of the mutations in class III is a glycine-to-aspartic acid missense mutation at codon 551 (G551D), which is located within the nucleotide binding domain. This mutation was found to have decreased nucleotide binding and reduced ATPase activity [53]. Vertex Pharmaceuticals developed ivacaftor, which is now in use for patients who have at least one G551D mutation. Ivacaftor increases the ion function of CFTR, which helps to normalize function of the bronchial epithelial cells in the lungs of patients [54]. This is an example of precision medicine, where the action of drug is specifically tailored to a specific patient population and exemplifies some of the shift seen in drug discovery over recent years, with a shift towards orphan/breakthrough/fast track indications [3].

6.5.3 Data Integration

The challenge discussed earlier in this chapter of correlating the genetic variation back to a phenotype still remains, but the landscape is starting to change. Many of the datasets that have been previously available have minimal clinical data associated with them, which reduces their utility. More recently there has been a move towards establishing cohorts with more complete and deeper clinical phenotype data, allied with genotypic data, such as Genomics England and the UK Biobank, which are broad disease/population resources, to others such as EpiPGX, which are more disease specific (in this case epilepsy). While these resources provide capabilities for the improved interpretation of variants involved in disease, when combined with Mendelian randomization approaches, they also support the potential to identify biomarkers and improve patient stratification.

Increasingly, these activities are seen as precompetitive, and there are now large consortia and public–private partnerships in place to combine datasets and work together to address complex problems and diseases, aiming to enable future drug discovery. As technologies and analytical techniques evolve, the door is opening to a more systematic application to an increasing number of complex diseases and questions. It is unlikely that these diseases will be driven purely by genetics alone and the ability to perform multivariate analysis, combining multiple data types using machine learning approaches, is increasingly being exploited to help us more fully understand disease mechanisms. Examples of this are the EU-funded public–private IMI projects AETIONOMY and PRECISEADS to use integrated analysis and machine learning approaches to define the molecular taxonomy of neurodegenerative and autoimmune diseases, respectively. Other examples are also emerging, as seen in coronary artery disease (CAD), where GWASs have identified large numbers of loci associated with CAD susceptibility. The challenge in this case is that the majority of the identified variants are in non-coding regions and are also co-inherited with hundreds of candidate regulatory variants. By integrating genomic, epigenomic, and transcriptomic profiling of cells and tissues, Miller et al. began to identify causal regulatory variation and understand the mechanisms by which these variants were associated with CAD risk [55].

The application of these approaches beyond oncology is required and underway. The previously described EU-funded IMI projects will lead to an increased understanding of the key drivers of disease and the stratification of 'common diseases' into discrete pathways, which will open up the drug target space for more effective and targeted therapies.

6.6 Conclusion

In order to reverse the decline in R&D productivity, the pharmaceutical industry has to reduce attrition rates and deliver more differentiated therapies. Genetics is a powerful tool that can significantly help to establish proof of causality in humans and provide information on the relative benefit and safety of modifying a target in humans, which can help to gain confidence in a target early, before the large investment of clinical trials has started.

While the evidence points towards genetics having an integral role in shaping a successful drug project, it is in of itself not a guarantee of success in drug discovery, nor can it be considered to be used in isolation. The developments in the field now mean that genetic data can be more efficiently generated and analysed, and this will support its application to drug R&D. New medicines were discovered when the genotypic knowledge was combined with other physiologic knowledge and technical feasibility [56]. However, beyond this there are other factors that need to go into the decision-making criteria, not least commercial viability.

However, as discussed in this chapter, knowledge of the causal gene/or mutation driving a disease rarely provides a clear molecular solution [57]. The need to be able to understand and interpret the data in the correct biological context is key to deriving maximum value from the use of genetics, and the downstream functional validation is crucial. In this context genetics and functional genomics and validation should be considered as a continuum. In fact the bottleneck in the industry today lies not in the ability to identify the genes, but being able to act on these in an efficient and pragmatic way and to build data packages that support uptake and investment as drug targets. In order to overcome this bottleneck, UCB and others have made a strategic investment in acquiring access to the required technologies to allow us to achieve this. It is anticipated that as these approaches and platforms are applied more systematically across our drug R&D pipeline, then they will help address the major challenges of attrition and differentiation.

References

1 Plenge, R.M. (2016). Disciplined approach to drug discovery and early development. *Sci. Transl. Med.* 8 (349): 349ps15.
2 Plenge, R.M., Scolnick, E.M., and Altschuler, D. (2013). Validating therapeutic targets through human genetics. *Nat. Rev. Drug Discov.* 12: 581–594.
3 Deloitte Centre for Health Solutions (2017) A New Future for R&D? Measuring the return from innovation 2017 www2.deloitte.com/content/dam/

Deloitte/uk/Documents/life-sciences-health-care/deloitte-uk-measuring-roi-pharma.pdf (accessed 12 December 2018).
4 Schulze, U., Ringel, M., Panier, V., and Baedeker, M. (2017). Value of 2016 FDA drug approvals: reversion to the mean? *Nat. Rev. Drug Discov.* 16: 78.
5 Hughes, J.P., Rees, S., Kalindjian, S.B., and Philpott, K.L. (2011). Principles of early drug discovery. *Br. J. Pharmacol.* 162 (6): 1239–1249.
6 Cook, D., Brown, D., Alexander, R. et al. (2014). Lessons learned from the fate of AstraZeneca's drug pipeline: a five-dimensional framework. *Nat. Rev. Drug Discov.* 13: 419–431.
7 Nelson, M.R., Tipney, H., Painter, J.L. et al. (2015). The support of human genetic evidence for approved drug indications. *Nat. Genet.* 47 (8): 856–860.
8 Business Wire® www.businesswire.com/news/home/20050309005392/en/IMS-Health-Reports-2004-Global-Pharmaceutical-Sales (accessed 12 December 2018).
9 Thomsen, S.K. and Gloyn, A.L. (2017). Human genetics as a model for target validation: finding new therapies for diabetes. *Diabetologia* 60 (6): 960–970.
10 Schubert, C.R., Xi, H.S., Wendland, J.R., and O'Donnell, P. (2014). Translating human genetics into novel treatment targets for schizophrenia. *Neuron* 84 (3): 537–541.
11 Wu, N.Q. and Li, J.J. (2014). PCSK9 gene mutations and low-density lipoprotein cholesterol. *Clin. Chimi. Acta* 431: 148–153.
12 Abifadel, M., Varret, M., Rabes, J.P. et al. (2003). Mutations in PCSK9 cause autosomal dominant hypercholesterolemia. *Nat Genet.* 34 (2): 154–156.
13 Kotowski, I.K., Pertsemlidis, A., Luke, A. et al. (2006). A spectrum of *PCSK9* alleles contributes to plasma levels of low-density lipoprotein cholesterol. *Am. J. Hum. Genet.* 78 (3): 410–422.
14 Irmer, D., Funk, J.O., and Blaukat, A. (2007). EGFR kinase domain mutations –
functional impact and relevance for lung cancer therapy. *Oncogene* 26 (39): 5693–5701.
15 Kobayashi, S., Boggon, T.J., Dayaram, T. et al. (2005). EGFR mutation and resistance of non-small-cell lung cancer to gefitinib. *N. Engl. J. Med.* 352 (8): 786–792.
16 Finlay, M.R., Anderton, M., Ashton, S. et al. (2014). Discovery of a potent and selective EGFR inhibitor (AZD9291) of both sensitizing and T790M resistance mutations that spares the wild type form of the receptor. *J. Med. Chem.* 57 (20): 8249–8267.
17 Manolio, T.A. (2010). Genome-wide association studies and assessment of the risk of disease. *N. Engl. J. Med.* 363 (2): 166–176.
18 Visscher, P.M., Wray, N.R., Zhang, Q. et al. (2017). 10 years of GWAS discovery: biology, function and translation. *Am. J. Hum. Genet.* 101 (1): 5–22.
19 Verstockt, B., Smith, K.G.C., and Lee, J.C. (2018). Genome-wide association studies in Crohn's disease: past, present, and future. *Clin. Transl. Immunol.* 7 (1): e1001.
20 Gallagher, M.D. and Chen-Plotkin, A.S. (2018). The post-GWAS era: from association to function. *Am. J. Hum. Genet.* 102 (5): 717–730.

21 Loos, R.J.F. and Yeo, G.S.H. (2014). The bigger picture of *FTO* – the first GWAS-identified obesity gene. *Nat. Rev. Endocrinol.* 10 (1): 51–61.
22 GTEx Consortium (2017). Genetic effects on gene expression across human tissues. *Nature* 550: 204–213.
23 Schendure, J. and Akey, J.M. (2015). The origins, determinants, and consequences of human mutations. *Science* 349 (6255): 1478–1483.
24 Bush, W.S. and Moore, J.H. (2012). Chapter 10: Genome-wide association studies. *PLoS Comput. Biol.* 8 (12): e1002822.
25 Al Hafid, N. and Christodoulou, J. (2015). Phenylketonuria: a review of current and future treatments. *Transl. Pediatr.* 4 (4): 304–317.
26 Yavropoulou, M.P., Xygonakis, C., Lolou, M. et al. (2014). The sclerostin story: from human genetics to the development of novel anabolic treatment for osteoporosis. *Hormones* 13 (4): 323–337.
27 Suen, P.K. and Qin, L. (2016). Sclerostin, an emerging therapeutic target for treating osteoporosis and osteoporotic fracture: a general review. *J. Orthop. Translat.* 4: 1–13.
28 Ribierre, T. and Baulac, S. (2016). mTOR pathway in familial focal epilepsies. *Oncotarget* 8 (4): 5674–5675.
29 Franz, D.N., Belousova, E., Sparagana, S. et al. (2014). Everolimus for subependymal giant cell astrocytoma in patients with tuberous sclerosis complex. *Lancet* 15 (13): 1513–1520.
30 Godard, P. and Page, M. (2016). PCAN: phenotype consensus analysis to support disease-gene association. *BMC Bioinformatics* 17 (1): 518.
31 Wray, N.R. and Gratten, J. (2018). Sizing up whole-genome sequencing studies of common diseases. *Nat. Genet.* 50: 635–637.
32 Jones, L. (2016). An industry perspective on drug target validation. *Expert Opin. Drug Discov.* 11 (7).
33 Kremer, L.S., Bader, D.M., and Prokisch, H. (2017). Genetic diagnosis of Mendelian disorders via RNA sequencing. *Nat. Commun.* 8: 15824.
34 Koscielny, G., Yaikhom, G., Iyer, V. et al. (2014). The International Mouse Phenotyping Consortium Web Portal, a unified point of access for knockout mice and related phenotyping data. *Nucleic Acids Res.* 42: D802–D809.
35 Willsey, J., Morris, M.T., Wang, S. et al. (2018). The psychiatric cell map initiative: a convergent systems biological approach to illuminating key molecular pathways in neuropsychiatric disorders. *Cell* 174: 505–520.
36 Krogan, N.J., Lippman, S., Agard, D.A. et al. (2015). The cancer cell map initiative: defining the hallmark networks of cancer. *Mol. Cell* 58 (4): 690–698.
37 Greene, C.S. and Voight, B.F. (2016). Pathway and Network-based strategies to translate genetic discoveries into effective therapies. *Hum. Mol. Genet.* 25 (2): 94–98.
38 Srivistava, P.K., van Eyll, J., Godard, P. et al. (2018). A systems-level framework for drug discovery identifies Csf1R as an anti-epileptic drug target. *Nat. Commun.* 9 (3561).
39 Lan, F., Lee, A.S., Liang, P. et al. (2013). Abnormal calcium handling properties underlie familial hypertrophic cardiomyopathy pathology in patient-specific induced pluripotent stem cells. *Cell Stem Cell* 12 (1): 101–113.

40 Sinner, M.F., Ellinor, P.T., Meitinger, T. et al. (2011). Genome-wide association studies of atrial fibrillation: past, present, and future. *Cardiovasc. Res.* 89 (4): 701–709.
41 Sinner, M.F., Tucker, N.R., Lunetta, K.L. et al. (2014). Integrating genetic, transcriptional, and functional analyses to identify five novel genes for atrial fibrillation. *Circulation* 130 (15): 1225–1235.
42 Adams, D., Cauquil, C., Labeyrie, C. et al. (2016). TTR kinetic stabilizers and TTR gene silencing: a new era in therapy for familial amyloidotic polyneuropathies. *Exp. Opin. Pharmacother.* 17 (6): 791–802.
43 Suhr, O.B., Coelho, T., Buades, J. et al. (2015). Efficacy and safety of patisiran for familial amyloidotic polyneuropathy: a phase II multi-dose study. *Orphanet. J. Rare Dis.* 10: 109.
44 Church, L.D. and McDermott, M.F. (2009). Canakinumab, a fully-human mAb against IL-1beta for the potential treatment of inflammatory disorders. *Curr. Opin. Mol. Ther.* 11 (1): 81–89.
45 Valeur, E., Gueret, S.M., Adihou, H. et al. (2017). New modalities for challenging targets in drug discovery. *Angew. Chem. Int. Ed.* 56 (35): 10294–10323.
46 Kola, I. and Bell, J. (2011). A call to reform the taxonomy of human disease. *Nat. Rev. Drug Discov.* 10: 641–642.
47 The Cancer Genome Atlas Research Network (2016). The molecular taxonomy of primary prostate cancer. *Cell* 163 (4): 1011–1025.
48 Wang, S., Cang, S., and Delong, L. (2016). Third-generation inhibitors targeting *EGFR* T790M mutation in advanced non-small cell lung cancer. *J. Hematol. Oncol.* 9: 34.
49 Senft, D., Leiserson, M.D.M., Ruppin, E., and Ronai, Z.A. (2017). Precision oncology: the road ahead. *Trends Mol. Med.* 23 (10): 874–898.
50 Chapman, P.B., Hauschild, A., Robert, C. et al. (2011). Improved survival with Vemurafenib in melanoma with BRAF V600E mutation. *N. Engl. J. Med.* 364: 2507–2516.
51 Eroglou, Z. and Ribas, A. (2016). Combination therapy with BRAF and MEK inhibitors for melanoma: latest evidence and place in therapy. *Ther. Adv. Med. Oncol.* 8 (1): 48–56.
52 Lavelle, G.M., White, M.M., Browne, N. et al. (2016). Animal models of cystic fibrosis pathology: phenotypic parallels and divergences. *Biomed. Res. Int.* 2016: 5258727.
53 Logan, J., Hiestand, D., Daram, P. et al. (1994). Cystic fibrosis transmembrane conductance regulator mutations that disrupt nucleotide binding. *J. Clin. Invest.* 94 (1): 228–236.
54 Condren, M.E. and Bradshaw, M.D. (2013). Ivacaftor: a novel gene-based therapeutic approach for cystic fibrosis. *J. Pediatr. Pharmacol. Ther.* 18 (1): 8–13.

55 Miller, C.L., Pjanic, M., Wang, T. et al. (2016). Integrative functional genomics identifies regulatory mechanisms at coronary artery disease loci. *Nat. Commun.* 8 (7): 12092.

56 Bai, J.P.F., Melas, I.N., Hur, J., and Guo, E. (2017). Advances in omics for informed pharmaceutical research and development in the era of systems medicine. *Exp. Opin. Drug Discov.* 13 (1).

57 Swinney, D.C. and Xia, S. (2014). The discovery of medicines for rare disease. *Future Med. Chem.* 6 (9): 987–1002.

7

Elucidating Target Biology and Drug Mechanism of Action Across Human Cell-Based Model Systems

John C. Dawson and Neil O. Carragher

The University of Edinburgh, Cancer Research UK Edinburgh Centre, MRC Institute of Genetics and Molecular Medicine, Crewe Road South, Edinburgh, Scotland, EH4 2XR, United Kingdom

7.1 Introduction

Recent analysis of drug approval rates between 2003 and 2011 indicates that, across all human therapeutic areas, approximately, only 10% of drug candidates that undergo initial clinical evaluation in phase I trials are successful in transitioning through further phases of clinical development to complete regulatory approval [1]. This data is consistent with a previous retrospective study conducted on clinical trial data collected between 1991 and 2000 indicating a similar success rate of 11% from first-in-human studies to drug approval [2]. Given that the approximately 90% of all candidate drugs failing during clinical development represent the most promising drug candidates developed by the biopharmaceutical industry, which have cost many years of scientific research effort and billions of dollars of investment, such high failure rates highlight the limitation of current preclinical drug discovery models to predict clinical success. Identifying the underlying causes of attrition during clinical development is key to evolving preclinical drug discovery and drug development models towards greater clinical success rates. High attrition across clinical development programs is a consequence of multiple contributing factors, which include but are not limited to the following: (i) suboptimal pharmacokinetics and absorption, distribution, metabolism, and excretion (ADME), (ii) lack of sufficient safety and efficacy, (iii) competing commercial interests, (iv) market competition, and (v) patent protection expiry. As the drug discovery process has evolved, the number of failures of small molecule drug candidates due to poor pharmacokinetic profiles appears to have diminished in recent years; however, this has been accompanied by a shift towards increased failure rates due to efficacy and safety issues [3]. While control and optimization of physicochemical properties of candidate drugs is clearly important with regard to achieving clinical success, significant progress has been made in this area, and recent analysis suggests that current drug discovery strategies mitigate for such issues and further optimization in this regard may be unlikely to have a significant effect on attrition in clinical development [3]. Overall, analysis indicates that further evolution of the drug

Target Discovery and Validation: Methods and Strategies for Drug Discovery,
First Edition. Edited by Alleyn T. Plowright.

discovery process is required to address the most pertinent issue of predicting safety and efficacy-related failures in the clinic [1, 2, 4, 5].

Further in-depth analysis across clinical development stages indicated that compared with commercial decisions not to file for approval (18%) and lack of clinical efficacy (54%), safety was least likely to cause attrition in phase III (9%), perhaps due to significant adverse events identified earlier in drug development [1]. A number of areas have also begun to address predictive toxicology in preclinical drug discovery using *in silico*, functional, and comparative genomic approaches [6]. In addition, recent developments in primary and induced pluripotent stem cell (iPSC)-derived human hepatocyte cell culture models, following iterative testing and optimization, confirm their ability to predict many cases of drug-induced liver injury observed in the clinic [7–9]. Similar approaches using stem cell-derived cardiomyocytes to engineer novel two-dimensional (2D) and three-dimensional (3D) cardiac tissue provide new integrated physiological models for assessing multiple cardiotoxic liabilities [10–12]. In contrast to the development of more robust evaluations of physicochemical properties and safety assessment during preclinical development, the evolution of preclinical models that more effectively predict clinical efficacy of novel therapeutic targets and drug candidates is lagging behind. This failure to make any significant improvements in prediction of clinical efficacy may in part be due to the complexity and lack of understanding of many human diseases combined with an over reliance on traditional approaches and established preclinical models, which while optimized for speed and cost poorly predict clinical response [13]. In many complex diseases broad heterogeneity of disease mechanism between distinct patients also contributes to high attrition in clinical development. Such heterogeneity highlights the needs for personalized medicine strategies, which utilize predictive biomarkers to stratify patient subgroups, which are most likely to respond to targeted therapy. Advances in next-generation sequencing (NGS) and classification of patients into molecularly defined subgroups, *in vitro* pharmacogenomics studies across well-characterized human-derived cell line or organoid panels, and the design of clinical diagnostic tests that evaluate the abundance or activation state of therapeutic targets all support personalized medicine strategies. Further development of predictive biomarkers at genetic, proteomic, metabolomic, and phenotypic levels to enable in-depth characterization of individual patient disease combined with development of the necessary computational and statistical approaches to integrate such data into a predictive score that will inform the most appropriate treatment course represents emerging areas of personalized medicine.

Analysis of specific therapy areas indicates that oncology is a particularly challenging area for drug development with only one in eight drugs entering clinical development in phase I achieving US Food and Drug Administration (FDA) approval and a 1 in 15 success rate when these candidate drugs are under evaluation in secondary oncology indications [1]. Regulatory approval of drug candidates is one measure of success of the drug discovery and development process; however, the impact that approved drugs have on patient survival and quality of life and the sustainability of healthcare provision across the wider patient population perhaps represent more important success metrics. Further meta-analyses of clinically meaningful efficacy on some of the most commonly used approved drugs have found that efficacy was often established based on surrogate outcomes in clinical trials and not on more relevant patient-oriented outcomes [14]. This analysis further highlights that a significant proportion of approved medications demonstrate relatively little efficacy with only 11 out of 17 of them showing a minimal clinically important difference [14]. A further study concentrated upon the analysis of 48 cancer drugs approved by the European Medicines Agency (EMA) between 2009 and 2013 across 68 cancer indications [15]. Clinical efficacy was determined by the European Society for Medical Oncology Magnitude of Clinical Benefit Scale (ESMO-MCBS). The results of this study reported that of 68 cancer indications with EMA approval, and with a median of 5.4 years follow-up (minimum 3.3 years, maximum 8.1 years), only 35 (51%) demonstrated a significant improvement in survival or quality of life, while 33 (49%) remained uncertain. Of 23 indications associated with a survival benefit that could be scored with the ESMO-MCBS tool, the benefit was judged to be clinically meaningful in less than half (11/23, 48%) [15].

These results starkly highlight current limitations and challenges in predicting which drugs and which drug targets will translate into clinically meaningful efficacy. The evolution of many complex human diseases has generated multiple biological redundancies in the genetics, pathway signalling, and pathophysiology of disease progression, thus counteracting the efficacy of new targeted therapeutics. Many of the complexities in the molecular pathology of human disease are now becoming elucidated and catalogued by advances in the application and bioinformatics analysis of NGS data acquired on individual patients. In cases of single gene disorders and mechanistic investigation of rare disorders, NGS has successfully identified specific genes or candidate gene variants associated with the clinical condition, thereby providing valuable information to inform the design of new specific therapies, biomarkers, and preclinical disease models [16]. The application of such clinical data to inform preclinical drug discovery strategies is often referred to as 'reverse translation' or 'back-translation' of clinical findings (e.g. Genome Wide Association Studies [GWAS], multi-omics analyses) into preclinical models, and this topic is discussed further in Chapter 6.

In more complex multifactorial and heterogeneous diseases, however, elucidation of the key therapeutic targets and reverse engineering of relevant disease models is not so simple. For example, whole genome sequencing of many solid tumours has revealed remarkable molecular heterogeneity and adaptation within and between patients presenting substantial challenges to the identification and prediction of targeted therapeutic strategies, which will eradicate or significantly alter the course of disease progression. Tumours may have many somatic mutations, not all of them are driver mutations, and the majority are in fact 'passenger' mutations that do not contribute to primary tumour pathogenicity or inform drug target hypotheses. However, these passenger mutations may confer additional survival advantages under the selective pressures of drug treatment and promote clonal evolution during therapy, providing opportunities for drug resistance to occur [17]. The optimal therapeutic strategy for treating complex heterogeneous disease remains unclear; strategies that target molecularly well-defined patient subgroups to guide personalized medicine, have the potential to be pathway independent, or form a component part of multi-targeted drug combination therapy may help overcome this complexity. Thus predicting the key therapeutic targets underpinning clinical outcomes in complex heterogeneous disease requires thorough analysis that embrace disease heterogeneity and can place drug mechanism of action (MOA) or individual target activity within the context of complex high-dimensional genetic, transcriptomic, and proteomic pathway datasets. This systems-level approach to understanding target biology within the disease-relevant context is becoming realized with new advances in human cell-based assay technologies, which can integrate with advances in molecular biology and bioinformatics to guide target validation studies [18, 19].

In this article we outline several recent state-of-the-art advances in functional biology tools and methodology and how they combine with new developments in human cell-based disease models to support a more comprehensive and informative analysis of target activity and drug MOA at phenotypic and pathway levels. We discuss how these platforms begin to address the significant challenges associated with disease complexity and the lack of biological understanding underpinning many disease areas of unmet therapeutic need. By recapitulating the biological complexity and uncertainties of human disease, we describe how these new advances are enabling a more empirical, evidence-led approach to functional target identification and validation under appropriate context. Finally, we describe how data provided from new phenotypic and pathway profiling technologies in human cell-based models can complement and combine with other emerging technologies including bioinformatics, chemoinformatics, chemical proteomics, and emerging computational methods to build a new robust systems analysis, which leverages more relevant and informative approaches for validation of novel therapeutic targets for human disease.

7.2 Advances in Human Cell-Based Model Development

Despite increasing research and development investments in the biopharmaceutical industry resulting in greater numbers of higher quality drug candidates, many of the most common human disorders (Alzheimer's, motor neuron diseases, solid tumours) remain unmet areas of urgent therapeutic need. In such diseases many promising new drug candidates developed using well-established preclinical models to demonstrate proof of concept did not demonstrate clinical efficacy. These observations highlight a critical gap in preclinical tests, which effectively predict clinical outcomes.

Preclinical drug discovery is currently undergoing a renaissance thanks to the convergence of a number of new breakthrough technologies that enable comprehensive evaluations of target biology and drug MOA under more physiologically relevant human cell and tissue context. These breakthrough technologies include iPSC models, clustered regularly interspaced short palindromic repeats and CRISPR-associated protein 9 (CRISPR/Cas) genome editing, 3D *ex vivo* tissue, and organoid models derived directly from patient samples coupled with new

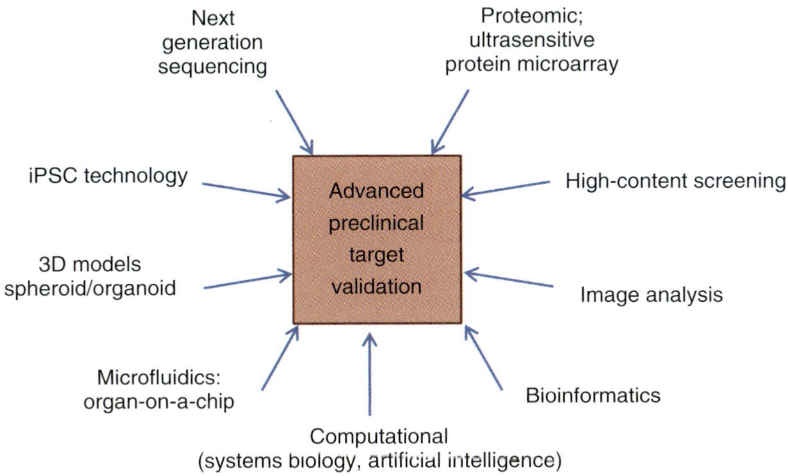

Figure 7.1 Convergence of new technologies to advance preclinical target validation. New technologies which are well placed to support an evidence-led platform for target validation and drug mechanism of action studies under more disease-relevant and information-rich context.

microfluidic and organ-on-a-chip devices. In addition, ever more sophisticated imaging and image analysis tools to capture complex disease phenotypes and new advances in ultrasensitive genomic and proteomic platforms linked to sophisticated bioinformatics machine learning and new evolving theoretical and technical advances in computational and artificial intelligence approaches for exploiting complex datasets are transforming this area (Figure 7.1). Such key breakthrough technologies are well placed to enhance target validation and drug MOA studies in a more disease-relevant and information-rich context with a view to more accurately predicting clinical efficacy. These technologies and their relevance to target validation and drug discovery are further outlined below.

7.2.1 Next-Generation Sequencing (NGS)

As previously discussed the increasingly widespread application of NGS profiling of human populations, specific patient cohorts and clinical biopsy specimens has transformed our understanding of the genetic basis of many complex diseases [16]. Recent genomic sequencing analyses of pancreatic cancer patient samples have revealed a complex mutational landscape with four common oncogenic events in well-known cancer genes (KRAS, TP53, SMAD4, and CDKN2A) in most pancreatic cancers and a low prevalence for mutations in gene products that are readily targetable through conventional therapeutic modalities [20]. This may explain the failure of the majority of clinical trials to show any meaningful survival benefit in pancreatic cancer, except in small patient subgroups [21]. Similarly, whole genome sequencing of oesophageal cancer patient biopsies illustrates a highly heterogeneous disease characterized by frequent large-scale genomic rearrangements, copy number alterations, and co-amplification of multiple receptor tyrosine kinases and mitogenic signalling pathways with limited number of mutations in actionable oncogenic drivers, which lie outwith the tumour suppressor protein family [22]. However, mutational signatures reveal three distinct molecular subtypes of oesophageal adenocarcinoma, which may help guide future patient stratification if effective and well-characterized therapeutic classes can be identified [22]. This new knowledge on the molecular basis of diseases can be used to guide the selection and design of new human cell line panels and organoid models, which represent the heterogeneity of disease for target validation studies and profiling the selectivity of hit compounds from compound screens. In addition new advances in precise genome editing (e.g. CRISPR) allow the custom design of isogenic models representing specific mutations and clinical subtypes of disease. Testing target hypotheses in such well-controlled isogenic cell line models provide robust evidence of genetic susceptibilities to target intervention that can help guide subsequent disease positioning and patient selection strategies that aim to maximize clinical response rates.

7.2.2 CRISPR Genome Editing

The discovery and development of CRISPR/Cas9 technology, as a highly efficient, fast, and low-cost gene editing tool applicable across many mammalian cell systems has opened up new avenues for developing cheaper, faster, and more translatable *in vitro* and *in vivo* models of human diseases [23, 24]. As already described applications of CRISPR include design of genetically engineered cell panels that incorporate specific driver mutations of disease and/or represent the complex heterogeneity of multiple genetic mutations associated with disease within individual patients or between distinct patients. The precise nature of the CRISPR editing also enables 'knockout' and 'knock-in' of catalytically inactive putative therapeutic targets in human cells. In addition, modified versions of the CRISPR/Cas9 system have also been developed, which recruit inducible transcriptional co-regulators that selectively activate or repress target genes [25]. Thus CRISPR gene editing can directly test the functional impact of different therapeutic targeting strategies including inhibition of enzyme activity, destabilization of protein levels, or activation of transcription across high-quality human and animal *in vitro* and *in vivo* models with high levels of precision and efficiency not previously possible. For more information on CRISPR, see Chapter 9.

7.2.3 Induced Pluripotent Stem Cell Biology

Although primary human and patient-derived *ex vivo* and organoid models are considered to be highly disease relevant for target validation and drug testing studies, the availability of the relevant tissue is a limiting factor for studying many human diseases, most notably neurodegenerative, liver, and cardiac disorders. In addition, the ability to scale up and expand primary tissue-derived models while still maintaining the relevant, genomic, epigenetic, and tissue architecture of the original tissue also remains a substantial challenge [26]. A major breakthrough in the ability to develop multiple tissue type-specific human cell-based models, including patient-derived cell assays at scale, has been achieved through the development of iPSC technology [27]. Human iPSC models exhibit several advantages over immortalized cell lines as a platform for target validation and drug testing. iPSCs can be derived from any patient in unlimited quantities and can be reprogrammed into many different tissue-specific cell types. They can represent normal healthy or diseased primary cells with a mostly stable genotype compared to transformed cell lines, and they possess an intrinsic capacity for self-renewal, facilitating their propagation and expansion for preclinical testing. Importantly, iPSCs are amenable to detailed genetic analysis and *in vitro* phenotypic characterization and also to new gene editing (CRISPR) technologies. Thus iPSC models provide a new exciting opportunity for modelling human disease *in vitro* and directly linking phenotype to genotype and validation of target hypotheses under appropriate species and tissue context [28].

7.2.4 3D Cell and Organoid Models

The most common approaches for culturing cells and modelling disease *in vitro* using cell-based assays are dependent on traditional 2D cell culture protocols. Such 2D cell culture methods were originally developed for convenience and low costs and have a number of disadvantages including poor representation of mechanical forces exerted on cells *in vivo*; inaccurate recapitulation of exposure to nutrients, oxygen, and ions and drug exposures within tissues; and compromised cell–cell and cell–extracellular matrix (ECM) interactions relative to *in vivo* tissue. Many options for new 3D *in vitro* and *ex vivo* models that better represent *in vivo* tissue biology are rapidly emerging as a consequence of new developments in *ex vivo* tissue culture, biomaterial scaffolds, and cell culture consumables that all support 3D cell culture [29]. Such developments include organoids that maintain stem cell and other primary tissue microenvironment niche factors to sustain *ex vivo* tissue cultures, which self-organize into 3D mini-organs [30, 31]. Organoids can be generated from both healthy and disease tissues providing opportunities to model normal human tissue homeostasis and disease pathology. With particular relevance to target discovery, target validation, and drug discovery applications, organoids can be expanded indefinitely while faithfully maintaining genomic stability and tissue identity. Organoid cultures are compatible with many functional cell biology techniques including CRISPR genome editing, compound library screening, and image-based phenotypic analysis to support target validation studies within appropriate 3D tissue and genomic context [32]. Recently, the development of a panel of patient-derived oesophageal adenocarcinoma (OAC) organoid cultures has been demonstrated to recapitulate the complex morphology and genomic and transcriptomic heterogeneity of OAC disease and has been applied to medium-throughput screening to reveal new therapeutic targets [33]. In another example, a 96-well human iPSC-derived cardiac organoid assay was utilized to optimize environmental parameters, including ECM, metabolic substrate, and growth factor conditions, which enhance cardiac tissue, viability, and function to create a new model system and uncover novel therapeutic strategies for cardiovascular disease [34]. Significant developments have taken place in 3D mono-cell culture and multicellular culture to create 3D spheroid microtissues, which are readily compatible with both custom design and standard multi-well plates, fluorescent reporters, and microscopic imaging techniques of phenotypic response [13] (Figure 7.2). Such spheroid cultures recapitulate 3D cell–cell communication, poor drug penetration, and hypoxic microenvironments within tissue [35]. Recent development of oligocortical spheroids derived from human iPSCs that demonstrate molecular and phenotypic features consistent with maturing oligodendrocytes and myelination of neurons provides a new *in vitro* platform for the discovery and validation of new therapeutic targets for demyelinating neurodegenerative conditions such as multiple sclerosis [36].

The application of 3D scaffolds incorporating different types of natural or synthetic biomaterials for cell culture each has their own advantages and limitations. Biologically derived 3D scaffold materials or natural hydrogels commonly include ECM proteins such as collagen, laminin, fibrin, and hyaluronic acid and *in vivo* derived ECM preparations such as Matrigel, which readily interact with cell–ECM receptors such as integrins to recapitulate cell–ECM communication observed *in vivo* [37]. Synthetically derived matrices, including polyvinyl alcohol (PVA), polylactide-co-glycolide (PLG), polycaprolactone (PLA), and polyethylene glycol (PEG) hydrogels, provide additional advantages in scalability and batch control and also offer more flexibility for tuning chemical composition and mechanical properties to more accurately recapitulate different tissue types and physiological and pathophysiological conditions such as muscle contraction and fibrosis [38]. The poor penetration and perfusion of drugs into 3D *in vitro* models can present limitations for drug testing and screening, but it also presents new opportunities to mimic fibrotic and poorly vascularized tissues associated with several diseases in which poor drug perfusion contributes to poor clinical efficacy [39, 40]. Such models can then be used to explore new therapeutic strategies and targets that promote drug perfusion [41]. Thus, culturing cells in 3D *in vitro* models can support the formation of multicellular tissue architectures and cell–cell and cell–ECM biochemical signalling that are more similar to *in vivo* settings and that support more accurate multicellular differentiation and function for preclinical testing.

7.2.5 Microfluidic and Organ-on-a-Chip Devices

Although the advantages of 3D model systems over 2D cell culture systems in terms of physiological and disease relevance are apparent, many established and emerging 3D models still exhibit significant limitations with regard to both utility for robust drug discovery applications and ability to truly recapitulate the pathophysiology of complex human disease [42]. The next generation of 2D and 3D *in vitro* cell-based models for more predictive target identification, validation, and drug discovery is likely to be derived from continued development of microfluidic and organ-on-a-chip devices. Such devices progress 2D and 3D cell culture studies away from the constraints of standard cell culture consumables. The design of truly novel devices for 3D culture that more accurately recapitulate tissue architecture, perfusion, and mechanical forces, representative of healthy and disease tissues, will require ingenuity and partnership between clinicians, pathologists, and cell biologists and micro-engineering design and manufacture

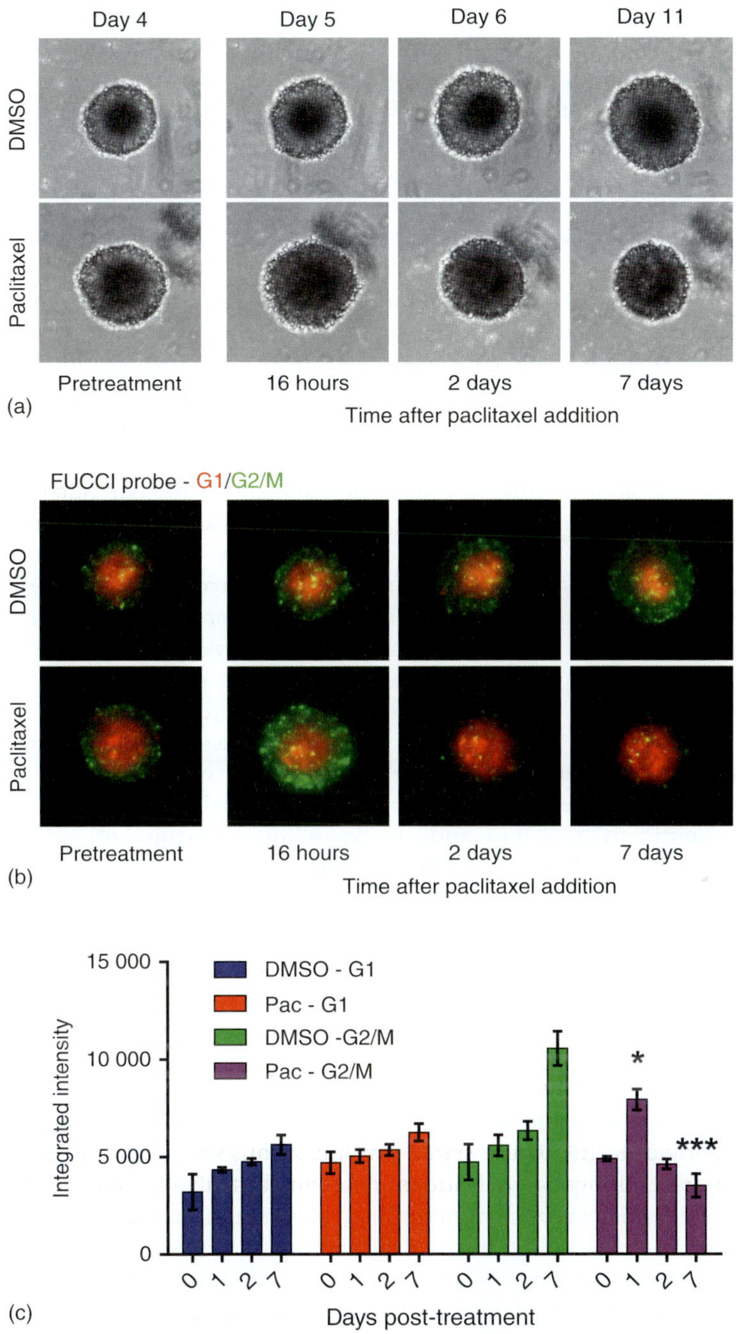

Figure 7.2 3D spheroid assays. Mouse squamous cell carcinoma (SCC) expressing a FUCCI cell cycle reporter cultured as spheroids. (a) Phase contrast images of SCC spheroids. (b) Fluorescence images of FUCCI cell cycle reporter reveals that cells in different stages of the cell cycle are found in different parts on the spheroid and respond differently to paclitaxel treatment. (c) Quantification of FUCCI probe expression. Mean ± SEM is shown, $n = 3$, for statistical analysis Dimethyl sulfoxide (DMSO) versus paclitaxel (Pac), * $p < 0.05$, *** $p < 0.001$.

capabilities. The production of miniaturized microfluidic perfusion systems that permit long-term *in vitro* growth of cells and compound dosing in 3D formats with the potential to scale up for large studies is beginning to be realized. Such developments include microfabricated devices with channels for supporting a 3D nerve-on-a-chip organoid platform [43] and 3D air–liquid interface models of intestinal, kidney, vascular, and lung disorders as exemplified by the OrganoPlate platform [44]. These models are compatible with existing automated liquid handling platforms and image-based phenotypic analysis of clinically relevant end points to support hit identification and target validation studies at scale (Figure 7.3). In addition, lower-throughput but more biologically complex organ-on-a-chip assay formats have been developed including a multi-organ chip comprising liver, tumour, and bone marrow cell lines [45], a two-organ-chip model emulating human type 2 diabetes mellitus to study pancreatic islet–liver crosstalk based on insulin and glucose regulation [46], and a four-organ-chip system that models human liver, skin, intestine, and kidney [47]. The advantage of these systems is that they offer a means of modelling and manipulating complex tissue microenvironments and the communication between distinct tissues, which exists *in vivo*. These systems are reported to produce levels of tissue and organ functionality that are not possible with conventional 2D or 3D cell models and thus through further experimental development and iterative re-engineering offer the hope of improved predictivity of clinical outcomes.

7.2.6 *In Vivo* Imaging

The increasing adoption of imaging technologies across preclinical drug discovery applications continues to evolve at a rapid rate with new advances in optics and robotic microscopes and an expanding repertoire of optical contrast agents, including functional live cell reporters to monitor enzyme activity in live cell and *in vivo* tissue microenvironments [48]. Together, such developments are contributing to highly dynamic and quantitative read-outs of target biology and drug MOA across preclinical models at cell, tissue, and whole organism levels [48]. The application of intravital optical imaging with techniques such as fluorescent protein photoswitching, photoactivation, bimolecular fluorescence complementation (BiFC), fluorescence recovery after photobleaching (FRAP), and fluorescence resonance energy transfer (FRET) provides precise and quantifiable functional read-outs of target activity and cell phenotype within live *in vivo* tissue microenvironments [48]. Low-resolution whole-body imaging techniques, such as luminescence-based approaches, have long been used in drug discovery to monitor disease progression and regression rates in preclinical rodent models during drug treatment [49, 50]. While such longitudinal whole-body imaging techniques provide valuable information on disease perturbation and/or target activity from fewer animals at significant cost savings compared with traditional preclinical methods, they provide limited information at single cell or subcellular resolution to inform a more in-depth evaluation of target biology. The integration of new optical biosensors of target activity combined with intravital imaging techniques including implantation of imaging windows provides unparalleled cellular, subcellular, and single molecule

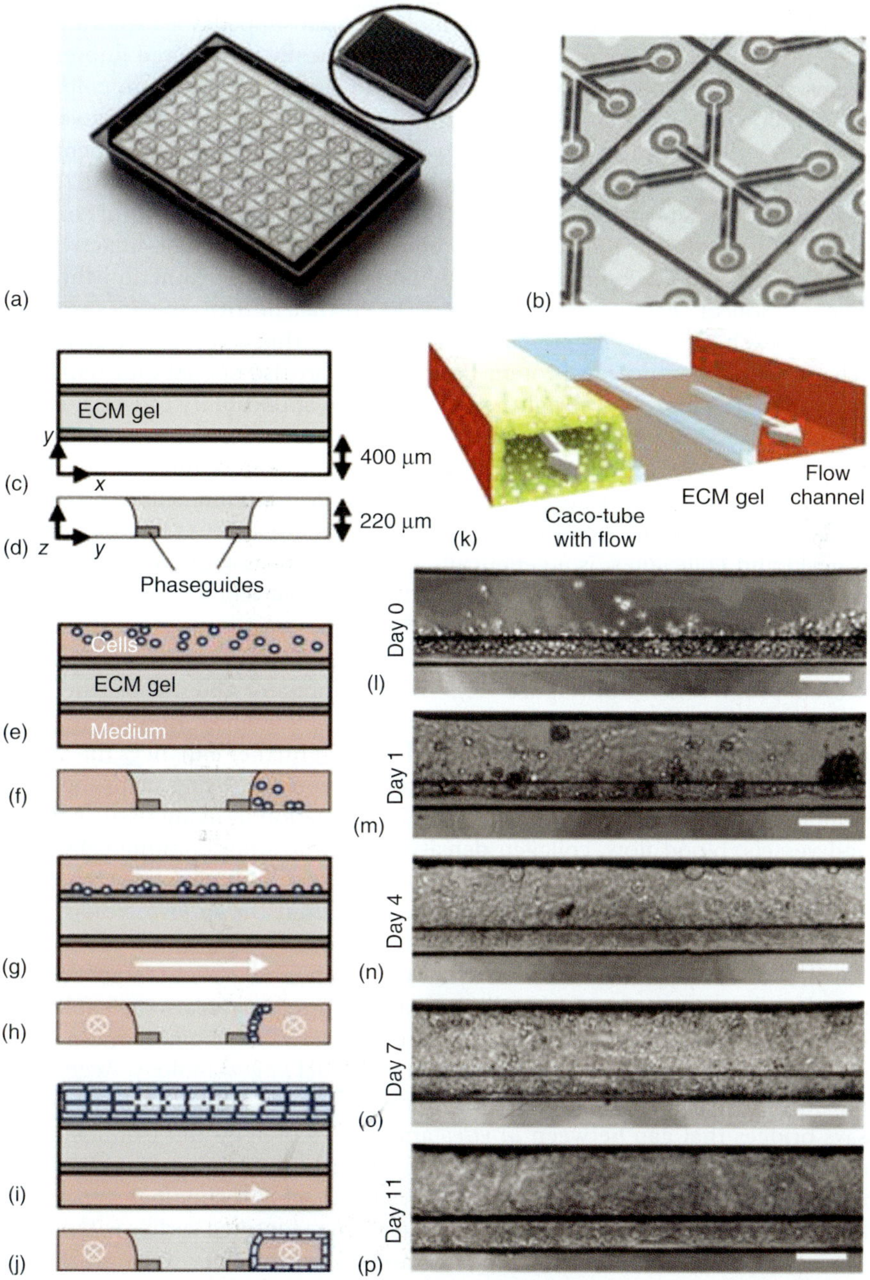

Figure 7.3 Emerging microfluidic assay formats. Overview of the method and microtitre plate format for modelling intestinal tubules in the OrganoPlate platform from Mimetas. Source: Reproduced from Trietsch et al. 2017 [44].

resolution of drug target activity within a live *in vivo* microenvironment [48]. Specific examples of optical imaging technologies that support the exploration of therapeutic target biology include the use of genetically engineered fluorescent proteins that are photoswitchable from dark to bright or from one colour to another following excitation at a specific wavelength [51]. Such photoactivatable probes can be used in live cell and *in vivo* systems to track cell movement and monitor protein target stability, and subcellular diffusion dynamics [52, 53]. FRAP offers an alternative approach for monitoring protein diffusion and dynamic intracellular processes. Chromophore-assisted light inactivation (CALI) is a specific technique for locally perturbing protein function through the generation of reactive oxygen species (ROS) that destroy specific proteins following excitation of an attached fluorophore. This approach provides a mechanism for inactivating protein targets with precise spatial and temporal control [54]. The efficiency, brightness, and *in vivo* applicability of FRET-based biosensors can be employed to monitor multiple aspects of target activity including protein–protein interactions, enzyme activity, and subcellular localization, allowing dynamic quantification of drug-target activity within cells and tissues. The fluorescence ubiquitination cell cycle indicator (FUCCI), developed by Miyawaki and colleagues, is a genetically encoded, two-colour (red and green) indicator that allows kinetic analysis of cell division at single-cell level within a live cell population [55]. FUCCI reporters can be used *in vitro* or *in vivo* to dynamically monitor the impact of target inhibition and drug exposure upon cell cycle progression [55] (Figure 7.2). The development and use of label-free imaging techniques such as coherent anti-stokes Raman scattering (CARS) microscopy and second harmonic generation (SHG) further enhances the ability of researchers to investigate the *in vivo* microenvironment. Using such label-free techniques allows visualization of structural information in living tissue such as blood vessels, blood flow, collagen density, and infiltrating immune cells [56]. Label-free imaging techniques when multiplexed with fluorescent reporters can provide much more contextual information about the *in vivo* biology of a disease.

Furthermore, the quantification of dynamic cell phenotypes and target activity *in vivo* using the same imaging methods and reagents that can also be applied to *in vitro* cell cultures provides new opportunities to reverse engineer more complex cell-based assay systems, which accurately model *in vivo* biology. Accurately modelling the dynamics of cell and target biology that exist *in vivo* into cell-based assays bridges that gap between *in vitro* and *in vivo* biology and frontloads the complexities of disease into earlier stages of target validation and drug discovery applications. Using such state-of-the-art *in vivo* imaging technologies may also allow deficient or ineffective targets and drugs to be identified earlier in the drug discovery pipeline, thereby reducing costs associated with late-stage preclinical and clinical failure [57].

7.2.7 High-Content Imaging

The continued development of automated high-throughput microscope platforms integrated with new optical probes and automated image analysis software tools has transformed the application of image-based phenotypic screening in cell-based assays and small model organisms [58]. With image analysis software capable of extracting several hundred measurements per cell from each image, researchers can detect and quantify subtle phenotypic changes that would otherwise be missed by manual analysis or traditional single end point assays. These developments have stimulated a new field of functional biology called high-content analysis [59, 60]. High-content analysis can replace the traditional manual analysis and subjective interpretation of cell, tissue, and whole organism phenotypic response following chemical or genetic perturbation with more robust quantitative phenotypic measurements. The development of validated image-based assays and automated image analysis protocols recording phenotypic response, which are transferable between laboratories, are well positioned to enhance experimental reproducibility in the biological sciences. Thus, further development and increased adoption of such quantitative phenotypic methods may help address previous reports of poor reproducibility of preclinical research related to target validation [61]. A further advantage of automated microscopic imaging over other cell-based assay platforms is the provision of spatial resolution in x, y, and z dimensions. This allows the development of cell-based models and screening assays towards more complex and disease-relevant heterogeneous co-cultures (Figure 7.4) and 3D models. The parallel assessment of target perturbation or drug response on adjacent normal and disease cell phenotypes within a single assay co-culture system provides valuable additional information of target biology across distinct cell types, which would normally coexist together in tissues and organs *in vivo*. Thus, relative to standard monoculture of single-cell lines, mixed co-culture cell models are expected to more accurately reflect outcomes within *in vivo* tissue microenvironments (Figure 7.4). Further integration of high-content imaging capabilities with new human iPSC technology, 3D multicellular models, and microfluidic devices promise to further increase disease relevance and provide additional information to better inform early target identification and validation studies.

7.3 Multiparametric High-Content Phenotypic Profiling of Target Biology and Drug Mechanism of Action

Integration of high-content imaging assays with the latest advances in multiparametric image analysis, multivariate statistics, machine learning, and new image informatics resources enables sophisticated classification of cell phenotypes across assay systems at scale. The advances in multiparametric high-content imaging enable the generation of a phenotypic fingerprint for every chemical and genetic perturbation tested to support a new discipline of phenotypic profiling to compare similarities and dissimilarities between distinct targets and drug MOA within cell, tissue, and small model organism systems [62–66]. It is anticipated that further development of these methods will better inform target identification, hit identification, and hit-to-lead medicinal chemistry programs

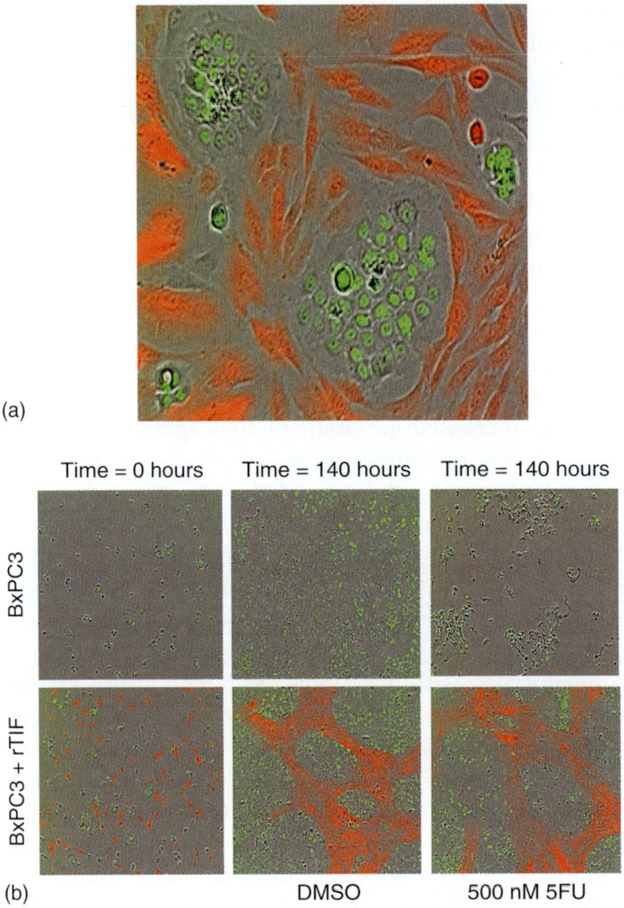

Figure 7.4 High-content co-culture assays. (a) Tumour cells (BxPC3) are labelled with NucLight (Essen Bio.) and red fluorescent protein expressing telomerase reverse transcriptase immortalised fibroblasts (rTIFs) are Telomerase reverse transcriptase (TERT)-immortalized dermal fibroblasts labelled with red fluorescent protein (RFP). (b) Tumour cells are protected from 5-FU-mediated cytotoxicity in this co-culture assay compared with monoculture of tumour cells alone.

in relevant models of disease. We outline below new opportunities provided by recent developments in multiparametric high-content imaging and image informatics with regard to functional annotation of genes and drug MOA within the context of intact cell-based assay systems. Image-based phenotypic measurements from cell-based assays can be recorded as an average of whole-well/cell population measurements or individual single-cell measurements. Individual single-cell measurements can provide significantly more detailed information on cell heterogeneity and classify distinct cell subpopulations for more precise phenotypic analysis [67]. Cell subpopulation analysis is important in understanding the heterogeneity within clonal cell populations arising in response to drug exposure, which can be a driver of clonal selection and therapeutic resistance.

New high-content imaging methods calculating phenotypic heterogeneity are thus highly relevant to the monitoring of disease evolution following pharmacological intervention and evaluation of longer-term duration of effective responses to targeted therapy [67]. The evolution of high-content image-based phenotypic profiling methods monitoring cell heterogeneity and classification of subpopulation responses at the single-cell level are now poised to support the development of more complex and clinically relevant heterogeneous and multicellular models for automated cell-based screening.

However, the challenge remains in how to optimally process complex multiparametric imaging data of phenotypic response to enable key decision-making to support advancement of target identification, validation, and medicinal chemistry activities. In 2004, Perlman et al. published the landmark paper describing the use of compound 'fingerprints' derived from multiparametric high-content phenotypic measurements. It was shown that compounds with known similar MOAs induced similar cell morphologies and thus similar multiparametric high-content phenotypic fingerprints [65]. Further development of high-content phenotypic profiling assays combined with multivariate statistics and machine learning methods demonstrated utility in the prediction of compound MOA based upon similar multiparametric phenotypic fingerprints with well-annotated reference compound sets [62, 65, 68–71] (Figure 7.5). Recent application of deep learning convolutional neural network (CNN) methods applied directly to the raw image data as the input into an appropriate classifier appears to perform well in the classification of cell phenotypes [72], and several groups have reported increased accuracy of CNN classifiers on high-content imaging data over approaches using extracted morphological measurements [73]. It remains to be seen how development of deep learning approaches to high-content imaging datasets evolves across different high-content assay model systems relative to traditional image analysis-based feature extraction and data normalization methods.

7.3.1 High-Content Cell Painting in Functional Genomics

The abovementioned examples of high-content profiling studies have employed a variety of distinct image-based assay formats, which make use of various combinations of fluorescent protein stains, DNA binding dyes, labelled antibodies, and engineered fluorescent reporter cell lines to create the raw image datasets for subsequent image analysis and phenotypic classification. Gustafsdottir et al. described the development of a relatively low-cost multiplex cytological profiling assay that 'paints the cell' with multiple fluorescent dyes to obtain quantitative phenotypic profiles of cell morphology without the need for specific antibody labelling or genetically engineered probes [74]. The optimized 'cell painting' assay multiplexes six fluorescent dyes, imaged in five spectral channels, to reveal eight broadly relevant cellular components or organelles. An automated image analysis software package, such as CellProfiler, can be applied to the cell painting assay to identify individual cells and calculate up to 1500 morphological feature measurements (e.g. various measures of size, shape, texture, intensity) to produce a rich profile that is suitable for the detection of subtle cellular phenotypes [63].

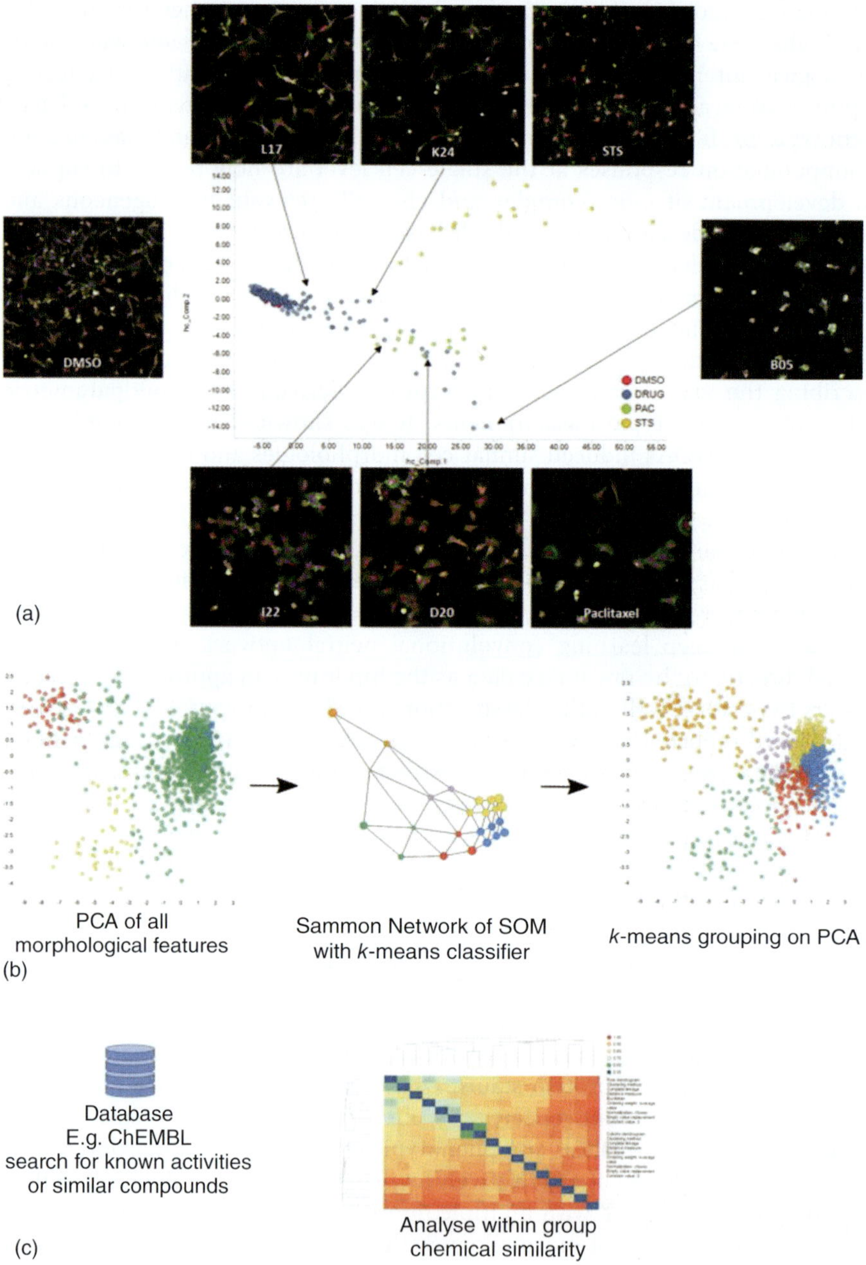

Figure 7.5 High-content phenotypic and chemical clustering. (a) Principal component analysis (PCA) and examples of phenotypic drug responses in a squamous cell carcinoma cell line. Principal components 1 and 2 are plotted accounting for >75% of the total variance. (b) Example workflow of phenotypic clustering and subsequent chemical structure analysis from Spotfire High Content Analyser software utilizing; PCA, Self-organizing map (SOM) and *k*-means clustering. (c) Use of chemical databases such as ChEMBL or structural chemical similarity analysis within phenotypic groups to identify or predict mechanism of action.

In a pilot screen of bioactive compounds, the assay detected a range of cellular phenotypes and the multiparametric phenotypic profiles were used to cluster compounds with similar annotated protein targets or chemical structure [63]. The cell painting assay can be applied to achieve a number of goals including categorization of the phenotypic impact of chemical or genetic perturbations and grouping chemical structure and/or genes with similar phenotypic profiles into functional pathways. A recent study evaluated if human genes can be functionally annotated using a cell painting assay to morphologically profile cDNA constructs. Results demonstrated that 50% of the 220 genes tested yielded detectable morphological profiles, which group into biologically meaningful gene clusters consistent with known functional annotation (e.g. the RAS-RAF-MEK-ERK cascade) [75]. These results provide proof of principle that multiparametric high-content phenotypic profiling assays may help assign function to the estimated 38% of genes in the human genome with unknown function [76] and identify new roles for functionally annotated genes [75]. Thus, multiparametric high-content cell painting assays can be used to morphologically characterize therapeutic target activity within physiologically relevant cell models.

7.3.2 Integration of Multiparametric High-Content Imaging with Chemoinformatics

The use of high-content phenotypic profiling to cluster compounds with similar phenotypic profiles integrated with known compound target selectivity data can be used to further elucidate target activity and on- or off-target activities of individual compounds within intact cell-based systems. Phenotypic clusters, which are enriched with compounds representing a specific target class, can be used to assign target hypotheses to phenotypically similar small molecules with unknown target activity (Figure 7.5). For example, a high-content imaging study generated phenotypic fingerprints to cluster mechanistically similar compounds using a Markov clustering algorithm, and then each compound cluster was analysed for enrichment of individual targets and gene sets to facilitate MOA analysis [77]. Individual target annotations for compounds were obtained from public and commercial drug target databases such as ChEMBL, DrugBank, GVK (GOSTAR), Integrity, and Metabase. Gene set enrichments were obtained from the following databases: BioSystems, Metabase, Integrity, Metabase pathway-derived gene sets (Metabase noodles), and Gene Go Ontologies [77].

7.3.3 Guiding Chemical Design and Target Selectivity from Multiparametric High-Content Analysis

The study of chemical structure–activity relationships (SARs) is a fundamental principle used by medicinal chemists to determine which structural motifs are required for effective drug target engagement, target selectivity, and phenotypic response. In theory, compounds with analogous chemical structures will bind the same or similar protein targets, a principle that is used to develop multiple derivatives of a compound hit from a screening assay, which may exhibit improved potency and selectivity properties. Young et al. provided one of the earliest studies integrating multiparametric high-content phenotypic profiles with chemical structure and predicted protein binding activities and determined that compounds with comparable chemical structures produce similar phenotypic fingerprints [78]. In this study they screened the human cervical cancer cell line (HeLa) with a small molecule compound library of 6547 compounds and performed factor analysis on 36 features to produce a phenotypic fingerprint for each compound. Similarity between chemical structures was performed by defining the molecular structure through radial atom neighbours followed by the construction of a structure similarity matrix by calculating the Tanimoto distance metric between the compounds. Two similarity matrices, one for phenotypic fingerprints and one for chemical structure, were clustered by similarity, which, when cross referenced, revealed phenotypic clusters that match up to groups of structurally similar compounds indicating that a relationship between chemical structure and multiparametric high-content phenotypic profiles can be obtained [78] (Figure 7.5). However, for some phenotypic clusters such as cytotoxicity, the concordance between phenotypic and chemical similarity was reduced compared with other more morphologically defined phenotypes. These studies also demonstrated that high-content phenotypes correlate better with predicted compound targets than with the compound structures themselves. These results provide early evidence for the effectiveness of multiparametric high-content profiling assays to predict targets based on phenotypic similarity between unknown and target-annotated compound sets. The study further indicates that small modifications in chemical structure are often associated with large phenotypic differences. This may possibly be due to amplified sensitivity of cell-based assay systems to modification of ligand–target interactions and potential for obtaining sharp activity cliffs arising from multiple mechanisms associated with cell permeability ($c\text{Log}\,P/D$-mediated), subcellular distribution, cell transport mechanisms, membrane interactions, etc. [79].

Despite the challenges, collective experience and reports from pharmaceutical and academic drug discovery groups indicate that cell-based phenotypic assays can support SAR if sufficient effort is taken in the design, validation, operation, and analysis of the phenotypic assay [80–83]. For example, results from a complex co-culture model of primary human endothelial and stromal progenitor cells, incorporating multiparametric high-content analysis of angiogenesis with chemoinformatics, identified novel compound scaffolds and enabled hit expansion with clear evidence of compound SAR [80]. In addition, iterative screening of small compound libraries across a well-defined suite of cancer cell line viability and high-content apoptosis, cell proliferation, and cell migration assays guided the design of novel, potent, and highly selective kinase inhibitors [82, 83].

7.4 Target-Annotated Compound Libraries for Phenotypic Screening and MOA Determination

It has become increasingly clear that our lack of understanding of the target biology underpinning many complex human diseases and knowledge gaps in the biological function of a significant proportion of the proteome [76] combined with a dearth of well-characterized and selective tool compounds [84] represent major limiting factors in our ability to effectively validate new drug targets. The application of high-quality chemical probes and well-characterized target-annotated compound libraries that encompass several structurally distinct molecules against each target class is highly valuable for target identification studies across phenotypic screening assays (see Chapter 1 for more details). Target-annotated tool compound sets have proven useful for in-depth assessment of the function of specific targets and, as described above, also support the elucidation of target hypotheses of novel compound hits by phenotypic profiling [77]. Initiatives such as the Structural Genomics Consortium (https://www.thesgc.org) and resources such as the Chemical Probes Portal (http://www.chemicalprobes.org/) provide and identify high-quality chemical probes for target validation. However, the scale of these initiatives is limited to small compound sets and narrow areas of biological target space. Thus, further investments and new technologies that accelerate the generation of pharmacological or genetic tools that precisely perturb target activity in complex *in vitro* and *in vivo* models are required. The development of publicly available and commercial chemoinformatics resources and drug target databases such as ChEMBL, which can assign target prediction to large compound sets, has proven valuable for compound MOA prediction from phenotypic screening [77, 78]. Similarly the availability of annotated phenotypic toolbox compounds from pharmaceutical industry open innovation initiatives (AstraZeneca Target Innovation, https://openinnovation.astrazeneca.com/target-innovation.html; Phenomics Discovery Initiative-Janssen Pharmaceuticals, http://npsc.ac.uk/pdi; Lilly-OIDD Emerging Biology program, https://openinnovation.lilly.com/dd/) or from commercial sources (Bioascent Phenotypic Toolbox, https://compoundcloud.bioascent.com/phenotypic-toolbox) supports exploration of target biology across broad varieties of cell and small model organism models of disease. Further investment in the development and distribution of larger target-annotated tool compound libraries, which provide references for classifying the MOA of phenotypic hit compounds and explore novel biological target space across new emerging human cell-based models is urgently needed.

7.5 Quantitative Pathway Profiling Across New Model Systems

Putative therapeutic targets do not work in isolation but are part of complex signalling networks operating within cells and are controlled by genetic, epigenetic, and environmental factors. The plasticity of cell behaviour and disease evolution often means that it is easy for disease cells to bypass the consequences of target perturbation through redundant and adaptive signalling mechanisms. Large-scale genetic, epigenetic, and proteomic analyses of patient samples highlight the substantial heterogeneity in disease within and between patients. Many complex human disorders are driven by derangements in multiple intracellular signalling pathways enhancing the ability of a diseased cell to rapidly and dynamically rewire its signalling circuitry following treatment with single pathway blocking agents, leading to ineffective treatment and/or therapeutic resistance [85]. For example, corticosteroids represent the primary pharmaceutical ingredient in prescribed anti-inflammatory medicines. However resistance to corticosteroid treatment of chronic inflammatory disease is a common problem, and thus understanding the pathways and mechanisms implicated in corticosteroid resistance will be valuable in identifying new therapeutic targets that can be combined with steroid therapy [86]. In addition, networks and pathway switching enable rapid tumour evolution and therapeutic evasion. Thus, new approaches are required to understand cancer cell signalling networks and 'driver' pathways that promote tumour progression to guide selection of the optimal drug–target combinations that collapse the communication between survival signalling networks across tumour types and thus reduce the likelihood of therapeutic evasion and recurrence. Thus placing target hypotheses within the correct context of pathway networks and anticipated resistance mechanisms *in vivo* is critically important to predicting success of therapeutic outcome in patient disease settings.

New advances in genomic and proteomic technologies (e.g. NGS, mass spectrometry, protein microarray technologies) that operate at multicellular and single-cell levels, combined with bioinformatics and computational approaches (systems biology and artificial intelligence), are advancing the knowledge base of target activity within integrated pathway networks. For example, the non-receptor tyrosine kinase, focal adhesion kinase (FAK), has for decades been implicated as a therapeutic target for cancer cell migration and metastasis by virtue of its role in mediating turnover of integrin linked focal adhesions that control cell adhesion. However, recent studies incorporating cytokine profiling and pathway network analysis have subsequently identified that FAK translocates to sub-adhesion complexes within the cell nucleus where it plays important roles in dictating gene expression and cytokine secretion profiles governing immune response and cancer cell survival [87, 88].

7.5.1 Pathway Profiling at the Gene Transcription Level

Recent technical advances in transcriptomic and post-translational pathway profiling approaches have substantially improved sensitivity and throughput and thus have become more applicable to drug MOA and target validation studies across complex human cell-based assays. Gene transcription-based profiling of mRNA using NGS platforms and whole genome expression arrays provide a comprehensive overview of gene activity in biological samples. Common applications of gene transcription profiling include genome-wide differential expression studies across samples to support disease classification, protein function, and drug MOA analysis. The Connectivity Map project exemplifies new bioinformatics approaches to support a systematic comparative analysis of gene expression profiles [89]. Connectivity Map combines a catalogue of gene expression profiles from large panels of compound perturbed samples with computational and statistical methods to support similarity profiling of gene expression patterns to infer compound MOA [89]. A proof-of-concept study was applied to identify the MOA of the natural product compound, gedunin, which possessed poorly characterized anticancer activity. Gene transcription profiles obtained from treating LNCaP prostate cancer cells with gedunin for six hours were subsequently used to query the Connectivity Map database, which identified high similarity with multiple HSP90 inhibitors; subsequent studies further confirmed HSP90 as a target of gedunin [90].

Recent technical advances in gene expression profiling include the development of more cost-effective gene expression methods for higher-throughput applications such as the L1000™ platform. L1000 is based upon the rapid quantification of 978 landmark gene transcripts in 384-well plate format and a computational model to infer expression across the wider genome [91, 92]. A recent study has applied supervised machine learning methods to L1000 data to correlate mRNA profiles following drug treatments with gene knockout experiments to predict targets for compounds [93]. More details on Connectivity Map and L1000 are described in Chapter 11.

The testing of a compound across large panels of genetically distinct cell lines followed by correlation of drug sensitivity profiles with basal gene expression patterns across cells can also be used to reveal specific target hypothesis. For example, cancer cell line sensitivity to the compound BRD5468 correlated with high expression of the monoglyceride lipase (MGLL) [94]. Treatment with the MGLL inhibitor, JZL184, or shRNA knockdown of MGLL attenuated the activity of BRD5468 confirming MGLL as the primary target for cancer cytotoxicity effects [94]. While many such cell panel sensitivity studies have been restricted to basic cell viability assays across large cancer cell panels, new advances in iPSC technology and high-content phenotypic assay development are well placed to progress drug sensitivity and transcriptomic profiling across new disease areas and phenotypes.

While gene transcription profiling has proven effective in elucidation of compound MOA, success is dependent upon the use of appropriate biological assays where the relevant target pathway for any given compound is activated within the appropriate pathway context. A further dependency is the cross referencing to a comprehensive and well-annotated reference set of transcriptomic signatures also generated under the appropriate biological context. Thus, further application of high-throughput transcriptomic profiling applied to either well-annotated MOA reference compound libraries or CRISPR-engineered cell panels where specific proteins have been systematically knocked out would provide a compendium of gene signatures. This would serve as valuable reference tools for understanding target biology and revealing drug-target MOA.

7.5.2 Dynamic Post-Translational Pathway Profiling Across Dose–Response and Time-Series Studies

While transcriptomic profiling has proven valuable in understating drug MOA and identification of new therapeutic targets, small molecule compounds, peptides, and antibody-based therapeutics typically target proteins, and it is the activation state of protein targets that dictates therapeutic responses. In contrast to mass spectrometry, antibody-based protein microarray technologies provide the combined advantages of high sensitivity, high throughput, and high quantification at a relatively low cost. Reverse phase protein array (RPPA) is an antibody-based proteomic methodology for simultaneous measurement of the abundance of multiple proteins and post-translational modifications across large sample sets [95]. Recent advances in RPPA technology include more sophisticated sample handling, quality control, certified quality affinity reagents, and optical detection, including planar waveguide detection systems that provide femtomole to zeptomole sensitivity in protein analyte detection in formats suitable for medium- to high-throughput applications [95, 96]. A typical RPPA platform incorporates the following core processes: preparation of total protein extracts from cell culture, *in vivo*, or clinical tissue samples. Protein extracts are then printed onto a nitrocellulose or a hydrophobic chip surface as individual sample spots. Immobilized protein sample spots on the microarray are then incubated with monospecific antibodies to detect individual proteins or their post-translationally modified forms (Figure 7.6). Using a similar approach Mischel and colleagues [97] performed single-cell phosphoproteomic analysis

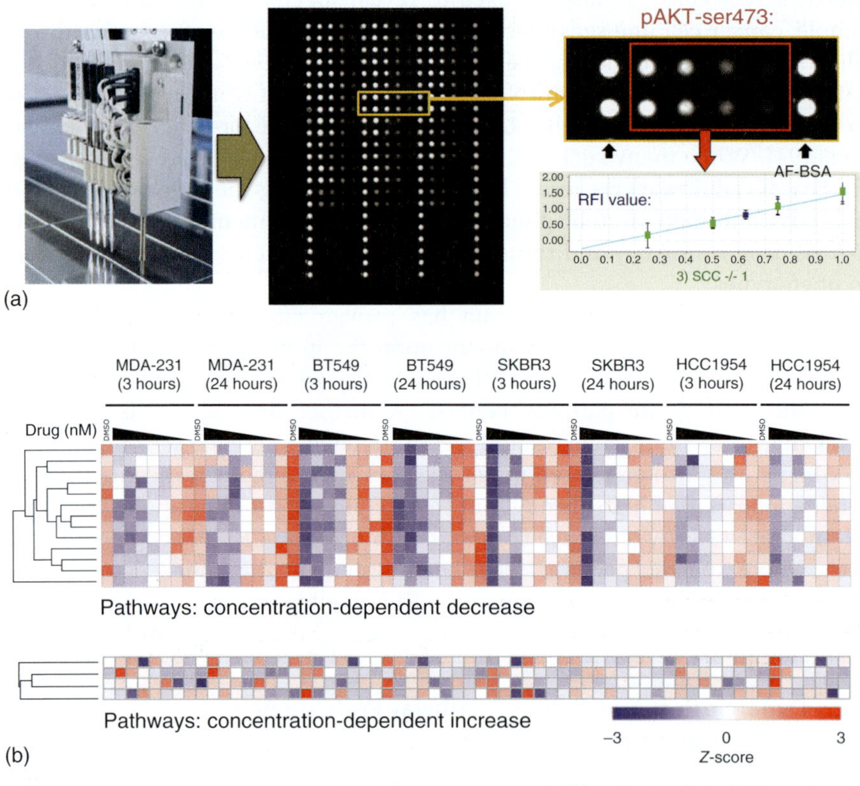

Figure 7.6 Reverse phase protein array (RPPA) platform. (a) Printing of protein extracts on solid surface microarrays for fluorescent antibody-mediated detection of protein analytes. (b) Application of RPPA across a panel of human breast cancer cell lines following compound treatment at 3 and 24 hour time points to identify potential pharmacodynamic pathway biomarkers and compensatory or resistance pathways following target intervention.

using a quantitative, antibody-based protein microarray platform integrated with a microfluidic device called the single-cell barcode chip (SCBC) [98]. The SCBC surpasses RPPA in sensitivity and ability to assay multiple proteins in small numbers of cells per chip. The SCBC platform has been applied to a model of drug resistance in brain cancer to identify pathways of resistance following treatment with an inhibitor of the mTOR kinase [97]. To generate a clinically relevant model of mTOR kinase inhibitor resistance, mice bearing patient-derived human glioblastoma (GBM) xenografts were treated with CC214-2, an ATP-competitive mTOR kinase inhibitor that crosses the blood brain barrier. Initial response to CC214-2 was characterized by decreased Ki-67 labelling in GBM, a measure of tumour cell proliferation, as detected by immunohistochemistry (IHC) analysis and was concordant with inhibition of mTORC1 and mTORC2. However, by day 27 following treatment, rapid tumour regrowth occurred with concomitant increases in glucose uptake and tumour volume, reactivation of mTORC1 and mTORC2 signalling, and marked increase in Ki-67 labelling, thus modelling the clinical scenario of resistance [97]. The SCBC platform was applied to cells dissociated from GBM xenografts during the responsive phase, and onset of resistance phase following inhibitor treatment and phosphoprotein data was subsequently mined with a systems-based computational approach to detect changes in multiple signalling nodes early and late in the course of resistance development [97]. The development of such ultrasensitive and high-throughput antibody-based protein microarray capabilities facilitates large-scale multiplex analysis of dynamic pathway signalling following target interventions. Such pathway profiling includes quantification of the level of low abundant proteins and post-translational epitopes across very small samples including *in vitro*, preclinical, or clinical biopsies. Thus, protein microarray technologies are particularly suited to studying the regulation and downstream pathway effects of target perturbation in miniaturized cell assays including human primary cell models. Dynamic profiling of post-translational pathway networks at sequential time points following target intervention can thus support the identification of drug resistance mechanisms to place target hypothesis within the context of dynamic pathway signalling networks, which can contribute to therapeutic resistance (Figure 7.6b). Compensatory and redundant post-translational mechanisms identified in preclinical and clinical material following target intervention can be mapped to public or proprietary drug–target databases to generate new drug combination or new target hypotheses, which may counteract dynamic pathway rewiring and therapeutic resistance. The characterization of drug resistance pathway mechanisms in clinical samples can also support reverse engineering of biochemical or cell-based screening assays, which recapitulate clinical resistance mechanisms to identify further novel drug resistance targets. Routine application of high-throughput protein microarray methods using relevant human cell-based models during early drug discovery phases (e.g. target validation, evaluation of hit series through to lead identification, lead optimization and evaluation of drug candidates) can provide a more comprehensive and unbiased pharmacodynamic assessment of drug MOA under the relevant biological context. This information will enable a more informative triage of target assessment and drug MOA to inform on subsequent investments and guide more optimal preclinical and clinical development strategies within the context of integrated signalling pathway networks.

7.6 Conclusions

New breakthroughs in genomics, proteomics, imaging, and informatics tools are converging with advances in cell-based assay technologies to enable in-depth exploration of target biology and drug MOA across complex human cell- and tissue-based models of disease. Such advances are well placed to support a new generation of functional *in vitro* and *in vivo* biological studies, which combine robust hypothesis testing and hypothesis generation to enable a more in-depth and unbiased evaluation of target biology under relevant tissue and disease context. The application of automated image acquisition, image analysis, and transcriptomic and proteomic pathway profiling technologies with well-validated quality control procedures removes subjectivity and supports more quantitative and reproducible evaluation of drug–target hypotheses across academic and industrial sectors. Such advances support multiple drug discovery operating models including target-based, phenotypic, chemocentric, and drug repurposing through robust functional characterization of drug–target mechanisms under appropriate biological context.

Recent retrospective reviews analysing drug attrition rates during clinical development and the respective merits and limitations of phenotypic drug discovery versus target-directed drug discovery strategies [1, 2, 99–101] do not yet reflect the widespread implementation of modern advances to target validation and drug MOA across new emerging human cell-based model systems described in this chapter. It therefore remains to be seen how each of these technical advances individually and collectively will impact upon future drug attrition rates in late-stage clinical development and the overall number of approved first-in-class medicines against new therapeutic targets. However, to maximize impact of these new breakthrough technologies and the adoption of alternative strategies to target identification and validation requires dedicated investment and bold decisions to replace more established and cost-effective preclinical models and drug discovery strategies.

The development of screening assays and preclinical models, which accurately predict clinical outcomes, is a significant challenge, which has to date not yet received the required investments from translational funding bodies, industry, and life science investors in order to reduce high attrition rates during late-stage clinical development. The development of preclinical models and associated technologies that support reverse translation studies (see Chapter 6 for more details) to improve clinical relevance and prediction of efficacy will be most effectively addressed through precompetitive academic–industry–clinical partnerships to share data and knowledge, which link closely to clinical insights and treatment outcomes. Such partnerships should also bridge disciplines to exploit new technical breakthroughs and the evolving integration of the biological sciences with micro-engineering, physics, mathematics, and advanced

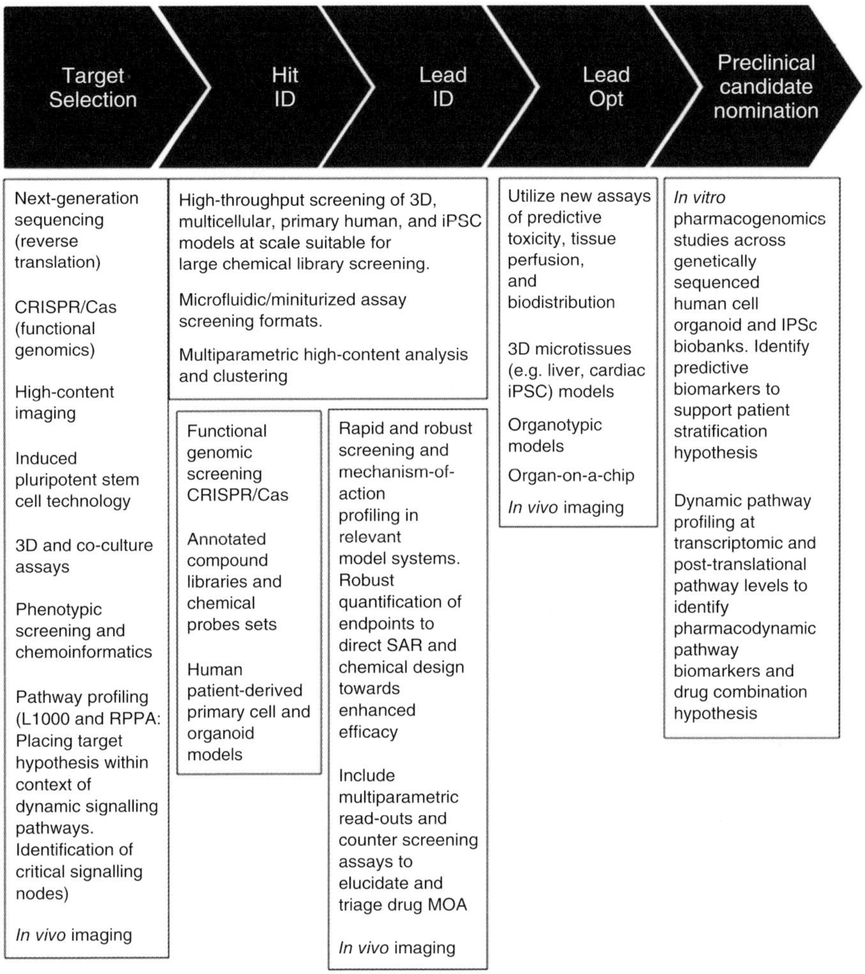

Figure 7.7 Integration of new target validation technologies to enhance the drug project operating model.

computational analysis. Through combined multidisciplinary efforts we can exploit new advances in technology and incorporate these into updated drug project operating models, which support more robust target validation and better informed preclinical and clinical development strategies (Figure 7.7).

References

1 Hay, M., Thomas, D.W., Craighead, J.L. et al. (2014). Clinical development success rates for investigational drugs. *Nat. Biotechnol.* 32 (1): 40–51.

2 Kola, I. and Landis, J. (2004). Can the pharmaceutical industry reduce attrition rates? *Nat. Rev. Drug Discovery* 3 (8): 711–715.

3 Waring, M.J., Arrowsmith, J., Leach, A.R. et al. (2015). An analysis of the attrition of drug candidates from four major pharmaceutical companies. *Nat. Rev. Drug Discovery* 14 (7): 475–486.
4 Bunnage, M.E. (2011). Getting pharmaceutical R&D back on target. *Nat. Chem. Biol.* 7 (6): 335–339.
5 Gupta, R. (2017). Clinical success versus attrition of investigational pharmaceuticals: a vignette. *Crit. Rev. Ther. Drug Carrier Syst.* 34 (6): 527–549.
6 Zhang, L., Mchale, C.M., Greene, N. et al. (2014). Emerging approaches in predictive toxicology. *Environ. Mol. Mutagen.* 55 (9): 679–688.
7 O'brien, P.J., Irwin, W., Diaz, D. et al. (2006). High concordance of drug-induced human hepatotoxicity with in vitro cytotoxicity measured in a novel cell-based model using high content screening. *Arch. Toxicol.* 80 (9): 580–604.
8 Pilling, J., Garside, H., and Ainscow, E. (2010). Development of a quantitative 96-well method to image glycogen storage in primary rat hepatocytes. *Mol. Cell. Biochem.* 341 (1–2): 73–78.
9 Szkolnicka, D., Farnworth, S.L., Lucendo-Villarin, B. et al. (2014). Accurate prediction of drug-induced liver injury using stem cell-derived populations. *Stem Cells Transl. Med.* 3 (2): 141–148.
10 Clements, M., Millar, V., Williams, A.S., and Kalinka, S. (2015). Bridging functional and structural cardiotoxicity assays using human embryonic stem cell-derived cardiomyocytes for a more comprehensive risk assessment. *Toxicol. Sci.* 148 (1): 241–260.
11 Ma, Z., Wang, J., Loskill, P. et al. (2015). Self-organizing human cardiac microchambers mediated by geometric confinement. *Nat. Commun.* 6: 7413.
12 Schaaf, S., Shibamiya, A., Mewe, M. et al. (2011). Human engineered heart tissue as a versatile tool in basic research and preclinical toxicology. *PLoS One* 6 (10): e26397.
13 Kelm, J.M., Timmins, N.E., Brown, C.J. et al. (2003). Method for generation of homogeneous multicellular tumor spheroids applicable to a wide variety of cell types. *Biotechnol. Bioeng.* 83 (2): 173–180.
14 Leucht, S., Helfer, B., Gartlehner, G., and Davis, J.M. (2015). How effective are common medications: a perspective based on meta-analyses of major drugs. *BMC Med.* 13: 253.
15 Davis, C., Naci, H., Gurpinar, E. et al. (2017). Availability of evidence of benefits on overall survival and quality of life of cancer drugs approved by European Medicines Agency: retrospective cohort study of drug approvals 2009–13. *BMJ* 359: j4530.
16 Mcdermott, U. (2015). Next-generation sequencing and empowering personalised cancer medicine. *Drug Discovery Today* 20 (12): 1470–1475.
17 Kruglyak, K.M., Lin, E., and Ong, F.S. (2014). Next-generation sequencing in precision oncology: challenges and opportunities. *Expert Rev. Mol. Diagn.* 14 (6): 635–637.
18 Wang, I.M., Stone, D.J., Nickle, D. et al. (2013). Systems biology approach for new target and biomarker identification. *Curr. Top. Microbiol. Immunol.* 363: 169–199.

19 Zhao, S. and Iyengar, R. (2012). Systems pharmacology: network analysis to identify multiscale mechanisms of drug action. *Annu. Rev. Pharmacol. Toxicol.* 52: 505–521.
20 Bailey, P., Chang, D.K., Nones, K. et al. (2016). Genomic analyses identify molecular subtypes of pancreatic cancer. *Nature* 531 (7592): 47–52.
21 Dreyer, S.B., Chang, D.K., Bailey, P., and Biankin, A.V. (2017). Pancreatic Cancer Genomes: Implications for Clinical Management and Therapeutic Development. *Clin. Cancer Res.* 23 (7): 1638–1646.
22 Secrier, M., Li, X., De Silva, N. et al. (2016). Mutational signatures in esophageal adenocarcinoma define etiologically distinct subgroups with therapeutic relevance. *Nat. Genet.* 48 (10): 1131–1141.
23 Cong, L., Ran, F.A., Cox, D. et al. (2013). Multiplex genome engineering using CRISPR/Cas systems. *Science* 339 (6121): 819–823.
24 O'duibhir, E., Carragher, N.O., and Pollard, S.M. (2017). Accelerating glioblastoma drug discovery: convergence of patient-derived models, genome editing and phenotypic screening. *Mol. Cell. Neurosci.* 80: 198–207.
25 Larson, M.H., Gilbert, L.A., Wang, X. et al. (2013). CRISPR interference (CRISPRi) for sequence-specific control of gene expression. *Nat. Protoc.* 8 (11): 2180–2196.
26 Nestor, C.E., Ottaviano, R., Reinhardt, D. et al. (2015). Rapid reprogramming of epigenetic and transcriptional profiles in mammalian culture systems. *Genome Biol.* 16: 11.
27 Takahashi, K. and Yamanaka, S. (2006). Induction of pluripotent stem cells from mouse embryonic and adult fibroblast cultures by defined factors. *Cell* 126 (4): 663–676.
28 Landgren, H. and Sartipy, P. (2014). Can stem-cell-derived models revolutionize drug discovery? *Expert Opin. Drug Discovery* 9 (1): 9–13.
29 Carragher, N., Piccinini, F., Tesei, A. et al. (2018). Concerns, challenges and promises of high-content analysis of 3D cellular models. *Nat. Rev. Drug Discovery* 17 (8): 606.
30 Osakada, F., Ikeda, H., Sasai, Y., and Takahashi, M. (2009). Stepwise differentiation of pluripotent stem cells into retinal cells. *Nat. Protoc.* 4 (6): 811–824.
31 Sato, T., Vries, R.G., Snippert, H.J. et al. (2009). Single Lgr5 stem cells build crypt-villus structures in vitro without a mesenchymal niche. *Nature* 459 (7244): 262–265.
32 Rios, A.C. and Clevers, H. (2018). Imaging organoids: a bright future ahead. *Nat. Methods* 15 (1): 24–26.
33 Li, X., Francies, H.E., Secrier, M. et al. (2018). Organoid cultures recapitulate esophageal adenocarcinoma heterogeneity providing a model for clonality studies and precision therapeutics. *Nat. Commun.* 9 (1): 2983.
34 Mills, R.J., Titmarsh, D.M., Koenig, X. et al. (2017). Functional screening in human cardiac organoids reveals a metabolic mechanism for cardiomyocyte cell cycle arrest. *Proc. Natl. Acad. Sci. U.S.A.* 114 (40): E8372–E8381.
35 Wenzel, C., Riefke, B., Gründemann, S. et al. (2014). 3D high-content screening for the identification of compounds that target cells in dormant tumor spheroid regions. *Exp. Cell. Res.* 323 (1): 131–143.

36 Madhavan, M., Nevin, Z.S., Shick, H.E. et al. (2018). Induction of myelinating oligodendrocytes in human cortical spheroids. *Nat. Methods* 15 (9): 700–706.
37 Verhulsel, M., Vignes, M., Descroix, S. et al. (2014). A review of microfabrication and hydrogel engineering for micro-organs on chips. *Biomaterials* 35 (6): 1816–1832.
38 Rimann, M. and Graf-Hausner, U. (2012). Synthetic 3D multicellular systems for drug development. *Curr. Opin. Biotechnol.* 23 (5): 803–809.
39 Olive, K.P., Jacobetz, M.A., Davidson, C.J. et al. (2009). Inhibition of Hedgehog signaling enhances delivery of chemotherapy in a mouse model of pancreatic cancer. *Science* 324 (5933): 1457–1461.
40 Smyth, M.J., Pietersz, G.A., and Mckenzie, I.F. (1987). Use of vasoactive agents to increase tumor perfusion and the antitumor efficacy of drug-monoclonal antibody conjugates. *J. Natl. Cancer Inst.* 79 (6): 1367–1373.
41 Nobis, M., Mcghee, E.J., Morton, J.P. et al. (2013). Intravital FLIM-FRET imaging reveals dasatinib-induced spatial control of src in pancreatic cancer. *Cancer Res.* 73 (15): 4674–4686.
42 Horvath, P., Aulner, N., Bickle, M. et al. (2016). Screening out irrelevant cell-based models of disease. *Nat. Rev. Drug Discovery* 15 (11): 751–769.
43 Curley, J.L. and Moore, M.J. (2011). Facile micropatterning of dual hydrogel systems for 3D models of neurite outgrowth. *J. Biomed. Mater. Res. Part A* 99 (4): 532–543.
44 Trietsch, S.J., Naumovska, E., Kurek, D. et al. (2017). Membrane-free culture and real-time barrier integrity assessment of perfused intestinal epithelium tubes. *Nat. Commun.* 8 (1): 262.
45 Sung, J.H., Kam, C., and Shuler, M.L. (2010). A microfluidic device for a pharmacokinetic-pharmacodynamic (PK-PD) model on a chip. *Lab Chip* 10 (4): 446–455.
46 Bauer, S., Wennberg Huldt, C., Kanebratt, K.P. et al. (2017). Functional coupling of human pancreatic islets and liver spheroids on-a-chip: towards a novel human ex vivo type 2 diabetes model. *Sci. Rep.* 7 (1): 14620.
47 Maschmeyer, I., Lorenz, A.K., Schimek, K. et al. (2015). A four-organ-chip for interconnected long-term co-culture of human intestine, liver, skin and kidney equivalents. *Lab Chip* 15 (12): 2688–2699.
48 Conway, J.R., Carragher, N.O., and Timpson, P. (2014). Developments in preclinical cancer imaging: innovating the discovery of therapeutics. *Nat. Rev. Cancer* 14 (5): 314–328.
49 Bremer, C., Tung, C.H., and Weissleder, R. (2001). In vivo molecular target assessment of matrix metalloproteinase inhibition. *Nat. Med.* 7 (6): 743–748.
50 Contag, P.R. (2002). Whole-animal cellular and molecular imaging to accelerate drug development. *Drug Discovery Today* 7 (10): 555–562.
51 Agasti, S.S., Kohler, R.H., Liong, M. et al. (2013). Dual imaging and photoactivated nanoprobe for controlled cell tracking. *Small* 9 (2): 222–227.
52 Wang, X., He, L., Wu, Y.I. et al. (2010). Light-mediated activation reveals a key role for Rac in collective guidance of cell movement in vivo. *Nat. Cell Biol.* 12 (6): 591–597.

53 Canel, M., Serrels, A., Miller, D. et al. (2010). Quantitative in vivo imaging of the effects of inhibiting integrin signaling via Src and FAK on cancer cell movement: effects on E-cadherin dynamics. *Cancer Res.* 70 (22): 9413–9422.

54 Bulina, M.E., Lukyanov, K.A., Britanova, O.V. et al. (2006). Chromophore-assisted light inactivation (CALI) using the phototoxic fluorescent protein KillerRed. *Nat. Protoc.* 1 (2): 947–953.

55 Sakaue-Sawano, A., Kurokawa, H., Morimura, T. et al. (2008). Visualizing spatiotemporal dynamics of multicellular cell-cycle progression. *Cell* 132 (3): 487–498.

56 Lee, M., Downes, A., Chau, Y.Y. et al. (2015). In vivo imaging of the tumor and its associated microenvironment using combined CARS / 2-photon microscopy. *Intravital* 4 (1): e1055430.

57 Scannell, J.W. and Bosley, J. (2016). When quality beats quantity: decision theory, drug discovery, and the reproducibility crisis. *PLoS One* 11 (2): e0147215.

58 Boutros, M., Heigwer, F., and Laufer, C. (2015). Microscopy-based high-content screening. *Cell* 163 (6): 1314–1325.

59 Bickle, M. (2010). The beautiful cell: high-content screening in drug discovery. *Anal. Bioanal. Chem.* 398 (1): 219–226.

60 Taylor, D.L., Woo, E.S., and Giuliano, K.A. (2001). Real-time molecular and cellular analysis: the new frontier of drug discovery. *Curr. Opin. Biotechnol.* 12 (1): 75–81.

61 Prinz, F., Schlange, T., and Asadullah, K. (2011). Believe it or not: how much can we rely on published data on potential drug targets? *Nat. Rev. Drug Discovery* 10 (9): 712.

62 Caie, P.D., Walls, R.E., Ingleston-Orme, A. et al. (2010). High-content phenotypic profiling of drug response signatures across distinct cancer cells. *Mol. Cancer Ther.* 9 (6): 1913–1926.

63 Bray, M.A., Singh, S., Han, H. et al. (2016). Cell painting, a high-content image-based assay for morphological profiling using multiplexed fluorescent dyes. *Nat. Protoc.* 11 (9): 1757–1774.

64 Bray, M.A., Gustafsdottir, S.M., Rohban, M.H. et al. (2017). A dataset of images and morphological profiles of 30 000 small-molecule treatments using the cell painting assay. *GigaScience* 6 (12): 1–5.

65 Perlman, Z.E., Slack, M.D., Feng, Y. et al. (2004). Multidimensional drug profiling by automated microscopy. *Science* 306 (5699): 1194–1198.

66 Wahlby, C., Kamentsky, L., Liu, Z.H. et al. (2012). An image analysis toolbox for high-throughput C. *elegans* assays. *Nat. Methods* 9 (7): 714–716.

67 Gough, A., Stern, A.M., Maier, J. et al. (2017). Biologically relevant heterogeneity: metrics and practical insights. *SLAS Discov.* 22 (3): 213–237.

68 Feng, Y., Mitchison, T.J., Bender, A. et al. (2009). Multi-parameter phenotypic profiling: using cellular effects to characterize small-molecule compounds. *Nat. Rev. Drug Discovery* 8 (7): 567–578.

69 Smith, K. and Horvath, P. (2014). Active learning strategies for phenotypic profiling of high-content screens. *J. Biomol. Screen.* 19 (5): 685–695.

70 Tanaka, M., Bateman, R., Rauh, D. et al. (2005). An unbiased cell morphology-based screen for new, biologically active small molecules. *PLoS Biol.* 3 (5): e128.

71 Ljosa, V., Caie, P.D., Ter Horst, R. et al. (2013). Comparison of methods for image-based profiling of cellular morphological responses to small-molecule treatment. *J. Biomol. Screen.* 18 (10): 1321–1329.

72 Godinez, W.J., Hossain, I., Lazic, S.E. et al. (2017). A multi-scale convolutional neural network for phenotyping high-content cellular images. *Bioinformatics* 33 (13): 2010–2019.

73 Kraus, O.Z., Grys, B.T., Ba, J. et al. (2017). Automated analysis of high-content microscopy data with deep learning. *Mol. Syst. Biol.* 13 (4): 924.

74 Gustafsdottir, S.M., Ljosa, V., Sokolnicki, K.L. et al. (2013). Multiplex cytological profiling assay to measure diverse cellular states. *PLoS One* 8 (12): e80999.

75 Rohban, M.H., Singh, S., Wu, X. et al. (2017). Systematic morphological profiling of human gene and allele function via cell painting. *eLife* 6.

76 Santos, R., Ursu, O., Gaulton, A. et al. (2017). A comprehensive map of molecular drug targets. *Nat. Rev. Drug Discovery* 16 (1): 19–34.

77 Reisen, F., Sauty De Chalon, A., Pfeifer, M. et al. (2015). Linking phenotypes and modes of action through high-content screen fingerprints. *Assay Drug Dev. Technol.* 13 (7): 415–427.

78 Young, D.W., Bender, A., Hoyt, J. et al. (2008). Integrating high-content screening and ligand-target prediction to identify mechanism of action. *Nat. Chem. Biol.* 4 (1): 59–68.

79 Warchal, S.J., Unciti-Broceta, A., and Carragher, N.O. (2016). Next-generation phenotypic screening. *Future Med. Chem.* 8 (11): 1331–1347.

80 Lee, J.A., Uhlik, M.T., Moxham, C.M. et al. (2012). Modern phenotypic drug discovery is a viable, neoclassic pharma strategy. *J. Med. Chem.* 55 (10): 4527–4538.

81 Gough, W., Hulkower, K.I., Lynch, R. et al. (2011). A quantitative, facile, and high-throughput image-based cell migration method is a robust alternative to the scratch assay. *J. Biomol. Screen.* 16 (2): 155–163.

82 Fraser, C., Dawson, J.C., Dowling, R. et al. (2016). Rapid discovery and structure-activity relationships of pyrazolopyrimidines that potently suppress breast cancer cell growth via SRC kinase inhibition with exceptional selectivity over ABL kinase. *J. Med. Chem.* 59 (10): 4697–4710.

83 Fraser, C., Carragher, N.O., and Unciti-Broceta, A. (2016). eCF309: a potent, highly-selective, cell-active mTOR inhibitor. *MedChemComm* https://doi.org/10.1039/C5MD00493D.

84 Edwards, A.M., Bountra, C., Kerr, D.J., and Willson, T.M. (2009). Open access chemical and clinical probes to support drug discovery. *Nat. Chem. Biol.* 5 (7): 436–440.

85 Lam, F.C. and Yaffe, M.B. (2016). Kicking genomic profiling to the curb: how re-wiring the phosphoproteome can explain treatment resistance in glioma. *Cancer Cell* 29 (4): 435–436.

86 Rodriguez, J.M., Monsalves-Alvarez, M., Henriquez, S. et al. (2016). Glucocorticoid resistance in chronic diseases. *Steroids* 115: 182–192.
87 Serrels, A., Lund, T., Serrels, B. et al. (2015). Nuclear FAK controls chemokine transcription, Tregs, and evasion of anti-tumor immunity. *Cell* 163 (1): 160–173.
88 Serrels, B., Mcgivern, N., Canel, M. et al. (2017). IL-33 and ST2 mediate FAK-dependent antitumor immune evasion through transcriptional networks. *Sci. Signal.* 10 (508).
89 Lamb, J., Crawford, E.D., Peck, D. et al. (2006). The connectivity map: using gene-expression signatures to connect small molecules, genes, and disease. *Science* 313 (5795): 1929–1935.
90 Hieronymus, H., Lamb, J., Ross, K.N. et al. (2006). Gene expression signature-based chemical genomic prediction identifies a novel class of HSP90 pathway modulators. *Cancer Cell* 10 (4): 321–330.
91 Liu, C., Su, J., Yang, F. et al. (2015). Compound signature detection on LINCS L1000 big data. *Mol. Biosyst.* 11 (3): 714–722.
92 Subramanian, A., Narayan, R., Corsello, S.M. et al. (2017). A next generation connectivity map: L1000 platform and the first 1,000,000 profiles. *Cell* 171 (6): 1437–1452.e17.
93 Pabon, N.A., Xia, Y., Estabrooks, S.K. et al. (2018). bioRxiv preprint first posted online 25 January 2018. https://doi.org/10.1101/254367.
94 Rees, M.G., Seashore-Ludlow, B., Cheah, J.H. et al. (2016). Correlating chemical sensitivity and basal gene expression reveals mechanism of action. *Nat. Chem. Biol.* 12 (2): 109–116.
95 Akbani, R., Becker, K.F., Carragher, N. et al. (2014). Realizing the promise of reverse phase protein arrays for clinical, translational, and basic research: a workshop report: the RPPA (Reverse Phase Protein Array) society. *Mol. Cell. Proteomics* 13 (7): 1625–1643.
96 Hellstrom, C., Dodig-Crnkovic, T., Hong, M.G. et al. (2017). High-density serum/plasma reverse phase protein arrays. *Methods Mol. Biol.* 1619: 229–238.
97 Wei, W., Shin, Y.S., Xue, M. et al. (2016). Single-cell phosphoproteomics resolves adaptive signaling dynamics and informs targeted combination therapy in glioblastoma. *Cancer Cell* 29 (4): 563–573.
98 Shi, Q., Qin, L., Wei, W. et al. (2012). Single-cell proteomic chip for profiling intracellular signaling pathways in single tumor cells. *Proc. Natl. Acad. Sci. U.S.A.* 109 (2): 419–424.
99 Moffat, J.G., Rudolph, J., and Bailey, D. (2014). Phenotypic screening in cancer drug discovery - past, present and future. *Nat. Rev. Drug Discovery* 13 (8): 588–602.
100 Eder, J., Sedrani, R., and Wiesmann, C. (2014). The discovery of first-in-class drugs: origins and evolution. *Nat. Rev. Drug Discovery* 13 (8): 577–587.
101 Swinney, D.C. and Anthony, J. (2011). How were new medicines discovered? *Nat. Rev. Drug Discovery* 10 (7): 507–519.

8

Cell Biology Methods in Target Validation

Manfred Koegl and Simon Wöhrle

Boehringer Ingelheim RCV GmbH & Co KG, Belghofergasse 15 Vienna, 1221, Austria

8.1 Introduction

The classical methods of target validation that are applied when no active compounds are yet available, such as RNA interference and clustered regularly interspaced short palindromic repeats (CRISPR)-based methods, are discussed elsewhere in this book (Chapter 9). This chapter will deal with a different problem: once a pharmaceutical agent, typically an antibody or a small molecule has been generated that can modulate a drug target *in vitro*, the question arises: does the compound exert the desired biological effects when added to cells in tissue culture, or to animals? Looking at this from the angle of the macroscopic response, one can rephrase the question: is there a causal relationship between the modulation of the target and the cellular response? In the following chapter, we will look at considerations and methods that have been applied to address and reliably answer this question:

1. We will discuss biomarkers to quantify the effect of a drug at different levels of resolution.
2. We will consider correlations of these biomarkers as a necessary consequence of cause–effect relationships, providing indirect proof for the mode of action of the drug.
3. We will discuss direct proof for a target being responsible for an observed response by introducing mutations in the presumptive drug target and/or by chemoproteomic approaches.

8.2 Biomarkers

The term biomarker encompasses, among other uses, parameters that change upon treatment of a cell or an organism with a pharmaceutical agent. To follow the effects of a drug on a cell, the availability of appropriate biomarkers is a prerequisite. In the following section, we will discern three types of biomarkers (Figure 8.1). This is by no means the only possible way to define biomarkers, but a useful one for the purpose of the discussion in this chapter.

Target Discovery and Validation: Methods and Strategies for Drug Discovery,
First Edition. Edited by Alleyn T. Plowright.

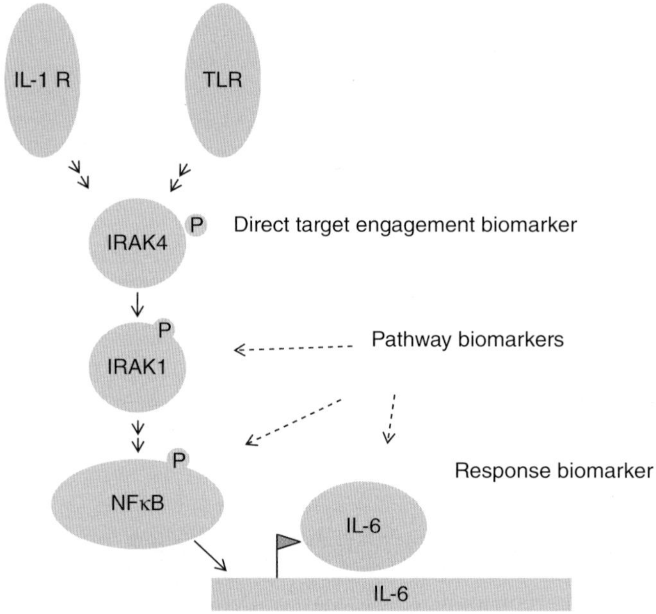

Figure 8.1 Three levels of biomarkers. The signal transduction pathway downstream of IL-1 and Toll-like receptors (TLR) is depicted. Engagement of these receptors results in the activation of IRAK4, which is the drug target of interest in this example, and also of IRAK1, which is assumed to be activated by phosphorylation through IRAK4; the transcription factor NF-κB, which gets phosphorylated and activated by kinases downstream of IRAK1; and an effector gene coding for IL-6. Autophosphorylation of IRAK4 is useful as a biomarker for its activation state and lends itself to use as a direct target engagement biomarker. The phosphorylation status of the IRAK1 and NF-κB are directly or indirectly regulated by IRAK4. Either of them can be used as a pathway biomarker. Finally, the mRNA or protein levels of IL-6 provide excellent response biomarkers.

8.2.1 Direct Target Engagement Biomarkers

We will refer to parameters that are expected to change immediately when a protein is bound by a drug as direct target engagement biomarkers. Such biomarkers provide a read-out for the activity of a pharmacological agent that is directly linked to the target itself. Naturally, the nature of such direct biomarkers depends to a large extent on the type of drug target that is engaged. For example:

- For covalently binding drugs, drug–protein adducts provide a convenient measure of target engagement.
- For kinases, the autophosphorylation that takes place on most activated kinases is an excellent target modulation biomarker. Autophosphorylation is preferable to the phosphorylation of other downstream substrates of the respective pathway, since the latter could be effected by other kinases and for this reason are not necessarily direct target engagement biomarkers. Kinases that are similar to the actual target typically are also the most likely off-targets for the inhibitor and often have overlapping substrates, complicating interpretation of data based on downstream kinase substrates. As a biomarker,

the typical autophosphorylation site of a kinase in its activation loop may be a good choice here. In the case of receptor tyrosine kinases such as the EGF receptor (EGFR), the autophosphorylation on multiple tyrosine residues is an excellent measure of the protein's activity.

- For some nuclear receptors, such as the androgen receptor, a change in subcellular localization can be a good direct read-out of target engagement. In the absence of a ligand, androgen receptor is primarily localized to the cytoplasm. Upon binding to an agonistic or antagonistic ligand, the receptor translocates to the nucleus, which can be visualized by GFP fusion proteins (Figure 8.2) [1]. Similarly, for G-protein-coupled receptors, receptor internalization can be a good biomarker of receptor activation [2].
- Assays measuring the displacement of a fluorescent or radioactive ligand from a target protein (e.g. as shown for CXCR4 [3]) can provide powerful direct target engagement biomarkers. Such assays are typically applied to transmembrane cell surface receptors or nuclear receptors.
- In other cases, protein degradation induced by drug binding is a good indicator of the drug meeting its target. This is the case, for example, with the oestrogen receptor when cells are treated with fulvestrant, which causes its degradation [4]. For drugs that are explicitly designed to cause the degradation of its target, such as proteolysis-targeting chimaeras (PROTACs) [5], disappearance of the drug target is the natural choice as a direct target engagement biomarker.

8.2.2 Indirect Target Engagement Biomarkers and Pathway Biomarkers

Modulation of a target's activity is a prerequisite for a pharmacological effect, but not a goal in itself. To elicit a biological response, the cellular process in which the target plays a role has to also be affected. However, this does not necessarily always need to be the case, e.g. in the case of redundant nodes of a pathway, in which inhibiting only one of two proteins serving overlapping functions only causes minor perturbations in the pathway. Hence, biomarkers are needed that measure the effect of modulating the target on the relevant cellular processes. We will refer to such biomarkers as indirect target engagement biomarkers or pathway biomarkers. For most practical purposes, the rule applies that the closer the biomarker is to the target, the better, since the opportunities for unexpected effects to interfere are lower.

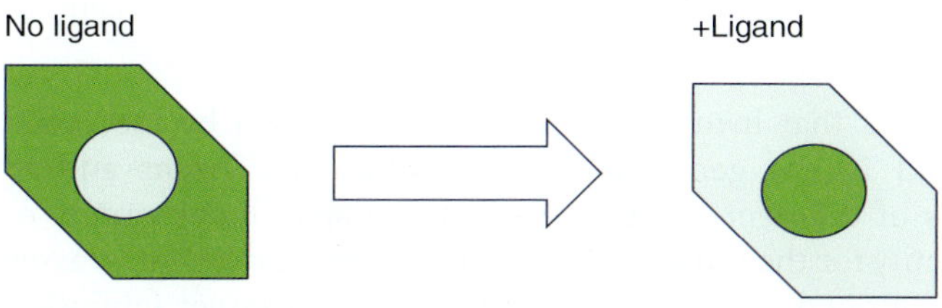

Figure 8.2 Ligand-induced nuclear translocation of a GFP fusion protein, such as the androgen receptor, as a direct target engagement biomarker.

In the case of the EGFR, biomarkers of pathway modulation include the measurement of Ras GTP loading, the phosphorylation of MEK/ERK, or the induction of transcriptional response genes such as DUSP6. In theory, the most proximal biomarkers would include the binding of signalling proteins to the receptor, such as GRB2 or PLCγ. In practice, such binding events are less useful than phosphorylation events since they are more difficult to be measured precisely and they are not direct evidence of pathway activation, in contrast to Ras GTP binding or activating phosphorylation marks on ERK or PI3K, which are directly linked to the activation of these proteins. For drug targets involved in transcriptional regulation, such as nuclear receptors or chromatin factors, the elevated or reduced expression of responsive genes or changes in chromatin modification marks provide useful pathway biomarkers, e.g. the regulation of histone 3 trimethylation at lysine 27 after inhibition of the methyltransferase EZH2 [6].

8.2.3 Response Biomarkers

Ultimately, the desired effect of a pharmaceutically active substance is an effect on cellular behaviour. In the case of cancer drugs, this can be the induction of cell death, e.g. by apoptosis. For such drugs, the dose-dependent induction of markers of apoptosis, for example, by the induction of caspase activity or the appearance of phosphatidylserine on the exterior sheet of the plasma membrane, can be used as biomarkers of drug response. In the case of anti-inflammatory drugs, the desired effect can be, for example, a reduction in the output of inflammatory cytokines such as interleukin 1 (IL-1), typically measured by ELISA or related methods. Throughout this chapter we will refer to biomarkers of cellular response as response biomarkers.

8.2.4 Correlation of Biomarkers

If assays for these three types of biomarkers are available, the response to modulating a drug target can be followed from the level of bimolecular drug–target interaction 'up' to the macroscopic response:

- *Target engagement biomarker*: Does the drug modulate its presumptive target's activity?
- *Pathway biomarker*: Does the modulation of target activity result in an altered pathway output?
- *Response biomarker*: Does the altered pathway output lead to a cellular response?

Drug discovery projects that involve compound optimization by medicinal chemistry efforts result in the generation of, at minimum, dozens and in some cases thousands of different compounds that can span many orders of magnitude in their affinity for the target. When measured using the three classes of biomarker assays described above, a causal relationship of target inhibition leading to a cellular response predicts that compounds that bind the target most potently (e.g. with a low IC_{50} value, as measured via the target engagement biomarker) will also modulate the pathway and response biomarkers most potently, while compounds that bind the target less potently will modulate the pathway and response biomarkers less potently. A plot of the IC_{50} values from the three types of biomarkers against each other will therefore show a clear correlation.

Figure 8.3 depicts a different example in which the correlation of biomarkers is excellent, inferring a causal relationship of the observed phenomena. The target in this example is BCL6, a transcriptional repressor protein that has been implicated as an oncogenic driver in lymphomas [7]. A series of compounds that bind to BCL6 and induce degradation of the protein was discovered in the course of a drug discovery project [8]. These compounds also inhibit the growth of the lymphoma cell line Farage in a semi-solid medium containing matrigel. A critical question to answer is then: are the binding of the compounds to BCL6, the degradation of BCL6, and the anti-proliferative effects causally connected? If this is the case, the measured potencies of the three phenomena should be clearly correlated. This is shown in Figure 8.3: Firstly, the affinity of binding of the compounds to BCL6 in cells is measured via monitoring the inhibition of BCL6 binding to its co-repressor protein NCoR1. Secondly, the potency of the compounds in inducing degradation of BCL6 is measured (Figure 8.3a). Thirdly, the potency of inhibiting proliferation is measured (Figure 8.3b). In this case, the excellent correlations ($R^2 = 0.8$ and 0.67, respectively) of both cellular biomarkers with the response biomarker are consistent with binding of the compounds to BCL6 inducing degradation of the protein and loss of BCL6 being responsible for the observed anti-proliferative effects. The assumption that the compounds' binding to BCL6 causes degradation of BCL6, which is incompatible with the growth of Farage cells, is supported by the data.

A second example is from the signalling pathway downstream of IL-1 and Toll-like receptors (TLR) highlighted earlier in this chapter. Firstly, the IC_{50} values of inhibitors of the kinase IRAK4 measured *in vitro* are plotted against the IC_{50} values measured with the target engagement biomarker in cells. Figure 8.4a shows a double logarithmic plot for such a relationship. There is a reasonable correlation apparent, indicating that the compounds reach and inhibit their target in cells.

To inhibit a pathway output by 50%, it may be necessary to inhibit the drug target to greater than 50%. A cellular response again only becomes apparent once the pathway is inhibited to greater than 50%. This leads to a parallel shift of the regression lines, which thus do not cross the origin. In the example in Figure 8.4b, which correlates the direct target engagement biomarker (autophosphorylation of IRAK4) with a pathway biomarker (phosphorylation of IRAK1), this shift is greater than 30-fold. This would indicate that almost complete inhibition of IRAK4 is required to shut down the activation of IRAK1 in these cells. However, in this example, the low correlation coefficient makes the alternative explanation at least equally likely, i.e. that inhibition of IRAK4 does not cause inhibition of the presumed downstream kinase IRAK1. The observed weak correlation may in this case also be explained by a cross-reactivity of the compounds with the two highly related kinases.

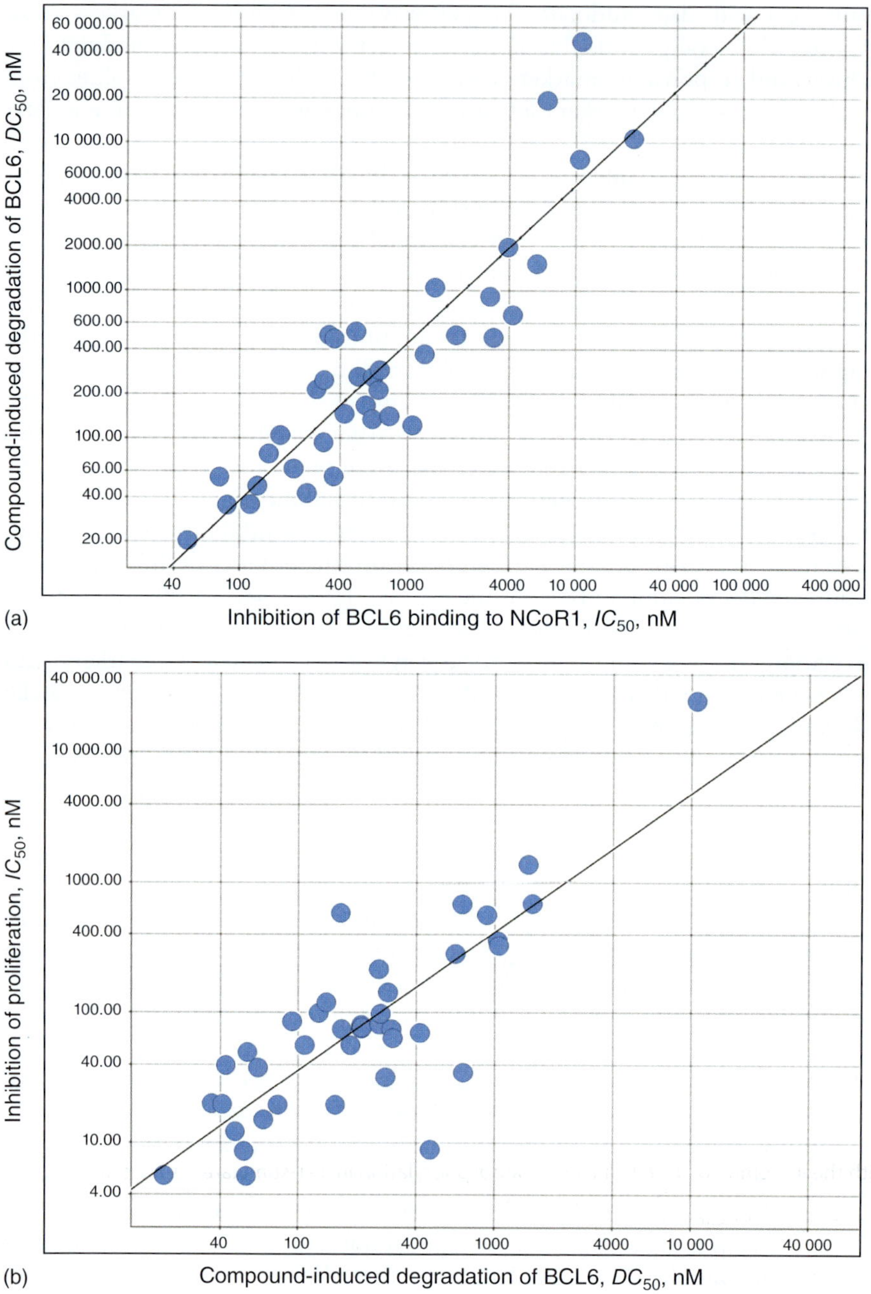

Figure 8.3 (a) The inhibition of the binding of BCL6 to its interaction partner NCoR1 as a measure for the compounds' potency in binding to BCL6 (in the absence of degradation) is plotted against DC_{50}s for compound induced degradation of BCL6. The interaction of NCoR1 to BCL6 is monitored in transiently transfected cells expressing tagged versions of the protein, followed by pulldown via the tag and quantitation of the binding partner. Correlation coefficient $R^2 = 0.8$. (b) Compound-induced degradation of BCL6 is plotted against the inhibition of proliferation in Farage cells grown in matrigel. DC_{50}, concentration of half maximal degradation. Correlation coefficient $R^2 = 0.67$.

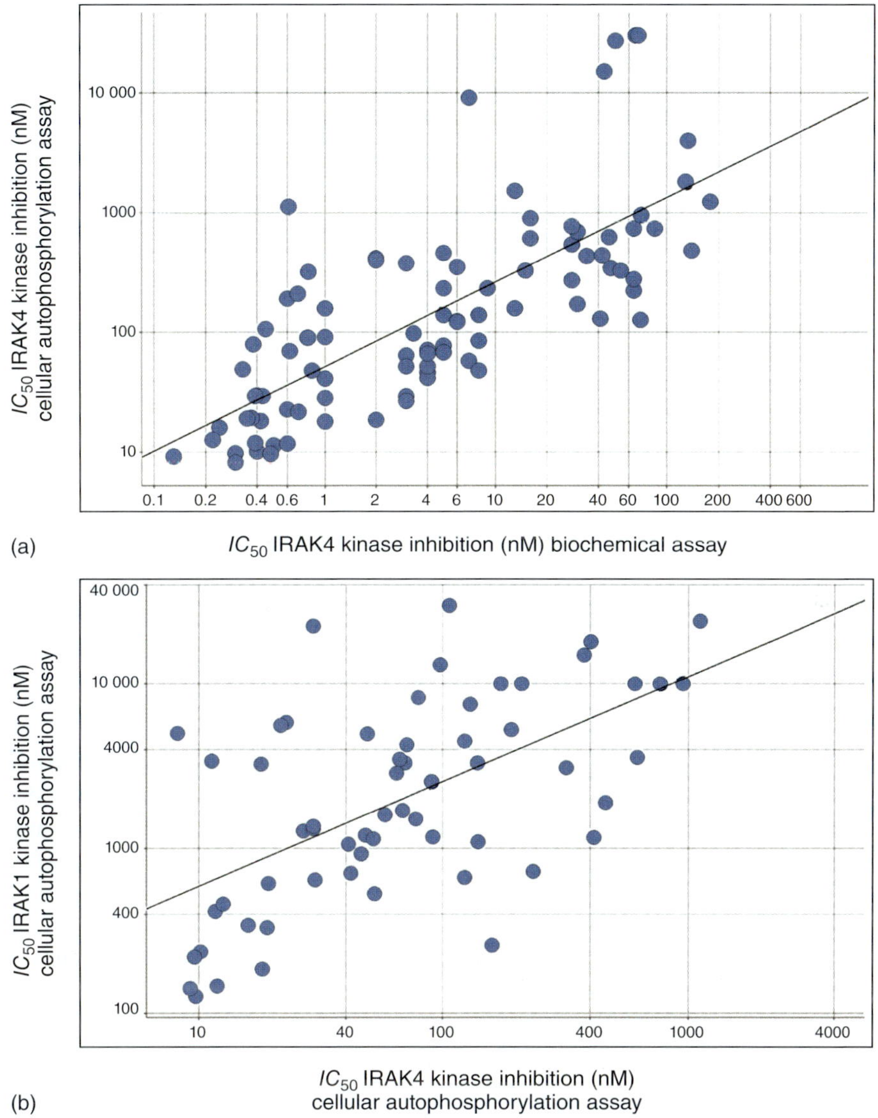

Figure 8.4 (a) Correlation of IC_{50} values for inhibition of IRAK4 in biochemical (cell-free) assays with the inhibition of IRAK4 kinase autophosphorylation in IL-1-stimulated A549 cells. Correlation coefficient $R^2 = 0.6$. (b) Correlation of IC_{50} values for inhibition of IRAK4 in IL-1-stimulated A549 cells as measured by autophosphorylation plotted against the IC_{50} values for inhibition of the presumed downstream target kinase IRAK1, also measured by autophosphorylation. The correlation coefficient of $R^2 = 0.35$ raises doubts as to whether the inhibition of IRAK4, as measured via IRAK4 autophosphorylation, necessarily causes an inhibition of IRAK1 activity in these cells. Note also the greater than 30-fold shift in the regression line: on average, 30 times more of the compound is required for inhibition of IRAK1 autophosphorylation than for IRAK4 autophosphorylation. (c) Lack of correlation of IRAK4 autophosphorylation with the phosphorylation of NF-κB in IL-1-stimulated A549 cells. In this case, it is extremely unlikely that an improvement of the potency of this compound series against IRAK4 will cause an improved inhibition of NF-κB phosphorylation.

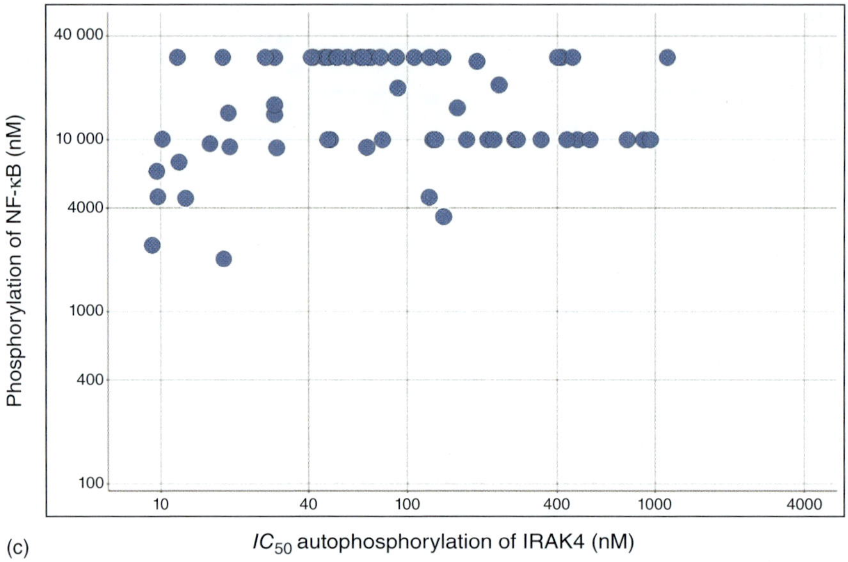

Figure 8.4 (*Continued*)

Finally, when the effects of the compound on IRAK4 are plotted against the presumptive downstream effect, in this case the activation of the pro-inflammatory transcription factor NF-κB by phosphorylation, no clear correlation is apparent (Figure 8.4c). The absence of this kind of correlation is reliable evidence that inhibition of the target cannot be the cause for the cellular responses observed. Instead, off-target effects take responsibility for any observed effects. This logic is obviously not applicable to the correlation from *in vitro* (cell-free) assays to cellular assays (Figure 8.4a). In this case, the correlation may be confounded by differences in plasma protein binding, cellular uptake and efflux or in the stability of the compound, to name a few. Where there is a lack of correlation of the three biomarkers that are measured in cells, there is no such reasoning and may signal the end of the project. In the context of drug discovery efforts, the lack of a correlation of the target engagement biomarker implies that optimization of the compound, resulting in more potent target engagement, cannot be expected to result in more potent target modulation or cellular response. Further improvement of the compounds is therefore futile, and further optimization efforts cannot be justified. However, one has to bear in mind that the connectivity of signalling pathways may be cell line dependent, such that the expected correlation may be evident in one cell line, but absent in another.

'Negative control compounds' that are very similar to an active compound in their chemical structure, but do not bind to the target, are useful controls to pinpoint the effect of a small molecule to a target. Such compounds which are most useful are those that only differ in their three-dimensional structure, but not in their chemical composition, i.e. pairs of enantiomers or diastereoisomers of compounds. For compounds that are different in structure but closely related, the negative control compounds typically differ by a few atoms only. In all cases, the inactivity of the inactive compound on all three biomarkers is a first step in linking a compound's effect to a cellular response. One has to bear in mind, however, that such negative control compounds are merely extreme cases of the kind of correlations discussed above and any conclusions taken from the comparison of a single pair of compounds are less reliable than those taken from larger numbers of compounds that span several orders of magnitude of potency.

8.3 Direct Evidence to Show That Modulation of a Target Leads to a Cellular Response

While the correlation of biomarkers is necessary to infer a causal relationship from target engagement to cellular response, it is not sufficient proof. Alternative explanations for such a correlation can be put forward, especially if the drug target is part of a family of proteins related in structure. For example, in the case of kinase inhibitors, a related kinase may be responsible for the correlation. The related kinase can be expected to have similar affinities as the actual target kinase for the group of compounds tested, leading to an apparently convincing correlation that is nevertheless not causal.

Also, at the beginning of a drug discovery project, a large group of compounds spanning orders of magnitude in their affinity for the target is hardly ever available. Thus, any conclusions based on the correlation of biomarkers can only be drawn long after significant investments in compound optimization have been made. Other methods are therefore required to answer the question whether target engagement has the desired consequences.

To prove that a target's inhibition is responsible for a response, the best evidence that can be obtained stems from genetic manipulation of the target that alters the cellular response. Two ways of manipulating a target will be discussed below:

1. The generation of artificially drug-sensitive versions of the target.
2. The generation of artificially drug-resistant versions of the target.

8.4 Direct Evidence That Target Modulation Is Responsible for Cellular Responses by Mutations Conferring Sensitivity to Existing Drugs

8.4.1 The 'Bump-and-Hole' Approach to Generate Sensitivity to Small Molecule Inhibitors

A critical step for any drug discovery project is to validate whether a cellular response to treatment with a small molecule is directly linked to pharmacological inhibition of the targeted protein and not the consequence of non-target-related (off-target) effects.

An elegant approach to link small molecule inhibition specifically to the desired target protein was first conceptually introduced for v-Src kinase by re-engineering of a small molecule–protein interface [9]. In this so-called

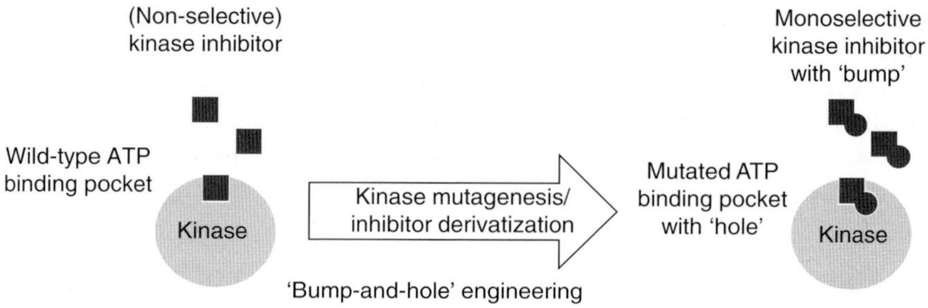

Figure 8.5 The 'bump-and-hole' approach to generate monoselectivity to small molecule inhibitors. A mutation in the small molecule binding site of a target protein is introduced, generating a 'hole' allowing a bulky derivative of the inhibitor to fit ('bump') into the extended target binding site.

'bump-and-hole' approach, depicted in Figure 8.5, a mutation in the ATP binding pocket was introduced whereby a large hydrophobic amino acid side chain was substituted with a smaller residue ('hole'). This renders the kinase susceptible to derivatives of the non-selective Src family inhibitor, PP1 [10], designed to fit the extended ATP binding pocket by addition of a large hydrophilic group ('bump').

Of note, the analogue-sensitive kinase mutant catalyses ATP with similar efficiency as the wild-type enzyme and therefore does not exhibit a loss-of-function phenotype that would impact on the cellular read-out of kinase function. Owing to steric hindrance, the modified, bulky kinase inhibitors are not compatible with the ATP binding scaffold of any kinase and thus represent monospecific inhibitors for the kinase target of interest [9]. While a potential off-target effect of the modified inhibitor can formally not be ruled out, this can be precisely monitored in cell models not harbouring the analogue-sensitive kinase mutant.

This concept has since been generalized for many protein kinases, making use of the conserved scaffold of the ATP binding pocket within the protein kinase family [11]. Thus, the 'bump-and-hole' approach can also be applied to kinase targets for which no tool inhibitors are available. This is exemplified for the putative cancer target RIOK1 [12]. Here, a substitution of methionine to alanine or glycine within the ATP binding pocket of the kinase allows binding of the PP1 analogue 1-NA-PP1, conferring a greater than 10-fold sensitization to 1-NA-PP1 treatment compared with RIOK1 wild-type parental cells in viability assays. This allows the effect of pharmacological inhibition to be mimicked, which is in contrast to genetic validation using CRISPR-mediated knockout or RNA interference methods (discussed in Chapter 9), that often lack precise temporal control over target inhibition.

The beauty of the approach is also highlighted by monospecific BCR-ABL inhibition using a PP1 analogue in leukaemia cell models driven by an analogue-sensitive BCR-ABL variant [13]. While monospecific BCR-ABL inhibition precisely phenocopies the efficacy of the clinically used BCR-ABL inhibitor Gleevec (imatinib) in BCR-ABL-driven B-cell acute lymphoblastic leukaemia models, it failed to similarly suppress myeloproliferative disorder progenitors dependent on KIT signalling, thus demonstrating that the clinical efficacy of Gleevec is in part attributed to its pleiotropic kinase selectivity profile.

In a reversed version of the concept, kinases can be turned resistant against a particular inhibitor by introducing a large amino acid that is not compatible with inhibitor binding, but does not overtly perturb kinase activity. In this way, isogenic cell pairs can be generated in which the wild-type kinase responds to an inhibitor, whereas the cell line expressing the mutant kinase does not. This approach has been applied to show that the response of a macrophage cell line to an inhibitor is due to the inhibition of SIK2. Expression of SIK2 bearing the bulky amino acid glutamine instead of threonine rendered these cells resistant to a rather promiscuous inhibitor, proving the point that SIK2 is responsible for the observed effects [14].

In addition to kinases, the 'bump-and-hole' concept has also been successfully applied to selectively target bromodomain-containing proteins. Here, analogous to the modification of the ATP binding pocket, a leucine residue within the binding site for acetylated lysine is substituted with a smaller alanine, creating a novel binding pocket for an ethyl derivative of the bromodomain inhibitor JQ1 [15]. As shown in Figure 8.6, introduction of this mutation to members of the bromo and extra-terminal (BET) protein family enables, for instance, to specifically address the function of single BET proteins, which is not possible with the promiscuous BET family inhibitor JQ1.

Thus, the 'bump-and-hole' approach constitutes a powerful technology to engineer monospecific small molecule inhibitors for functional validation of any kinase- and bromodomain-containing target protein. In the future, this concept might be further extended to other protein classes. With the emergence of the CRISPR/Cas9 technology, it has also become increasingly feasible to directly introduce the analogue-sensitizing mutations into the endogenous locus of any appropriate cell model. The generation of isogenic cells lines, which differ only in their sensitivity to the monospecific small molecule, allows to precisely

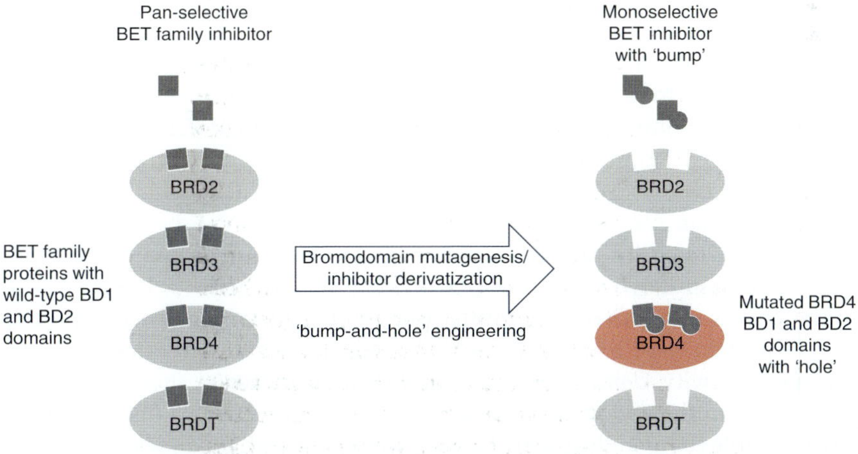

Figure 8.6 The 'bump-and-hole' approach to generate monoselectivity to pan-selective BET family inhibitors. A mutation in the BD1 and BD2 bromodomains of BRD4 generates monoselectivity to a bulky derivative of a pan-selective BET family inhibitor, allowing to selectively monitor the effects of BRD4 inhibition.

monitor the physiological consequences of pharmaceutical target inhibition versus potential off-target effects.

8.4.2 Chemogenomic Approaches for Inducible Degradation of Protein Targets

For many potential drug targets, in particular the highly sought-after novel, but thus less extensively studied targets, pharmacological agents that could be used as tool compounds do not exist. While RNAi- or CRISPR-based technologies have proven tremendously useful to identify and validate potential drug targets, e.g. for cancer therapy [16–18], it is often advantageous to be able to assess the effect of pharmacological inhibition of a potential drug target in the early stages of the drug development process. As mentioned previously, genomic knockdown/knockout strategies lack tight temporal control over target gene inhibition and do not allow to precisely mimic complex pharmacodynamic effects such as partial and short-lived target inhibition.

In the absence of a reasonably potent and selective tool compound, chemogenetic inducible degradation approaches have proven valuable to model pharmacological target inhibition. Two such concepts, degradation tag (dTAG)- and auxin-inducible degron (AID)-based methods, will be described in detail here. Both systems are based on degradation of the target protein of interest via engagement of the cellular E3 ubiquitin ligase and proteasome machinery using generic small molecules.

The AID system makes use of a proteasome-dependent degradation pathway present in plants that is controlled by Auxin family phytohormones [19]. Auxin binding to the F-box protein transport inhibitor response 1 (TIR1) leads to the assembly of an active Skp, Cullin, F-box (SCF)-containing complex. The SCF^{TIR1} complex targets proteins of the auxin or IAA (AUX/IAA) transcription repressor family for polyubiquitylation and subsequent degradation via the proteasome [20, 21] (see Figure 8.7).

The F-box protein TIR1, which determines substrate specificity for AUX/IAA proteins, is unique to plants. However, the SCF machinery is conserved across eukaryotes, and mammalian cells are therefore able to functionally incorporate TIR1 in their SCF complexes [22]. Expression of TIR1 in mammalian cells generates a novel SCF specificity for AUX/IAA proteins that is not matched by any mammalian protein. Auxin-inducible degradation can be conferred to any target protein of interest by fusion with an AID-compatible degron-tag. AUX/IAA protein-derived degron-tags are reasonably small (<10 kDa). Still, potential effects of a (N- or C-terminal) degron-tag fusion on the function of the target protein have to be thoroughly tested to avoid any interference with its biological activity. Using CRISPR-based knock-in strategies such tags can be easily inserted in the endogenous target gene locus, generating a fusion protein that is amenable to rapid degradation upon treatment with auxin with a half-life of 10–20 minutes [23].

The functionality of this system to assess acute inhibition for targets not (yet) trackable with pharmacological agents has been recently demonstrated for the transcription factor MYC [24], a protein deemed ‘undruggable’ despite its

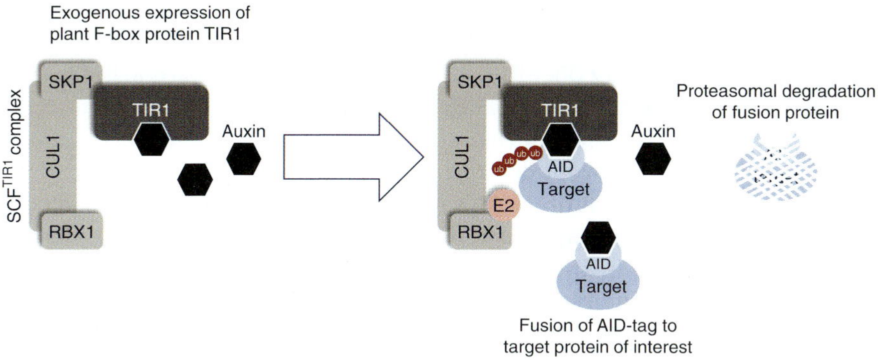

Figure 8.7 The auxin-inducible degradation (AID) system. Exogenously expressed plant F-box protein TIR1 is incorporated into mammalian SCF complexes. This generates a novel target specificity for proteins harbouring AID-degron tags. Auxin treatment leads to polyubiquitylation and subsequent degradation of the target protein–AID fusion via the proteasome.

discovery as a promising cancer target decades ago [25]. Direct versus indirect transcriptional functions of MYC have been difficult to dissect using RNAi or CRISPR approaches, and, in fact, MYC has been proposed to function rather as a global 'transcriptional amplifier' than a specific transcription factor due to its ubiquitous promoter occupancy [25, 26]. However, AID-tagging of MYC in a TIR1-expressing chronic myeloid leukaemia cell line allowed for auxin-inducible rapid degradation of MYC within minutes. Using this model system, combined with a sequencing method to quantify newly synthesized mRNA, Muhar et al. were able to define a set of direct MYC target genes and to highlight protein and nucleotide biosynthesis as key pathways downstream of MYC [24].

The dTAG system uses a very similar approach, but is entirely based on the endogenous ubiquitin ligase machinery and does not necessitate the generation of a cell line stably expressing an exogenous F-box protein. Instead, the dTAG approach uses a bispecific molecule that links the target protein to the proteasome machinery via concomitant engagement of the target protein and an E3 ubiquitin ligase. Such bispecific molecules are termed proteolysis-targeting chimeras (PROTACs), representing a novel class of small molecule inhibitors that catalytically facilitate degradation of the target protein of interest [27]. The concept has been successfully applied to cancer targets such as BRD4 [28, 29]. PROTACs cause the target protein to come into close proximity with the E3 ligase, thereby rendering the target protein an artificial substrate of the E3 ligase, resulting in its ubiquitylation and degradation via the proteasome machinery. Clearly, the concept relies on the availability of ligands to both the E3 ubiquitin ligase and the target protein. While generic binders to cereblon (CRBN), von Hippel–Lindau tumour suppressor (VHL), and other E3 ubiquitin ligases exist [30], often ligands selective for the target protein of interest are not available.

This limitation is addressed by the dTAG system, which introduces a generic ligand–target protein element to the PROTAC approach, by utilizing a bifunctional small molecule that simultaneously engages the E3 ligase cereblon (CRBN) and a mutant form of the FK506 binding protein FKBP12. The molecule termed dTAG consists of a selective ligand to CRBN and a binder to the phenylalanine-36 to valine variant of FKBP12 (FKBP12-F36V) [31] coupled via a carbon linker [32]. The selectivity for FKBP12-F36V over the endogenous form of the protein is critical to avoid any interference of the molecule with FKBP12-related functions. Analogous to the AID concept described above, this generates monospecificity for an exogenous target. Of note, the selectivity to FKBP12-F36V was achieved using the 'bump-and-hole' approach described earlier, based on non-selective FKBP family ligands [31]. The selectivity of the dTAG molecule is then, similar to the AID concept, conferred to any target protein of interest by fusion with the FKBP12-F36V variant (see Figure 8.8). The fusion protein can be introduced to the cell model of choice by exogenous expression. Subsequently, the endogenous target protein must be inactivated, for example, by CRISPR-mediated knockout of the gene, to be able to study the effect of acute loss of the target protein. Alternatively, the CRISPR technology can also be applied to directly engineer the FKBP12-F36V fusion into the endogenous target loci, thereby preserving the transcriptional regulation of the fused target protein.

The functionality of this approach was first demonstrated for the transcriptional activator ENL, highlighting its critical function as a driver of oncogenic growth in leukaemia cell models [32]. In this study, ectopic expression was used to introduce a FKBP12-F36V-ENL fusion protein to a leukaemia cell model, followed by CRISPR-mediated knockout of the endogenous ENL gene. Treatment with nanomolar concentrations of dTAG led to efficient degradation of FKBP12-F36V-fused ENL within 30 minutes, allowing the cellular responses to loss of ENL to be assessed with similar kinetics as a hypothetical small molecule inhibitor of ENL [32]. Similarly, the method has been applied to decipher the immediate effects on downstream signalling pathways upon dTAG-mediated targeted degradation of KRAS and MYC [33]. Of note, the dTAG molecule has pharmacological properties supporting *in vivo* testing of target proteins, for instance, in mouse xenograft models [33].

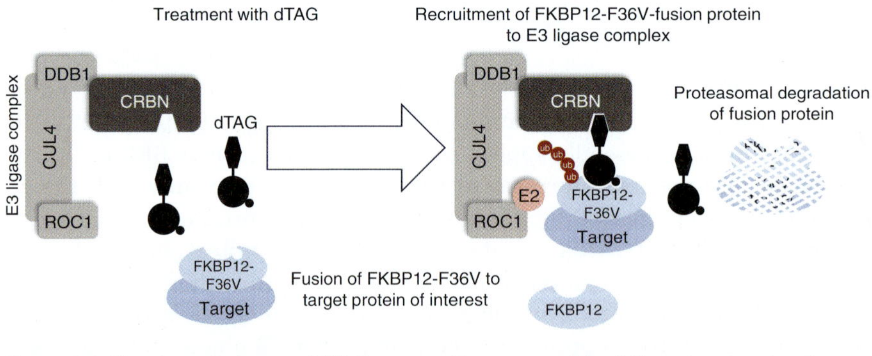

Figure 8.8 The degradation tag (dTAG) system. Treatment with a bifunctional molecule (dTAG) simultaneously engaging E3 ligase CRBN and a mutant form of FKBP12 (FKBP12-F36V) recruits FKBP12-F36V-fused target proteins to the proteasomal machinery, leading to degradation of the target protein. Endogenous FKBP12 is not affected due to the selectivity of dTAG for the mutated form of FKBP12.

The dTAG approach can also be applied to endogenous loci of target genes. Using CRISPR-mediated knock-in, our laboratory has engineered an oesophageal squamous cell carcinoma cell line harbouring a C-terminal insertion of the FKBP12-F36V sequence at the coactivator-associated arginine methyltransferase 1 (CARM1) gene locus. Treatment with dTAG led to a strong but not complete reduction of CARM1 protein levels in this model system, which did not interfere with proliferation of the cell line (Figure 8.9), in contrast to full genetic ablation of CARM1 by CRISPR knockout (not shown).

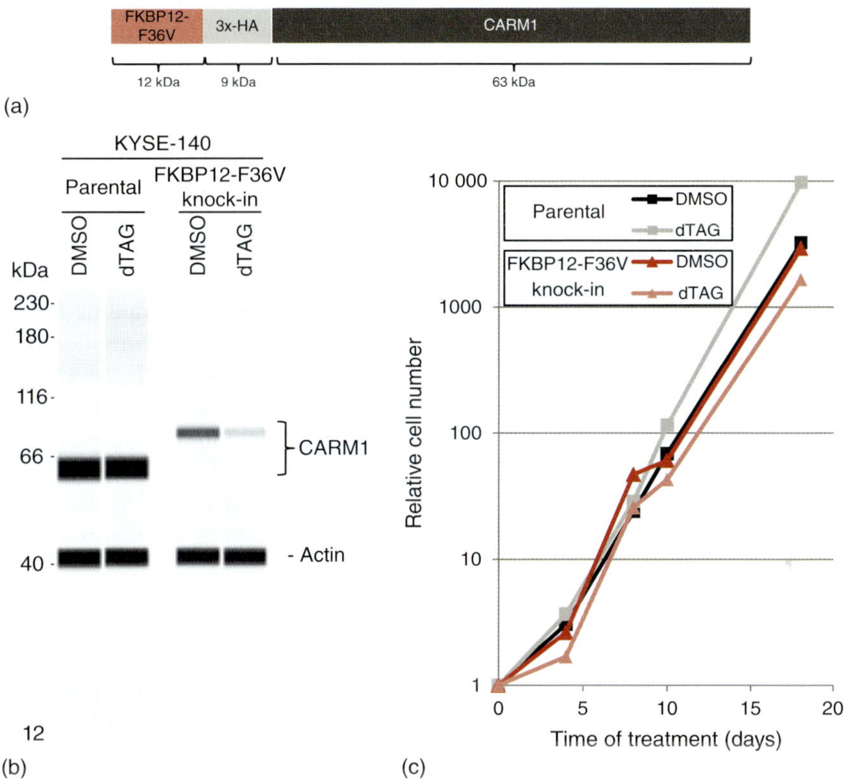

Figure 8.9 dTAG-mediated degradation of CARM1. (a) Schematic overview of the FKBP12-F36V fusion to CARM1 generated via CRISPR-mediated knock-in the oesophageal squamous cell carcinoma cell line KYSE-140. An additional human influenza haemagglutinin (HA)-tag is fused to the target protein along with FKBP12-F36V. (b) Treatment with dTAG (500 nM) led to (incomplete) degradation of FKBP12-F36V-fused CARM1 at 18 hours' post-treatment. In the parental cell line, dTAG treatment had no effect on protein levels of unedited, non-tagged CARM1. CARM1 and FKBP12-F36V-CARM1 were detected with anti-CARM1 antibody. Actin was used as a loading control. Note the lower expression levels of CARM1 in the knock-in cell line versus the parental control line. (c) Long-term treatment with dTAG did not lead to impaired proliferation in FKBP12-F36V-CARM1 knock-in cells. Parental and knock-in cell lines were treated with 1 μM of dTAG over a period of 18 days. Medium and compound were refreshed every three to five days and cell numbers were counted, split, and re-plated for long-term monitoring of cell proliferation. Source: Figure kindly provided by Katharina Ehrenhöfer-Wölfer (Boehringer Ingelheim, Vienna, Austria).

FKBP12 has a molecular weight of 12 kDa. As for the AID-tag, potential effects of the FKBP12-F36V fusion on target protein function, e.g. interference with binding partner interactions or changes in subcellular localization, have to be carefully monitored. Specific to the CRBN-based PROTAC molecules is that the CRBN binding moiety of the molecule on its own can engage endogenous proteins such as IKAROS family zinc-finger 1/3 (IKZF1/3), casein kinase 1α, or the translation termination factor GSPT1 and induce their degradation [34–37], irrespective of the FKBP12-F36V-targeting moiety. Similar off-target degradation effects have not been described for VHL-based PROTACs. However, potential off-target effects of dTAG treatment can be precisely monitored in parental isogenic cell models not harbouring the FKBP12-F36V fusion.

It is relevant to note that similarly to genomic knockdown/knockout strategies, targeted protein degradation in most cases does not resemble the mechanism of action for target inhibition with pharmacological agents. A protein may harbour multiple domains exerting different enzymatic or scaffolding functions. While dTAG and AID approaches affect the integrity of the target protein as a whole and thus block all (including potential unknown) protein functions, small molecule or biological agents typically selectively interfere with enzymatic functions or protein–protein interactions.

An example illustrating this discrepancy is the chromatin remodelling factor BRM (SMARCA2). BRM contains both an ATPase domain and a bromodomain, required to catalyse nucleosome repositioning and to interact with acetylated lysines respectively [38]. Using RNA interference approaches, BRM has been identified as a potential drug target in a subset of lung carcinomas [39]. However, pharmacological targeting of BRM with a small molecule inhibitor of the bromodomain fails to phenocopy the effects observed upon RNAi-mediated gene knockdown because the biologically relevant function of BRM as a cancer drug target is related to the ATPase domain [40].

In summary, both AID and dTAG represent generic approaches to pharmacological inhibition of basically any target protein of interest. It is of particular relevance for drug discovery research to be able to mimic the effects of dose-dependent target inhibition as well as different treatment schedules. The possibility to address such questions in the target validation stage of the drug development process prior to the availability of tool compound inhibitors might allow to better scrutinize and select relevant from poor drug targets and may help to limit the characteristically high attrition rate of drug development projects. The powerful genetic tools that are available now facilitate the implementation of these technologies in cellular models with high precision and reasonable effort. In the future, these approaches might be transferred to more complex and disease-relevant model systems such as organoid cultures or (in the case of dTAG) engineered mouse models.

8.5 Resistance Conferring Mutations

A mutation in the binding site of the target protein that prevents drug binding, but preserves the biological function of the target, confers resistance to the drug.

Thus, the comparison of two cell lines that differ only by the presence or absence of such a mutation allows pinpointing the effect of a drug to a particular target.

For anti-proliferative drugs, resistance-conferring mutations can be selected for in an unbiased manner by growing large numbers of cells in the presence of the drug and isolating resistant clones that continue to grow. To increase the chance of a resistance mutation occurring, the mutation rate of the cells can be artificially increased by chemical mutagenesis or irradiation of the cells. Multiple resistant clones are analysed by whole exome sequencing. Genes with a significantly increased mutation rate in resistant clones are candidates for being the sought for drug target. This approach has recently been successfully applied in proof-of-principle experiments in haploid cells to highlight the targets for two cytotoxic substances [41]. While this method is unbiased with respect to the target, one has to bear in mind that there are ways of generating resistance that bypass the need for mutations in the drug target, such as the up-regulation of enzymes that metabolize the drug or pump it out of the cell.

If a well-grounded assumption regarding the identity of the drug target exists, an easier way is to express mutagenized versions of the presumptive target ectopically in the cell. Different options exist to introduce mutations into the cDNA coding for the target:

- First, since in most cases the active (catalytic) site of the target will be known, a limited set of point mutations may be introduced that are expected or known to interfere with the binding of the target to the drug while preserving the function of the target and therefore lead to resistance.
- Second, the target cDNA can be randomly mutagenized. This can be done by propagation of the expression plasmid in error-prone strains of *Escherichia coli* or by amplification of the cDNA using error-prone PCR. Alternatively, the locus of the target can be subjected to dCas9-directed hypermutation [42] by use of a chemical mutagen such as *N*-ethyl-*N*-nitrosourea on the cells that have been transformed or transduced with the plasmid. In the latter case, mutagenesis will affect the complete genome and not only the target expressing plasmid. Thus, not all resistance-conferring mutations will reside in the ectopically expressed target, since other mutations affecting the activity of the respective pathway or drug uptake may also lead to resistance.
- Lastly, since the advent of gene synthesis, it has become possible to deliberately create libraries of the cDNA in which every codon is systematically altered to code for every other possible amino acid [43].

Thus mutagenized collections of expression constructs for the target in question can be expressed one by one in a cell line and examined for cellular responses to the drug (Figure 8.10).

If the drug in question induces cell death, this can be done using pooled libraries of plasmids directing expression of the mutagenized target cDNAs, as has been done, for example, with EGFR inhibitors and the T790M mutation [44]. Drug-resistant versions of the target will allow cells to survive lethal doses of the drug, leading to outgrowth of resistant closes under drug treatment. The isolation and analysis of the cDNA from surviving cells shows (i) if such mutations can be found, that the drug exerts its function via binding to the

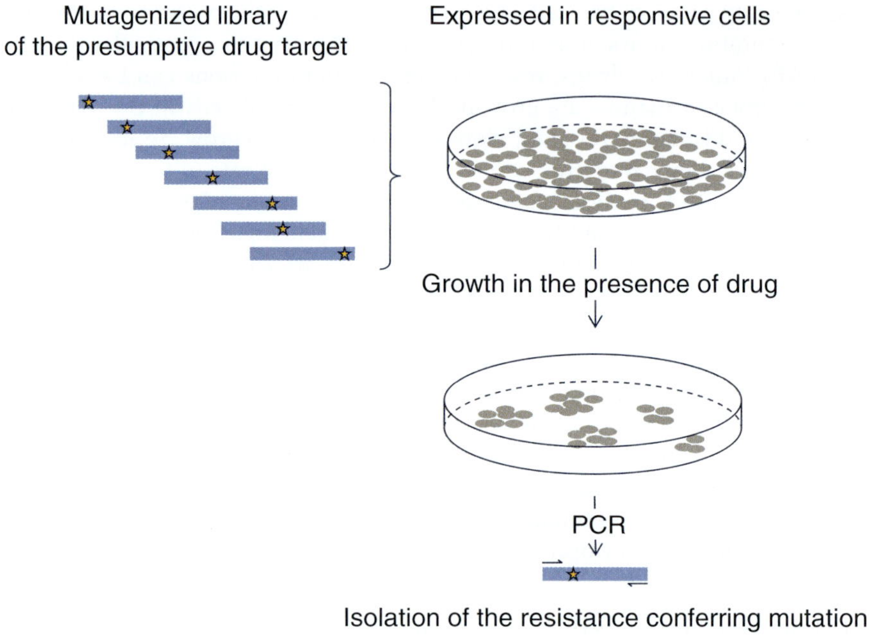

Figure 8.10 Selection of drug-resistant clones from a library of mutated cDNAs of the presumptive target proves that the presumptive drug target is indeed responsible for the anti-proliferative effect of the drug.

target, and (ii) which mutations the target confer resistance. In the case of the development of first-in-class inhibitor PT2399 of the transcription factor HIF2α, a mutation in the PAS domain of HIF2α was used to test if the inhibitor indeed works as expected [45]. Expression of the PAS domain-mutant version of HIF2α, but not of wild-type HIF2α, conferred resistance to PT2399 to cells, proving unequivocally that HIF2α is the relevant drug target for PT2399.

To complete a convincing data package, resistant conferring versions of the drug target can be tested *in vitro* for binding to the drug, the prediction being that they will show significantly reduced potency for drug binding.

The difficulty in these experiments is that the resistance-conferring mutations have to preserve the function of the protein in question, which can be challenging. In some cases, there is an elegant possibility to achieve this by exchanging the relevant domain of the target for a related one. Such domain swap experiments take advantage of the observation that despite distinct differences in the sequence and structure of protein domains of the same kind in different proteins, the essential function is often conserved. This has been shown for the bromodomain of BRD9 [46]. This domain can be inhibited by the small molecule BI-7273, whereas the bromodomain of BRD4 does not bind to this compound. In MV-4-11 leukaemia cells, which depend on BRD9 function, a chimaeric version of BRD9 that has its bromodomain replaced for the one of BRD4 can substitute for wild-type BRD9 and sustain proliferation. While the parental MV-4-11 cells were shown to be sensitive to BI-7273, cells expressing the chimaeric version

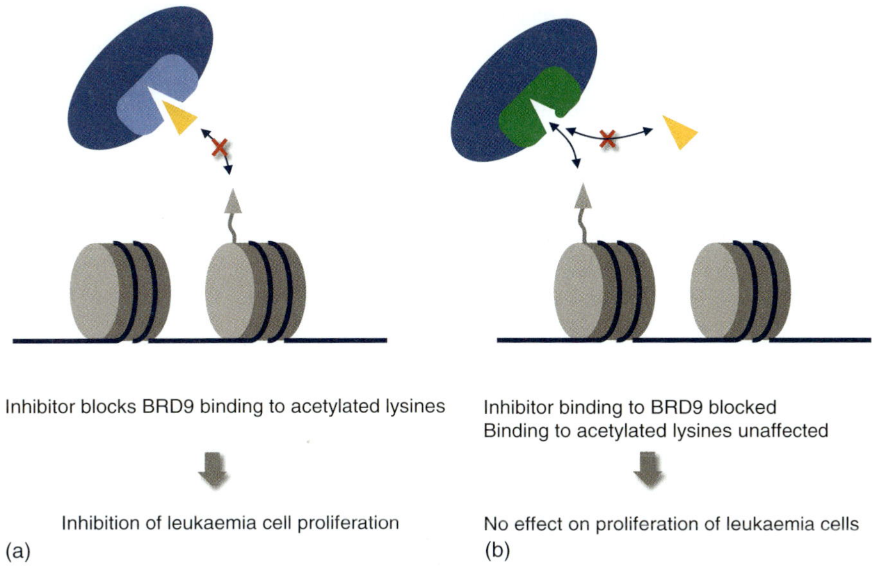

Figure 8.11 Swapping the bromodomain of BRD9 for the bromodomain of BRD4 does not affect bromodomain binding to acetylated lysines, but prevents inhibitor binding and anti-proliferative effects, thus proving on-target activity.

continue to proliferate unabated in the presence of this compound (Figure 8.11). Similarly, the methyltransferase domain of EZH2 can be replaced with the same domain from EZH1, causing resistance to an EZH2 selective inhibitor [46].

Validating a protein as a drug target has always been a challenge. The common saying that a target is not validated unless the respective drug shows efficacy in the clinic still applies. Remarkably, the major reasons for clinical failure of drug candidates are lack of efficacy and lack of therapeutic window, pointing to weaknesses in the underlying therapeutic concepts [47]. However, with the advent of RNA interference to knock down the expression of a target, the possibilities opened up by effective genome manipulation using CRISPR/Cas and the ability to do whole genome sequencing, for example, to find resistance-conferring mutations have made the task of validating a drug target significantly more straightforward. Together, these developments should reduce the risk of pursuing artefacts in drug discovery early on and help to reduce attrition rates in the clinic.

References

1 Marcelli, M., Stenoien, D.L., Szafran, A.T. et al. (2006). Quantifying effects of ligands on androgen receptor nuclear translocation, intranuclear dynamics, and solubility. *J. Cell. Biochem.* 98: 770–788.

2 Amarandi, R.M., Hjorto, G.M., Rosenkilde, M.M., and Karlshoj, S. (2016). Probing biased signaling in chemokine receptors. *Methods Enzymol.* 570: 155–186.

3 Van Hout, A., D'Huys, T., Oeyen, M. et al. (2017). Comparison of cell-based assays for the identification and evaluation of competitive CXCR4 inhibitors. *PLoS One* 12: e0176057.

4 McDonnell, D.P. and Wardell, S.E. (2010). The molecular mechanisms underlying the pharmacological actions of ER modulators: implications for new drug discovery in breast cancer. *Curr. Opin. Pharmacol.* 10: 620–628.

5 Neklesa, T.K., Winkler, J.D., and Crews, C.M. (2017). Targeted protein degradation by PROTACs. *Pharmacol. Ther.* 174: 138–144.

6 Knutson, S.K., Kawano, S., Minoshima, Y. et al. (2014). Selective inhibition of EZH2 by EPZ-6438 leads to potent antitumor activity in EZH2-mutant non-Hodgkin lymphoma. *Mol. Cancer Ther.* 13: 842–854.

7 Basso, K. and Dalla-Favera, R. (2012). Roles of BCL6 in normal and transformed germinal center B cells. *Immunol. Rev.* 247: 172–183.

8 Kerres, N., Steurer, S., Schlager, S. et al. (2017). Chemically induced degradation of the oncogenic transcription factor BCL6. *Cell Rep.* 20: 2860–2875.

9 Bishop, A.C., Shah, K., Liu, Y. et al. (1998). Design of allele-specific inhibitors to probe protein kinase signaling. *Curr. Biol.* 8: 257–266.

10 Hanke, J.H., Gardner, J.P., Dow, R.L. et al. (1996). Discovery of a novel, potent, and Src family-selective tyrosine kinase inhibitor. Study of Lck- and FynT-dependent T cell activation. *J. Biol. Chem.* 271: 695–701.

11 Bishop, A.C., Ubersax, J.A., Petsch, D.T. et al. (2000). A chemical switch for inhibitor-sensitive alleles of any protein kinase. *Nature* 407: 395–401.

12 Hormann, A., Hopfgartner, B., Kocher, T. et al. (2018). RIOK1 kinase activity is required for cell survival irrespective of MTAP status. *Oncotarget* 9: 28625–28637.

13 Wong, S., McLaughlin, J., Cheng, D. et al. (2004). Sole BCR-ABL inhibition is insufficient to eliminate all myeloproliferative disorder cell populations. *Proc. Natl. Acad. Sci. U.S.A.* 101: 17456–17461.

14 Clark, K., MacKenzie, K.F., Petkevicius, K. et al. (2012). Phosphorylation of CRTC3 by the salt-inducible kinases controls the interconversion of classically activated and regulatory macrophages. *Proc. Natl. Acad. Sci. U.S.A.* 109: 16986–16991.

15 Baud, M.G., Lin-Shiao, E., Cardote, T. et al. (2014). Chemical biology. A bump-and-hole approach to engineer controlled selectivity of BET bromodomain chemical probes. *Science* 346: 638–641.

16 McDonald, E.R. 3rd,, de Weck, A., Schlabach, M.R. et al. (2017). Project DRIVE: a compendium of cancer dependencies and synthetic lethal relationships uncovered by large-scale, deep RNAi screening. *Cell* 170: 577–592 e10.

17 Tsherniak, A., Vazquez, F., Montgomery, P.G. et al. (2017). Defining a cancer dependency map. *Cell* 170: 564–576 e16.

18 Zuber, J., Shi, J., Wang, E. et al. (2011). RNAi screen identifies Brd4 as a therapeutic target in acute myeloid leukaemia. *Nature* 478: 524–528.

19 Nishimura, K., Fukagawa, T., Takisawa, H. et al. (2009). An auxin-based degron system for the rapid depletion of proteins in nonplant cells. *Nat. Methods* 6: 917–922.

20 Kepinski, S. and Leyser, O. (2005). The *Arabidopsis* F-box protein TIR1 is an auxin receptor. *Nature* 435: 446–451.

21 Dharmasiri, N., Dharmasiri, S., and Estelle, M. (2005). The F-box protein TIR1 is an auxin receptor. *Nature* 435: 441–445.

22 Tan, X., Calderon-Villalobos, L.I., Sharon, M. et al. (2007). Mechanism of auxin perception by the TIR1 ubiquitin ligase. *Nature* 446: 640–645.

23 Natsume, T., Kiyomitsu, T., Saga, Y., and Kanemaki, M.T. (2016). Rapid protein depletion in human cells by auxin-inducible degron tagging with short homology donors. *Cell Rep.* 15: 210–218.

24 Muhar, M., Ebert, A., Neumann, T. et al. (2018). SLAM-seq defines direct gene-regulatory functions of the BRD4-MYC axis. *Science* 360: 800–805.

25 Dang, C.V. (2012). MYC on the path to cancer. *Cell* 149: 22–35.

26 Nie, Z., Hu, G., Wei, G. et al. (2012). c-Myc is a universal amplifier of expressed genes in lymphocytes and embryonic stem cells. *Cell* 151: 68–79.

27 Toure, M. and Crews, C.M. (2016). Small-molecule PROTACs: new approaches to protein degradation. *Angew. Chem. Int. Ed.* 55: 1966–1973.

28 Zengerle, M., Chan, K.H., and Ciulli, A. (2015). Selective small molecule induced degradation of the BET bromodomain protein BRD4. *ACS Chem. Biol.* 10: 1770–1777.

29 Winter, G.E., Buckley, D.L., Paulk, J. et al. (2015). DRUG DEVELOPMENT. Phthalimide conjugation as a strategy for in vivo target protein degradation. *Science* 348: 1376–1381.

30 Ottis, P. and Crews, C.M. (2017). Proteolysis-targeting chimeras: induced protein degradation as a therapeutic strategy. *ACS Chem. Biol.* 12: 892–898.

31 Clackson, T., Yang, W., Rozamus, L.W. et al. (1998). Redesigning an FKBP-ligand interface to generate chemical dimerizers with novel specificity. *Proc. Natl. Acad. Sci. U.S.A.* 95: 10437–10442.

32 Erb, M.A., Scott, T.G., Li, B.E. et al. (2017). Transcription control by the ENL YEATS domain in acute leukaemia. *Nature* 543: 270–274.

33 Nabet, B., Roberts, J.M., Buckley, D.L. et al. (2018). The dTAG system for immediate and target-specific protein degradation. *Nat. Chem. Biol.* 14: 431–441.

34 Kronke, J., Fink, E.C., Hollenbach, P.W. et al. (2015). Lenalidomide induces ubiquitination and degradation of CK1alpha in del(5q) MDS. *Nature* 523: 183–188.

35 Lu, G., Middleton, R.E., Sun, H. et al. (2014). The myeloma drug lenalidomide promotes the cereblon-dependent destruction of Ikaros proteins. *Science* 343: 305–309.

36 Kronke, J., Udeshi, N.D., Narla, A. et al. (2014). Lenalidomide causes selective degradation of IKZF1 and IKZF3 in multiple myeloma cells. *Science* 343: 301–305.

37 Ishoey, M., Chorn, S., Singh, N. et al. (2018). Translation termination factor GSPT1 is a phenotypically relevant off-target of heterobifunctional phthalimide degraders. *ACS Chem. Biol.* 13: 553–560.

38 St Pierre, R. and Kadoch, C. (2017). Mammalian SWI/SNF complexes in cancer: emerging therapeutic opportunities. *Curr. Opin. Genet. Dev.* 42: 56–67.

39 Oike, T., Ogiwara, H., Tominaga, Y. et al. (2013). A synthetic lethality-based strategy to treat cancers harboring a genetic deficiency in the chromatin remodeling factor BRG1. *Cancer Res.* 73: 5508–5518.

40 Vangamudi, B., Paul, T.A., Shah, P.K. et al. (2015). The SMARCA2/4 ATPase domain surpasses the bromodomain as a drug target in SWI/SNF mutant cancers: insights from cDNA rescue and PFI-3 inhibitor studies. *Cancer Res.* 75: 3865–3878.

41 Horn, M., Kroef, V., Allmeroth, K. et al. (2018). Unbiased compound-protein interface mapping and prediction of chemoresistance loci through forward genetics in haploid stem cells. *Oncotarget* 9: 9838–9851.

42 Hess, G.T., Fresard, L., Han, K. et al. (2016). Directed evolution using dCas9-targeted somatic hypermutation in mammalian cells. *Nat. Methods* 13: 1036–1042.

43 Li, A., Sun, Z., and Reetz, M.T. (2018). Solid-phase gene synthesis for mutant library construction: the future of directed evolution? *ChemBioChem* 19: 2023–2032.

44 Ercan, D., Zejnullahu, K., Yonesaka, K. et al. (2010). Amplification of EGFR T790M causes resistance to an irreversible EGFR inhibitor. *Oncogene* 29: 2346–2356.

45 Cho, H., Du, X., Rizzi, J.P. et al. (2016). On-target efficacy of a HIF2alpha antagonist in preclinical kidney cancer models. *Nature* 539: 107–111.

46 Hohmann, A.F., Martin, L.J., Minder, J.L. et al. (2016). Sensitivity and engineered resistance of myeloid leukemia cells to BRD9 inhibition. *Nat. Chem. Biol.* 12: 672–679.

47 Harrison, R.K. (2016). Phase II and phase III failures: 2013–2015. *Nat. Rev. Drug Discovery* 15: 817–818.

9

Genetic Manipulation/Modulation for Target Discovery and Validation

Christophe Lanneau [1], Georges Kalouche [1], Xinming Cai [2], Francois Lo-Presti [1], and Christoph Potting [3]

[1] Sanofi R&D, 1 Avenue Pierre, Brossolette, Chilly-Mazarin, 91380, France
[2] Sanofi R&D, 270 Albany Street, Cambridge, MA 02108, USA
[3] Sanofi-Aventis Deutschland GmbH, Industriepark Höchst, D-65926, Frankfurt-Am-Main, Germany

9.1 Introduction

Identifying and validating a molecular target remains a major challenge in drug discovery. The use of genetic manipulation technologies has increased constantly and is now of fundamental value for the identification as well as validation of novel drug targets and for the whole process of drug discovery. In particular, novel genetic manipulation technologies based on guided nucleases enable target discovery by genome-wide genetic screening with high specificity using disease-relevant models and read-outs and allow quick and precise disease model generation for early target validation (see also Chapter 7 for more details).

Genetic manipulation, i.e. the manipulation of the sequence of a gene, has been employed for decades, and random mutagenesis has been widely used to generate mutations and new microbial strains to investigate genotype–phenotype relations. The first targeted genetic manipulations were accomplished in yeast and mice in the 1980s [1–4] and relied on homologous recombination. However, recovery of recombinants still requires powerful selection, and the whole process can be very time consuming [5]. Besides a constant gain in experience and knowledge of genetic manipulation, manifestation of the enormous capabilities of today's genetic manipulation technologies would not have been possible without the scientific progress in other areas of biology such as the generation and curation of high-quality genomic data. While the availability of genomic data alone is enabling for biomedical research by facilitating the linkage of individual genes to diseases, it also sets the stage for a rational design of genetic manipulation reagents to allow highly specific targeting of disease loci. In particular for complex pathologies such as Parkinson's disease [6], where a host of genetic susceptibility factors interact with environmental risk factors, genomic data combined with modern genetic manipulation technologies can be very powerful and enables researchers to perform disease-gene interrogation studies in a fast, cost-effective, and precise manner. Modern genetic manipulation

Target Discovery and Validation: Methods and Strategies for Drug Discovery,
First Edition. Edited by Alleyn T. Plowright.

technologies based on transcription activator-like effector nucleases (TALENs) as well as zinc-finger nucleases (ZFNs) and clustered regularly interspaced short palindromic repeats (CRISPR) have become indispensable for biomedical research and drug discovery and are often referred to as 'gene editing' technologies reflecting their site specificity. When combining gene editing with complex cell-based models, including primary cells, induced pluripotent stem cells (iPSCs) or 3D models, along with powerful technologies such as flow cytometry and microfluidics, entirely new avenues are opening up to access, identify, and validate biomedically relevant targets. New areas of molecular biology can be explored such as the involvement of long non-coding RNAs (lncRNAs) in disease-relevant tissues including pancreatic beta cells [7] and the immune system [8]. Genetic screening is now possible at an unprecedented scale and speed as well as specificity but necessitates close interdisciplinary interactions of skilled molecular biologists, screening experts, and bioinformatics experts.

Among available technologies, the CRISPR/Cas technology is at present the tool of choice, and its flexibility enables researchers to explore novel biomedical terrain. This chapter discusses the development and principles of modern gene editing technologies with a focus on the CRISPR/Cas technology. Current methods and applications of the CRISPR/Cas technology will be outlined followed by key considerations for successful gene editing experiments. Further technology development will be covered and the impact of the CRISPR/Cas technology on target discovery and validation will be highlighted.

9.2 Overview of the Development of Leading Genetic Manipulation Technologies

9.2.1 RNAi, ZFNs, and TALENs

For more than a decade, RNA interference (RNAi) has brought a new approach to functional molecular screening. RNAi is a fast, flexible technology that is compatible with existing high-throughput systems and processes against the human genome to identify new drug targets and significantly advance experimental biology. RNAi does not act directly on the genome, but it is an endogenous post-transcriptional reaction to double-stranded RNA (dsRNA) that was originally discovered in *C. elegans* [9]. RNAi technologies have since proven to be able to control the gene expression in many eukaryotes, including humans [10]. The RNAi pathway is triggered by the presence of dsRNA, which is cleaved by Dicer (an RNase II enzyme) into microRNA (miRNA) or small interfering RNA (siRNA) (20–25 base pairs [bp] in length) with an extension of two nucleotides at the 3′ end. The heteroduplex of dsRNA is loaded onto the RNA-induced silencing complex (RISC) and used as a guide to identify complementary target mRNA via Watson–Crick base pairing to initiate RNA degradation [11].

Large-scale RNAi screens for cancer dependencies have recently been performed by multiple groups, providing systematic assessments of the effects of single gene knockdown on cell viability across a wide range of well-characterized cancer cell lines that are beginning to reflect the diversity of tumour types [12–14]. RNAi screening has led to the identification of genes such as the predisposition gene ALK on neuroblastoma as a candidate gene for HDAC8 inhibitors [15]. RNAi was also used in an *in vivo* setting via the delivery of pools of small hairpin RNAs (shRNAs) into mouse livers to identify the kinase MKK4 as a master regulator of liver regeneration [16]. Furthermore, RNAi has also been exploited on complex models such as *Wolbachia*–insect interactions [17]. Recently RNAi was also successfully engaged to probe the druggable genome for modifiers of α-synuclein levels and identify 60 promising targets [18]. The accessibility of commercially available well-validated human whole-genome RNAi libraries has made this approach more straightforward.

In 1980, Robert Roeder and Donald Brown discovered that the correct initiation of transcription requires the binding of a 40-kDa protein factor, also called factor A or transcription factor IIIA (TFIIIA) [19]. TFIIIA interacts with a 50 bp specific region, called the internal control region, and was the first eukaryotic transcription factor to be described. In 1982, Miller and Mertz discovered a repeated motif within TFIIIA, which was later called a zinc finger. The zinc-finger motif is now recognized as having a distinct principle of DNA recognition compared with the classical helix-turn-helix motifs found in previously described DNA-binding proteins [20]. Zinc fingers (which can be fused with a nuclease, a complex known as ZFN) bind to DNA as a tandem, with a polar surface to recognize different lengths of DNA (or RNA). Each finger domain has an analogous structure but differs through variations in key amino acid residues. This modular design allows a large number of combinational possibilities to interact with DNA (or even with RNA). One interesting possibility for the use of such ZFNs is the selective targeting of genetic differences in mutated or engineered cells. In 1994, Choo and Klug presented for the first time a protein containing a designed zinc finger that recognized a specific DNA sequence both *in vitro* and *in vivo* [21]. This proof of principle led to the appreciation of the potential of engineered zinc fingers for research as well as for therapeutic purposes and led to the foundation of the first biotech companies applying ZFNs.

Major applications of gene editing using ZFNs are based on the introduction of a site-specific DNA double-strand break (DSB) into the 'gene-of-interest' locus. All eukaryotic cells are able to repair DSBs via the homology-directed repair (HDR) or the non-homologous end-joining (NHEJ) DNA repair pathways. These repair pathways are highly conserved across a wide range of eukaryotic cell types as well as mammalian species, but not in HDR- and NHEJ-deficient prokaryotes where DSBs usually lead to organismal death. In eukaryotes, these mechanisms can be used to introduce mutations or artificial constructs at the site of the break, leading to a modification of the target gene. The most common application of ZFN-based genetic manipulation takes advantage of errors introduced during DNA repair that render a gene non-functional.

This approach has been applied in various species and cellular contexts to knock out specific genes in a single step without selection for the desired event and could presumably be applied in a vast range of biological models. Gene disruption has been used in mammalian somatic cell genetic engineering, in which the ZFN is transiently expressed followed by analysis of single-cell-derived clones [22, 23]. Since around the year 2000, researchers engaged in drug discovery exploited ZFNs to knock out genes to identify those that promote disease or to better understand the importance of multiple genes and protein interactions in order to design more sophisticated approaches to treatment [24]. With ZFNs, researchers have investigated the pathological role of genes in many species from rat [25, 26] to human, related to a range of pathologies such as renal injury [27, 28], hypertension [29], cancer [30, 31], and immune system disorders [32, 33]. ZFNs have also provided an opportunity to investigate epigenetic changes in mice [34] or human cells [35, 36].

TALENs, first described in the early 2000s, are artificial restriction enzymes generated by fusion of a DNA-binding domain, called transcription activator-like effector (TALE), with a nuclease domain. TALENs are based on a discovery made when *Xanthomonas*, a well-known plant pathogenic bacterium, was being investigated [37]. *Xanthomonas* produces proteins called TALEs that bind to specific DNA sequences in the infected plant and then affect expression of the targeted plant's gene. This bacterium causes a plant's cell to grow abnormally large. In 2007, researchers determined that *Xanthomonas* causes this phenotype through TALE's ability to bind to DNA, and in the next year they described the code for recognition of the target DNA by TALE proteins [38].

The breakthrough in the practical application of TALEs in genetic manipulation occurred when two discoveries were made. The first was that these protein units can easily be synthesized [39] and joined together to create synthetic TALEs that recognize and target any desired sequence of DNA. The second discovery was that an enzyme that cuts DNA, known as a nuclease, can be attached to the TALE [40]. This combination of a synthetic TALE with its attached nuclease is a TALEN. TALEN-mediated specific DNA cuts can be performed in living cells including cultured cells or stem cells, and scientists have demonstrated that it is a powerful gene editing tool for a wide range of cultured human cells [41–44].

As with ZFNs, TALENs have permitted the introduction of specific mutations in a number of model organisms such as zebrafish [45–47], frog [48], rat [49], and pig [50]. TALENs have primarily been used to knock out genes by using the NHEJ endogenous mechanism, but scientists also use a TALEN pair to double cut in the same chromosome in order to generate large deletions/inversions of chromosomal segments [50]. Similarly to ZFNs, TALENs have also been used for target engagement studies, for example, CCR5 in HIV infection [51] or in the cancer field [52–54]. Scientists have also used a collection of TALEN constructs to knock out 88 human genes associated with cardiomyopathies in iPSC-derived cardiomyocytes, illustrating the powerful combination of iPSCs and gene editing technologies for understanding the biological function of genes and the pathological significance of genetic variants in human cardiovascular diseases [55]. However there are still limitations to TALENs. Identification motifs are very challenging to construct due to spatial reorganization and are often unstable when cloned, and construction of the 2–3 kb of coding sequence per target further limits high-throughput screens and necessitates costly and time-consuming experiments (Figure 9.1).

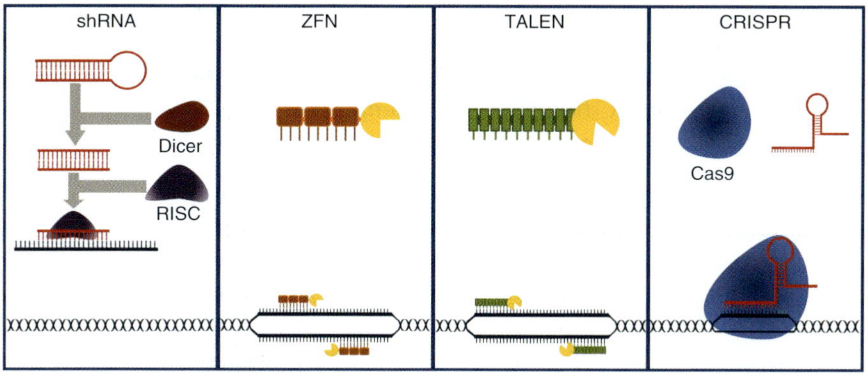

Figure 9.1 Schemes illustrating how shRNA, zinc-finger nuclease (ZFN), TALEN, and CRISPR act on RNA or DNA to elicit molecular modification. In contrast to shRNA that only binds to RNA to elicit RNA degradation but have no direct effect on the genome, ZFN dimer, TALEN dimer, and CRISPR reagents bind directly to DNA. ZFN and TALEN target sites consist of unique 'left' and 'right' half-binding sites separated by a spacer sequence (5–7 base pairs [bp] for ZFN and 12–20 bp for TALEN). Each zinc-finger domain (dark brown box) contacts with 3–4 bp, but individual TALE repeats (Green box) containing 33–35 amino acids recognize a single bp. Differing from ZFN and TALEN, CRISPR requires an RNA-based bridging element (red block), which confers the selectivity for the specific DNA sequence.

9.2.2 Clustered Regularly Interspaced Short Palindromic Repeats (CRISPR)

The development of the CRISPR/Cas technology to become an indispensable tool in biological research is based on years of basic science research [56]. The contribution from many scientists resulted in the transitioning of the CRISPR/Cas system from being recognized as a peculiar prokaryotic feature to a reprogrammable gene editing technology, which holds great promise and has the potential to revolutionize biomedical research. Important historic milestones will be outlined briefly below.

Although having already attracted attention earlier, only in 2002 did Ruud Jansen et al. [57] reveal that a family of repetitive DNA sequences in prokaryotes characterized by direct repeats varying in length between 21 and 37 bp is associated with a set of adjacently located genes. Due to these characteristics, they referred to the family of repetitive DNA sequences as the CRISPR and to the associated genes as **C**RISPR-**as**sociated (*cas*) genes. As CRISPR loci are present in prokaryotes, but absent in eukaryotes, and are derived from bacteriophage DNA, researchers started to hypothesize that CRISPR loci may constitute a bacterial immune system [58–61]. This hypothesis was corroborated by a study in 2007, which showed that CRISPR together with the associated *cas* genes provides acquired resistance against viruses in prokaryotes [62]. Subsequent studies focused on mechanistic aspects of the CRISPR/Cas system and revealed that among Cas-encoded proteins some have endonuclease activity and that DNA cleavage is key to bacterial immunity [63, 64]. The discoveries in 2012 that a Cas endonuclease can be guided by short CRISPR RNA (crRNA) transcripts in a ribonucleoprotein (RNP) complex to mediate specific programmable DNA cleavage for silencing of invading nucleic acids marked an important milestone in the development of the CRISPR/Cas system towards a powerful technology [65, 66]. While the endogenous CRISPR system required a bridging element, a trans-activating crRNA (tracrRNA), for complexing the crRNA with the Cas nuclease, the same studies showed that the system can be further simplified by fusing the tracrRNA with the crRNA in a single guide RNA (gRNA). Shortly after these discoveries, several studies in 2013 adapted the CRISPR/Cas system for gene editing in eukaryotic cells and thus paved the way for further development of the technology in multiple directions for a range of purposes [67–69].

9.3 Considerations for Designing and Interpreting CRISPR Experiments

9.3.1 Methodological Considerations for Genetic Manipulation by the CRISPR/Cas Technology

Building on the rapidly expanding wealth of knowledge on the CRISPR/Cas system, guidelines for the use of the system as a technology have emerged and enable scientists to generate gene manipulations/modifications in cells within a couple of weeks [70]. A few methodological considerations have to be made in order to achieve genetic manipulation with high precision. Several CRISPR/Cas systems have been identified in prokaryotes, and while classification efforts are ongoing, a common classification proposes three types (I–III) based on multiple features including the phylogenies of ubiquitous *cas* genes [71]. Each system comprises repetitive DNA sequences within a CRISPR array that are separated – 'interspaced' – by variable DNA sequences, known as spacers, each of which forms a functional unit with one DNA repeat. This unit encodes the crRNA which provides the specificity for the Cas nuclease for a DNA target via Watson–Crick base pairing. An additional feature is needed for the Cas nuclease in order to be accurately positioned at a DNA target region, and this is known as a protospacer adjacent motif (PAM), a short DNA motif next to the target sequence. The best characterized and most used system is the type II CRISPR system from *Streptococcus pyogenes*. In this case, the spacer element of the crRNA consists of 20 bp and, among *cas* genes, *cas9* encodes the effector nuclease, a 1366 amino acid protein that requires a 5′-NGG PAM site. Of note, Cas nucleases from other species may depend on different PAM sites and have a different molecular weight and cutting site [56]. To enable CRISPR/Cas-mediated genetic manipulation in mammalian cells, both Cas9 and a gRNA, a fusion of the crRNA and the tracrRNA, must be delivered to the cells (see Section 9.3.4 for more details). Design of the gRNA sequence to match a target sequence flanked by a PAM site in the mammalian genome can redirect Cas9 towards that specific locus. Once the Cas9/gRNA RNP complex has engaged the target locus, Cas9 can hydrolyse both DNA strands in the vicinity of the PAM site, resulting in a DSB. Of note, hydrolysis of the individual strands is mediated by distinct Cas9 domains opening up the possibility for single-strand modifications by engineering Cas9 enzymatic domains [65] (see further discussion below). Similar to other gene editing technologies, DSBs are subjected to endogenous DNA repair processes: either the NHEJ or the HDR processes. The outcome of DNA repair depends on whether NHEJ or HDR was used. Unless a repair template is present, DSBs will be repaired by NHEJ, which is an error-prone process and often introduces insertion/deletion (indel) mutations at the target locus. NHEJ-introduced indels in a gene may lead to frameshift mutations and premature termination codons (PTCs), thereby generating functional gene knockouts. The presence of a repair template, e.g. in the form of an exogenous DNA template consisting of an insertion sequence flanked by target gene homology arms, can redirect DNA repair towards HDR to generate precise genetic insertion manipulations albeit at lower frequencies compared with NHEJ. As the specificity of CRISPR/Cas-mediated gene editing depends on the gRNA and unwanted editing at off-target sites may present a pitfall, it appears obvious that the design of the gRNA is critical (see Section 9.3.3). Besides the gRNA design, Cas9 has also been a research focus to further minimize off-target editing. Cas9 consists of two catalytic domains, HNH and RuvC, each of which is responsible for cutting one of the two DNA strands at a gRNA target site. While the mutation of critical residues in both domains renders Cas9 catalytically dead, mutation of only one catalytic domain results in a nickase enzyme, and protocols are available describing a double-nicking strategy using the Cas9 nickase mutant with paired gRNAs to minimize off-target cleavage [70].

The described CRISPR/Cas technology thus enables genetic manipulations ranging from functional gene knockouts to precise template-mediated modifications such as single nucleotide mutations for probing causal genetic variations [70]. Practically, a common approach for a CRISPR/Cas editing experiment involves the following:

1. Design of gRNA by scanning the gene of interest for suitable target locations and selection of spacer sequences.
2. The gRNA and Cas9 are delivered to the cells.
3. Successful editing of the target gene has to be confirmed.

The gRNA design is key for efficient and specific editing, and multiple bioinformatic tools are available that help to design gRNAs.

A more detailed description of gRNA design will be discussed in Section 9.3.3 before additional important considerations for a successful application of the CRISPR/Cas technology are outlined.

9.3.2 Choosing a Cellular Model: Biological and Genomic Aspects

Editing the genome requires a good knowledge of the CRISPR/Cas methodology and of the targeted sequences. Genome editing also requires determination of the best biological model for testing a hypothesis. For CRISPR/Cas screening purposes, cell models must respect classical screening parameters (e.g. doubling time, culture conditions) and remain cultivable up to the functional analysis of the genome manipulation. The use of disease-relevant cells, e.g. primary cells, although successfully tested with CRISPR/Cas technology remains challenging, for example, in terms of cost and transfection efficiency compared with immortalized cells (see Chapter 7 for more details on human cell-based model systems to explore biology) [72, 73]. Furthermore, since CRISPR/Cas targets the genome, genetic stability after long-term passaging and genomic characteristics of the cell model are also essential parameters.

Cell lines used in CRISPR experiments are often derived from tumour cells with an atypical copy number of chromosomes. Some commonly used cells such as HEK293 and K-562 are pseudo triploid, meaning that these cells contain at least three copies of chromosome sets and therefore three copies of most gRNA targets. The number of chromosomes in HeLa (ATCC® CCL2™) cells can also vary including one fourth being abnormal chromosomes [74]. Gene editing becomes even more challenging with aneuploid cells since a designed gRNA target one, or multiple, or no copy of a gene or genomic sequence [75]. Due to the random action of NHEJ, target editing of all sequence copies may be incomplete or result in an altered structure. Thus determination of the cell ploidy is important for correct and efficient gene editing.

Recently, generation of mouse haploid embryonic stem cells (ESCs) spontaneously undergoing diploidization during differentiation steps revealed interesting perspectives in improving gene editing efficiencies [76]. Cells can be engineered at the haploid state, enabling efficient modification and higher targeting efficiency than with diploid ESCs.

As for polyploidy, copy number variations (CNVs), due to structural modification of the genome architecture, have implications for gene editing efficiency. CNVs can arise because of deletions or, more frequently, duplications of a gene or genomic regions encompassing multiple genes [77]. Both recurrent and non-recurrent CNVs are frequently associated with diseases and coincide with regions of chromosome instability [78, 79]. CRISPR/Cas screening in a region of CNV may lead to significant DNA damage [80]. The cell response correlates with both the increased number of genomic CNV and the total number of DNA cuts at target loci. This correlation is observed across the multiple chromosomal structural alterations and induces a decrease of physiological parameters such as cell proliferation [80].

The read-out of a screen based on loss-of-function approaches using CRISPR is often a phenotypic change. The absence of the expected phenotype may be due to poor efficiency but may also result from genetic redundancy or from genetic compensation. Their mechanisms of action are still incompletely understood and debated except for some key points. Genetic redundancy is often associated with essential genes. Paralog genes are derived from ancestral genes during evolution by duplication and often have unique functions, but some paralogs still maintain similar functions. Redundancy can also occur with genes from different origin but with convergent functions [81]. Thus, knockout of one gene may not always result in a phenotypic change since the other gene will compensate for the disruption by a similar function. Genetic compensation may also occur from mRNA decay due to mutated mRNA or inefficient translation [82]. This compensatory mechanism modifies the expression of genes involved in the same pathway to compensate the defect. While this phenomenon reduces the apparent efficiency of gene knockout in specific gene screening, combinatorial screens using orthologous CRISPR/Cas systems offer a way to discover new targets and redundant or compensatory genes [83].

A bioinformatic study of the reference sequence is necessary before using CRISPR/Cas. Ensembl [84] and RefSeq [85] databases provide reference sequences for a given gene and lists splicing variants and polymorphisms. However reference genomes are artificial assemblies of known (and sometimes predicted) sequences from different sample types. As shown for HeLa cells, reference sequences may largely diverge from primary transcript sequences, emphasizing the need to use the most relevant sequences [74]. FANTOM [86] is another interesting database, which relies on transcription start sites (TSS) annotations based on the cap analysis of gene expression (CAGE) technique. This latter database may be preferred specifically for CRISPRa and clustered regularly interspaced short palindromic repeats interference (CRISPRi) applications where using well-characterized TSS is necessary [87]. Annotations of the human genome are dynamic, and changes include discovery of new splicing variants and minor or major single nucleotide polymorphisms (SNPs) [87]. Thus it is necessary to adapt reference sequences to those probably present in the samples for SNPs or tissue (and cell)-specific splice variants. The development of next-generation sequencing (NGS) databases allows the retrieval of more and more cell model-specific primary transcript sequences. Another advantage of CRISPR/Cas technology is that generated mutated cells can be compared to the wild-type isogenic control. CRISPR/Cas can also be used for studying disease by engineering mutant disease-relevant cells and reverting these cells to a 'normal phenotype' by correcting the mutation [88]. Therefore, it is essential to check the cell characteristics (e.g. tissue origin, species, strain, or population-specific data) before their use in CRISPR/Cas experiments.

Alternative splicing moved the 'one gene–one protein' hypothesis to a 'one gene–(potentially) multiple transcripts and proteins'. These multiple transcripts, called splicing variants, occurring in approximately 95% of multi-exon genes [89] can generate the same protein as the main transcript. In many cases, these splicing variants can be non-coding variants and in other cases can generate proteins with different functions. Spliced variants can even produce proteins with opposite functions (e.g. pro- and anti-angiogenic VEGF-A, functional caspase 1 and inhibitory caspase 1 variants) [90–92]. Differential splicing is also involved in pathology or resistance towards existing medicines (for example, CD19 resistance against CART-19 immunotherapy) [93]. These alternative splicing events add complexity to the choice of CRISPR gRNAs, namely, whether a common or a specific exon has to be targeted depending on the studied function [94]. Specific exon targeting can be used to identify the exact role of a splicing variant as has been done for the M-line titin, an abundant protein in striated muscle [95]. Specific exon targeting can also be used for screening specific therapeutic compounds [93]. Alternative splicing also occurs for lncRNAs. CRISPR/Cas-mediated modulation of the lncRNA Xist splicing has recently shown that the short isoform of Xist is sufficient to induce X-chromosome inactivation [96].

Non-coding DNA represents 98% of the genome and contains many regulatory domains (e.g. promoters, enhancers). Application of CRISPR/Cas in this field represents a huge potential for new target discovery as revealed by the identification of novel enhancer elements [97] and lncRNA functions [98]. Unlike protein-coding genes, many lncRNAs act as molecular modulators of transcript-dependent and transcript-independent functions of their targets. While the RNAi method is highly efficient in invalidation studies of lncRNAs, CRISPR/Cas has a huge benefit in the research of lncRNAs, due to its in-cis regulative function. CRISPR/Cas provides new openings for further investigating the function of lncRNAs, revealing new functions and complex interactions [99].

Usually, for protein-coding genes, a gRNA is sufficient to invalidate a gene of interest since indels may disrupt the mRNA reading frame. However, because lncRNAs are less conserved between species and vary widely in their activity and action modes, gRNA design and effect evaluation are less easy due to an unpredictable effectiveness in other species models.

Despite these difficulties, CRISPR/Cas has proven efficient in elucidating novel functions for different lncRNAs. Compared with lncRNAs, miRNAs are relatively easy to knock out, and some results suggest that the knockout efficiency of miRNAs is higher than that of lncRNAs [100]. This may be attributed to the fact that miRNA genes are much smaller in size than lncRNAs, however, the number of potential PAM sites is smaller giving less flexibility to select potentially efficient gRNAs.

9.3.3 gRNA Design

The design of a gRNA is a critical process that determines the probability of success of any CRISPR/Cas editing experiment and builds on the integration of cell biology, genomics, and bioinformatics. Since the discovery of the basic requirements for a gRNA to target a precise location in the genome, that is, the recognition of a 20-nucleotide sequence adjacent to a PAM site, much knowledge has been gained and can help to improve on-target gene editing efficiency while decreasing the occurrence of artefacts and off-target effects.

9.3.3.1 Identification of Target Locations

The selection of target locations for the design of gRNA mainly depends on the intended CRISPR/Cas-induced modifications. While knock-in genetic perturbations considerably restrict gRNA design to the vicinity of the intended insertions, gene knockout studies are less restrictive. However, as loss-of-function experiments aim at attributing a particular phenotype to a given gene, strategic selection of locations for gRNA design is essential to avoid misleading interpretations.

NHEJ-mediated generation of indels in protein-coding sequences eventually produces frameshift mutations (Figure 9.2a) that disrupt the mRNA reading frame and often lead to the introduction of a PTC. The mutated transcript will either be degraded by a cytoplasmic mRNA quality control process, the nonsense-mediated decay (NMD) pathway, or will translate into an aberrant C-terminal truncated protein. Leveraging the rules of NMD for gRNA design provides the opportunity to restrict the production of truncated proteins with potentially unexpected effects as the NMD surveillance system will degrade

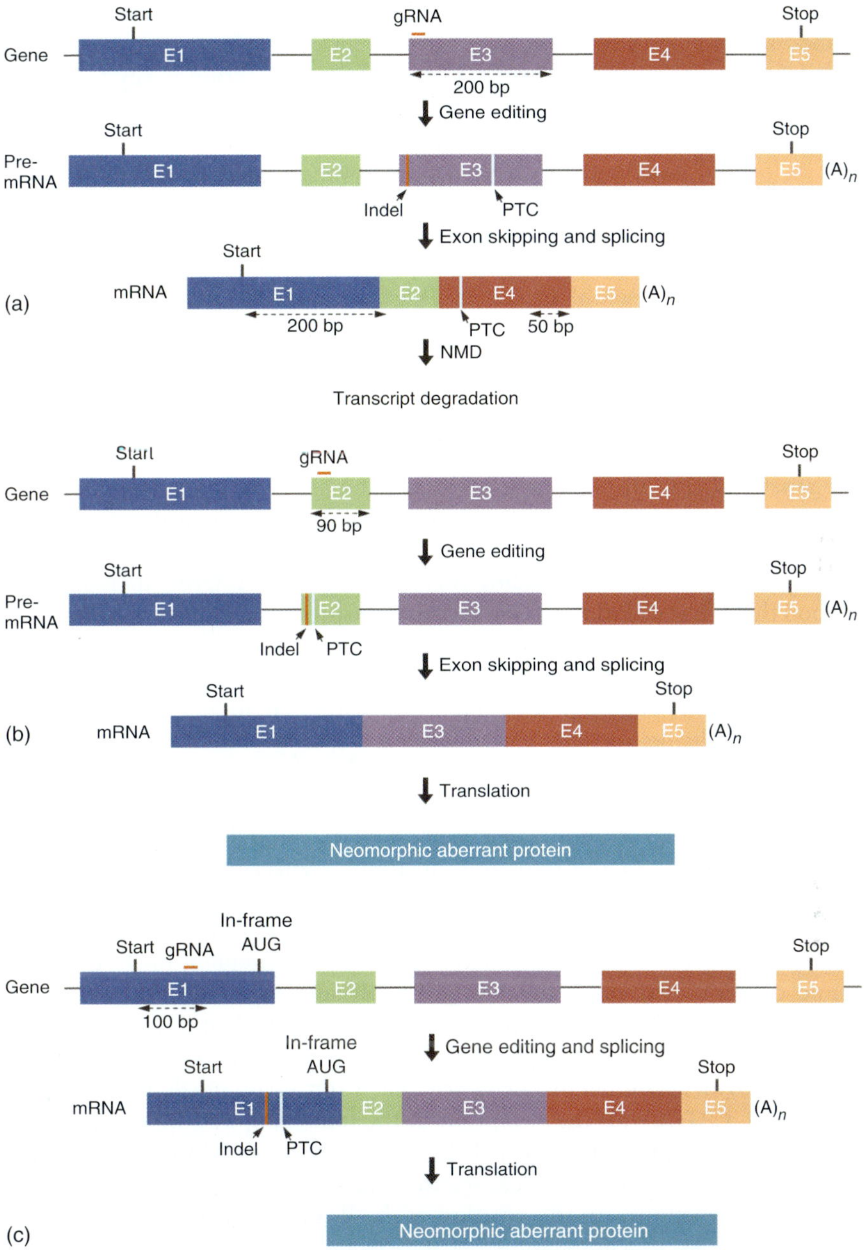

Figure 9.2 Potential gene editing outcomes depending on the target locations of the guide RNA (gRNA). (a) A gRNA targeting a non-symmetric exon and inducing a premature termination codon (PTC) in the same exon produces a frameshift by exon skipping and splicing of the remaining exons. The newly formed PTC, downstream of the first 200 nucleotides and 50 nucleotides upstream of the last exon junction, activates the nonsense-mediated decay (NMD) pathway, which leads to the transcript degradation. (b) A gRNA targeting a symmetric exon and inducing a PTC in the same exon allows in-frame deletion of the exon by exon skipping and splicing of the remaining exons. Maintenance of the mRNA reading frame could favour the translation of an aberrant protein. (c) A gRNA targeting the first 100 nucleotides downstream of the start codon favours reinitiation of translation at an in-frame AUG codon, resulting in the production of an aberrant protein.

the transcript after a pioneering round of translation [101]. Among a recently described set of rules governing NMD in human cells [102], the location of a PTC at least 50 nucleotides upstream of the last exon junction is key to trigger transcript degradation. Furthermore, NMD efficiency decreases for PTC positioned within 200 nucleotides downstream of the start codon. Therefore, a gRNA should be located sufficiently upstream of the last exon junction and outside the vicinity of the initiation codon to favour degradation of an mRNA bearing a PTC.

In order to probe gene functions, the selected target location sequences must be shared by all the protein-coding transcript variants. For that purpose, genome databases, such as Ensembl or RefSeq, give annotated transcripts produced from independent promotors or alternative splicing. However, overlapping exon sequences from all the available transcript variants may not exist or could greatly limit the extent of the gene regions selectable for gRNA design. Transcript categories and scores in Ensembl can help to identify and prioritize the most relevant transcripts based on supporting information. In addition, information about genetic alterations encountered in specific cell lines such as SNPs, copy number, or transcript variants may be obtained from large-scale sequencing datasets [103, 104] in order to tailor gRNA design to a specific cell model. Furthermore, targeting the 5′ coding region of a gene of interest increases the likelihood that a frameshift mutation disrupts the protein sequence and prevents the translation of a C-terminal truncated protein with potentially reduced or aberrant functions [105–107].

Recent studies revealed that CRISPR/Cas editing may induce the generation of alternative splicing variants through exon skipping [108–112], which may account for unintended consequences in gene knockout studies. At least two seemingly independent mechanisms could explain exon skipping. Firstly, Mou et al. observed large genomic deletions, which resulted in splice acceptor site removal, splicing of the remaining in-frame transcript and translation of an aberrant neomorphic protein, i.e. a protein with potentially deleterious dominant-negative or gain-of-function effects [110]. Accordingly, recent studies reported that CRISPR/Cas editing may indeed induce frequent on-target large genomic deletions extending over many kilobases [113]. Nonetheless, exon skipping is also observed in cell clones harbouring few nucleotide indels outside the intron–exon boundaries suggesting the existence of another mechanism. Sui et al. provided compelling evidence that exon skipping depends on the generation of a PTC, with the exception of the first exon, but did not occur as a result of an in-frame mutation [112]. This mechanism, which supports the hypothesis of a yet unknown nuclear scanning process, suggests different potential outcomes depending on the position of the PTC. A gRNA that induces the generation of a PTC in a non-symmetrical exon, i.e. an exon whose length is not a multiple of three nucleotides, would lead to the disruption of the reading frame by exon deletion potentially resulting in the activation of the NMD pathway and subsequent transcript degradation (Figure 9.2a). On the contrary, exon skipping induced by a PTC generated in a symmetrical exon would lead to maintenance of the reading frame and potentially the translation of a neomorphic aberrant protein (Figure 9.2b). Nonetheless, the precise location of a PTC induced by an indel cannot be predicted. An alternative strategy could consist of targeting a large exon whose deletion would significantly disturb the protein structure. In any case, alternative splicing induced by exon skipping exhorts to assess the consequences of gene editing at the transcriptional level.

Alternative translation initiation, a process contributing to proteome diversity, may also cause misleading results in gene knockout studies. According to the ribosome scanning mechanism, the 5′-proximal AUG triplet of an mRNA initiates translation. However, the first AUG may be bypassed if its nucleotide context deviates from the Kozak consensus sequence, leading to the initiation of translation at a downstream AUG, a mechanism known as 'leaky scanning' [114, 115]. A gRNA targeting the annotated translation initiation site (TIS) may disrupt the AUG triplet or an optimal surrounding sequence and consequently favours initiation of translation at a downstream start codon. An in-frame alternative TIS would result in the translation of an N-terminal protein variant with potentially distinct properties [116]. As a consequence, a gRNA should not target the TIS region in loss-of-function experiments to prevent generation of alternative start site variants. In addition, alternative TIS may arise from the resumption of ribosome scanning after termination of translation of a short upstream open reading frame (uORF). This reinitiation process depends on several variables such as the length of the uORF and the intercistronic sequence [117]. Studies showed that the uORF median size in human transcripts is about 50 nucleotides [118, 119]. Furthermore, the reinitiation efficiency of uORF lengthened to 100 nucleotides was largely reduced in experimental systems [120]. Therefore, a gRNA should target a location downstream of the first 100 nucleotides from the start codon to prevent reinitiation from an in-frame AUG and translation of an alternative protein (Figure 9.2c).

In summary, several complex mechanisms at the transcript-level, such as NMD, exon skipping, leaky scanning, and reinitiation of translation, are to be considered to identify target locations that prevent the generation of neomorphic aberrant proteins and potential biased phenotypic interpretations. An alternative strategy relies on using two gRNAs to remove the entire coding sequence of a gene of interest but involves an increased number of on-target and off-target cleavage sites, which may be associated with complex genomic rearrangements [121] and toxic cellular responses [80, 122, 123]. Furthermore, certain features may influence the efficiency to disrupt a gene function. In particular, protein-level annotations, such as protein domain, interspecies conservation, and disordered state, significantly impact the functional outcomes of gene editing as not only frameshift but also in-frame mutations may lead to loss of functions [124–126].

9.3.3.2 Selection of Spacer Sequences

Once target locations have been identified, 20 nucleotide spacer sequences are selected adjacent to a Cas9 NGG PAM site, which occurs on average every eight bp in the human genome. However, studies suggest that significant differences exist between gRNA abilities to efficiently and selectively disrupt a gene function. Defining the rules that govern gRNA mutagenesis activity has thus important implications to predict and control gene editing outcomes both in genome-wide screens and small-scale target validation studies.

Optimization of Spacer On-Target Activity A series of large-scale studies were performed to decipher the determinants that dictate mutagenesis efficiency. For that purpose, several methods and read-outs were employed to evaluate gRNA on-target activity, at the nucleic acid or the protein level, across a variety of cell types and organisms [105–107, 127–132]. These studies contributed to the identification of key parameters for improving gRNA design.

The results showed that spacers with a low or high GC content tended to be less active and suggested that GC percentages between 40% and 60% would be optimal to ensure high rates of mutagenesis [105, 107, 128, 130]. Furthermore, the presence of secondary structures in the spacer may adversely affect gene editing efficiency by either stabilizing the gRNA [130] or interfering with Cas9 activity [133]. Despite a high discrepancy in the spacer nucleotide preferences, most of the studies revealed that a guanine at the −1 position proximal to the PAM improves mutagenesis efficiency [105, 107, 127, 128, 131, 132], while the presence of an adenine seems to be unfavourable [128, 130]. A negative bias against thymine was also observed at the 3′ end of the spacer sequence, from positions −1 to −4, which may be explained by a decrease in gRNA expression as U-rich regions induce a termination signal for RNA polymerase III, which allows transcription of gRNAs delivered by lentivirus or plasmid vectors [105, 132, 134]. Thus, these findings underline the fact that some spacer nucleotide preferences observed in specific experimental conditions may not be extrapolated to other settings such as the delivery of *in vitro* transcribed gRNAs.

The nucleotide context surrounding the DNA cleavage site also impacts the repair process and gene editing efficiency. The microhomology-mediated end-joining mechanism differentiates itself from the NHEJ pathway by contributing to a subset of deletions that occur between microhomologous sequences flanking the cleavage site [135] and affects a gRNA ability to disrupt a gene function by inducing either out-of-frame or in-frame mutations [136, 137]. Furthermore, studies suggest that epigenetic features influence Cas9 binding and functioning. While DNA methylation and nucleosome occupancy seem to have an indirect or weak effect on cleavage efficiency [129, 134, 138], potentially because of the constant chromatin remodelling process, three-dimensional chromatin structures inhibit editing at specific target sites [139, 140]. In particular, gene editing efficiency was shown to be improved by RNA polymerase transcription activity as it dislodges the Cas9 complex from the DNA strand and favours the repair process [141]. These findings may explain the interrelation between chromatin state and editing outcomes.

Determination of Spacer Off-Target Activity Initial studies showed that Cas9 cleavage activity allows mismatches between the gRNA and the target genomic locus [129, 142] and depends on mismatch number, distribution, and location. Mismatches at the 5′ end of the spacer sequence are more tolerated than those within the 10–12 bp proximal to the PAM site, defined as the seed region. Furthermore, Cas9 specificity is influenced by the mismatch base nature [143] and the presence of non-symmetric pairings, or bulges, between the gRNA and the genomic locus [144]. Cas9 cleavage may also occur at alternative PAM sites albeit with low efficiency [129]. All these parameters that affect off-target activity have been studied by screening the activity of thousands of perfect match or mutated gRNAs targeting the CD33 gene [106]. Overall, the position and the base composition of the mismatches appear to be the major determinants of gRNA off-target activity.

Various techniques have been employed to accurately detect off-target sites. Chromatin immunoprecipitation sequencing (ChiP-seq) may provide information concerning the Cas9 binding profile [134, 145] but does not necessarily correlate with Cas9 cleavage, which usually requires a higher level of gRNA base pairing with the target sequence [146]. Unbiased cell-based approaches such as genome-wide, unbiased identification of DSBs enabled by SEQuencing (GUIDE-seq), which relies on the sequencing of captured oligonucleotides into DSB [121], or high-throughput genome-wide translocation sequencing (HTGTS), which is based on chromosomal translocation at DSB [147], were shown to be sensitive techniques that brought further insight into off-target site identification.

The experimental design can significantly increase gRNA specificity. Indeed, off-target modifications may be minimized by reducing the cell exposure to the CRISPR/Cas components [129] through either the delivery of the RNP complex, which is rapidly cleared from the cell [148], or the control of Cas9 expression by inducible promotors [149]. Furthermore, high-fidelity versions of Cas9, developed by rational design [150, 151] or unbiased screening [152], as well as gRNAs with truncated spacer sequences [121], can reduce the off-target activity but may also limit on-target efficiency [153]. Finally, optimizing the gRNA design by the use of predictive tools can help to improve specificity.

9.3.3.3 Predictive Tools

Several different tools have been developed for predicting gRNA on-target activity and a comparison of 36 of them has recently been described [154]. The most basic tools rely on the localization of PAM sites to identify spacer sequences. Based on the publicly available gRNA large-scale studies, computational design rules have been defined, and several groups have developed predictive algorithms. The tools based on these predictive algorithms incorporate one or multiple determinants that have been shown to modulate on-target activity. For example, CRISPR-ERA [155] provides a gRNA score that takes into account basic information such as the GC content, while CHOPCHOP [156] prioritizes a guanine at the −1 position proximal to the PAM. Lastly, machine learning-based tools have been used by training logistic regression models to improve predictability. As the tools were developed from gRNA features defined in specific experimental conditions, their performance may not be reproduced in other settings. For example, the Moreno-Mateos score [131], whose algorithm was trained on zebrafish data obtained from *in vitro* transcribed gRNA, does not translate well to the Doench score [106] that was developed from screens realized in a human cell line using gRNA delivered by lentiviruses [157]. While these models rely mostly on the spacer features, a recent predictive score that was obtained by training a machine learning model on two independent datasets [106, 124] and by combining spacer determinants to transcript-level (e.g. alternative transcript, NMD activation) and protein-level (e.g. domain structure, sequence conservation) annotations showed increased predictive power compared with the Doench score [125].

Most of the tools that predict on-target activity also evaluate potential off-target sites with calculated scores based on the identities and the positions of the mismatches. The currently available algorithms confer variable influence to different parameters such as each possible nucleotide change at each position, the succession of mismatches, or the distance to the PAM [157]. The cutting frequency determination (CFD) score, which is based on the largest dataset [106] and was shown to be the most accurate [157], evaluates the likelihood for a gRNA to induce cleavage at an off-target site. On the other hand, a gRNA specificity score, which aggregates all the potential off-target activities for a given gRNA, was implemented [129], and machine learning-based modelling approaches recently increased its predictive potential [158].

CRISPOR [159] is a useful web-based tool for target validation knockout studies that supports several predictive models. Based on recognition of the PAM sites in a target location sequence, spacers are identified and ranked by a specificity score, which predicts the overall gRNA off-target activity in a reference genome for up to four mismatches [129, 157]. The spacers that recognize unique locations in the genome and exhibit high specificity are characterized by a score value above 50. Furthermore, all the possible off-targets are sorted by the CFD score and annotated with their location in an exon, an intron, or an intergenic region. Both the efficiency scores from Doench et al. and Moreno-Mateos et al., as well as the microhomology score that predicts out-of-frame mutations, are displayed on the result page of the web-based tool to select spacers with higher gene disruption potential. In addition, information on genomic variants is provided and allows the exclusion of spacers targeting SNPs to prevent mismatches between the spacer and the target sequence.

While the currently available tools enable the selection of potentially efficient and selective gRNAs, integration of other relevant information such as the gene, the transcript and the protein structures, the generation of transcriptional variants, or the epigenetic features could help to further increase *in silico* predictability. Furthermore, the translatability of these tools, developed from data obtained in specific experimental conditions, to other biological models or CRISPR/Cas delivery methods is limited and would necessitate the accumulation and comparison of large sets of on-target and off-target gene editing data. Considering the predictive potential of the current computational tools, analysis of genome-wide screens or small-scale target validation studies should include results obtained from several different gRNAs to mitigate off-target effects and potential artefacts associated with gene editing. Beyond gRNA efficiency, future models may significantly improve the precision of the CRISPR/Cas technology by incorporating prediction of the specific gene editing outcomes obtained with a gRNA, as the repair process appears to be non-random and determined by the target sequence [137, 160].

9.3.4 Successful Application of the CRISPR/Cas Technology

9.3.4.1 Delivering CRISPR Reagents to Target Cells

Although the basic components (DNA, RNA, or protein) are the same whatever the choice of biological model, the method to deliver all components that are mandatory to edit genes varies broadly, and choosing the most suitable one for the planned experiment is critical for a successful approach. Delivery can be split into two major categories: delivery vehicle and cargo [220] (Figure 9.3). Regarding CRISPR/Cas9 cargos, there are three options that are commonly described: DNA plasmid encoding both the Cas9 protein and the gRNA, mRNA for Cas9 translation in combination with a separate gRNA, and Cas9 protein associated with gRNA (also named ribonucleoprotein [RNP] complex) [161].

Plasmids encoding Cas9 and gRNAs were the first cargos used to edit genomes for an *in vitro* purpose. Thanks to publicly available plasmid reagents through, for example Addgene, this approach was broadly adopted by academic groups. The academic community developed numerous plasmid modifications and protocol variations, but the former still typically contain shared features such as the use of genes conferring antibiotic resistance or fluorescent proteins for easy

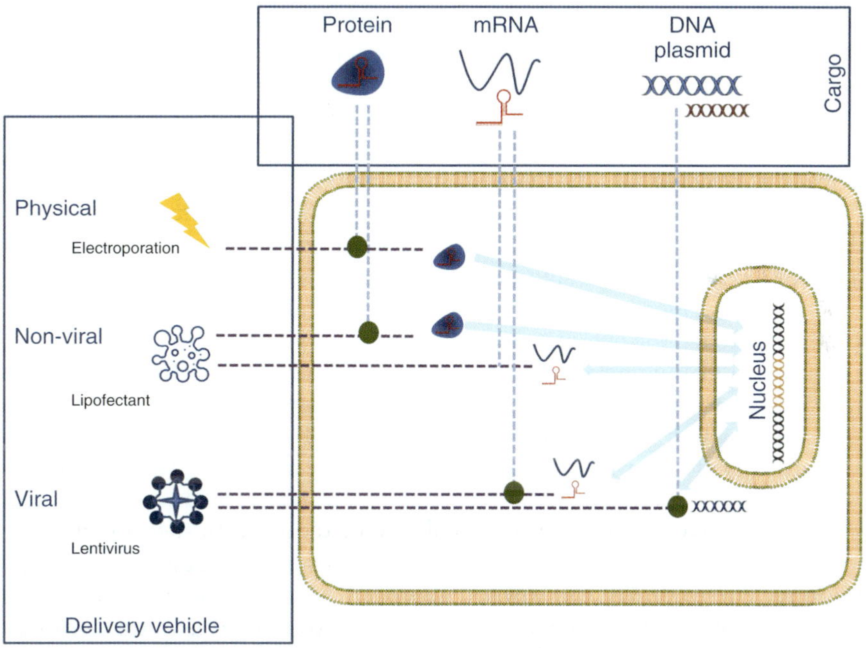

Figure 9.3 Schematic diagram depicting options for delivering gene editing components to cells. Each dotted blue line indicates those most used to successfully deliver cargo and edit specific genomic sites. Ribonucleoprotein complex of gRNA and Cas9 protein could be directly delivered to the nucleus with electroporation or lipofection. mRNA coding for Cas9 and gRNA could also be delivered by electroporation or lipofection but must be translated in the cytoplasm before acting on the genome. Delivering DNA coding for both gRNA and Cas9 is usually delivered with lentivirus but needs to first reach the nucleus to be transcribed to mRNA, exported to cytoplasm to be translated, and return to the nucleus to act on the genome.

visualization and/or selection. Plasmid reagents are easy to modify and produce at large scale, but the use of plasmids to express Cas9 and gRNA faces issues regarding the rate of component expression and how long they are present within the cell. Plasmid or viral delivery of Cas9 and gRNA(s) requires the use of the endogenous cellular transcription/translation machinery to generate functional Cas9/gRNA complexes, which results in a significant lag in peak Cas9 protein expression. Usually researchers use the same plasmid to co-express the protein Cas9 and gRNA. However, for expressing the protein from DNA, there is a need for the plasmid to enter the nucleus to be functionally linked to lag in function between Cas9 protein and gRNA (Figure 9.3). In the early days of using Cas9, researchers opted for plasmid genomic insertion. This artificial continuous expression of Cas9 is linked to a potential increase in off-target effects. To limit off-target effects and minimize the unwanted impact on the genome, researchers have investigated numerous solutions to induce transient Cas9 expression. First, placing an inducible promoter (the tetracycline operator, for example) upstream of the Cas9/dead Cas9 (dCas9) (see Section 9.4) sequence is a classical solution to achieve transient expression of genome editing basic components [80, 162]. This availability-on-demand approach was also used with the magnet system or light-sensitive protein, leading to a photoactivatable dCas9 system [163, 164]. Conditional genome editing can also be achieved by incorporating CRISPR with the Cre/loxP system, where Cre functions as a trigger to inactivate a loxP-flanked (floxed) allele via Cre/loxP-mediated recombination.

For drug discovery purposes, DNA plasmid cargo is still an option, but a straightforward method to produce the plasmid on a large scale and low cost still needs to be achieved. The DNA plasmid cargo is broadly used for screening purposes thanks to lentivirus vectorization. Coupling high infection rate with scale-up and parallelized approach for particle production, lentivirus-based gene editing is now the gold standard for running a CRISPR screen.

In vitro transcribed mRNA offers an attractive alternative to DNA. Once mRNA has reached the cytoplasm, translation can start instantaneously without the need to enter the nucleus (Figure 9.3). This feature that only needs a translation step creates an added value for the mRNA approach especially in efficacy in quiescent (where chromatin is highly compacted) or hard-to-transfect cells (lower quantity of material to transfect), reducing the potential risk of insertional mutagenesis. But such options are limited by the intracellular localization of mRNA during endocytosis. mRNA will be translocated into the endosome where the carrier of mRNA should facilitate endosomal escape via endosome disruption. For example, the mRNA approach was successfully achieved in cultured mouse cardiac fibroblasts via a cardiac-targeting sequence fused to a nine arginine-containing peptide. Results demonstrated the partial direct reprogramming of cardiac fibroblasts towards cardiomyocyte cells because of mRNA efficient transfection with low toxicity [165]. Direct delivery of Cas9-encoding mRNA as a cargo for CRISPR is still fairly low in drug discovery. This is partially due to the difficulty to produce large-scale high-quality mRNA coding for Cas9 and also to the availability of alternative solutions.

Cas9 RNPs are delivered as pre-existing functional gRNA/Cas9 protein hetero-complexes, ready to cleave the genome, with no need to be transcribed and translated, and which are quickly cleared from the cell via protein degradation pathways (Figure 9.3). There are two major advantages of the RNP complex compared to other cargos: Firstly, the extreme efficiency of the components to induce mutations in targeted genes. Secondly, rapid clearance of Cas9 RNPs from the cell may increase CRISPR specificity by reducing the time that Cas9 is available for off-target cleavage. The characteristics of RNPs make this type of cargo useful for CRISPR applications where limited expression of Cas9 is required such as knockout generation or DNA sequence insertion. If it is needed, selection is more difficult in the case of RNP complexes although gRNAs fused with fluorescent probes are commercially available. In terms of RNP complex delivery, usually three to five gRNAs are delivered in parallel, and cleavage efficiency is typically higher and more specific than when gRNAs are expressed from a plasmid. However, standard assays (see next paragraph) to confirm gene editing can be used for rapid comparison of gRNA efficiencies to choose the most optimal gRNA, in terms of both efficiency and specificity [70]. The RNP cargo is now a mature option, commercially available, and widely used to knock out genes especially for target validation. The major issue for RNP is the delivery of the complex and the cost of purified Cas9. The RNP complex can be used for multiple target invalidation experiments in parallel but still limited for large-scale screening.

The delivery vehicle used will often be strongly impacted by the choice of cargo due to packaging capabilities. Vehicles used to deliver the gene editing system cargo can be classified into three general groups: physical delivery, viral vectors, and non-viral vectors (Figure 9.3).

The most common physical delivery method is electroporation especially for *in vitro* purposes. Other methods such as osmotic shock delivery are currently under investigation [166]. Even though microinjection is quite efficient, this delivery lacks throughput and is time consuming [167].

Viral delivery vectors include specifically engineered non-integrative adeno-associated virus (AAV) and integrative lentivirus vehicles. AAV is not really well suitable for *in vitro* purposes due to lack of genomic insertion but can be used in non-proliferating cell models. For difficult-to-transfect cell lines or primary cells, lentiviral vectors are preferred. Lentivirus delivery is now the most popular delivery system for CRISPR screening. It allows gRNA barcoding simplifying the deconvolution of the screen results. Non-integrative lentivirus particles are now commercially available, opening the way to deliver the RNA coding for Cas9 with appropriate gRNAs with a high efficiency while preserving original cell phenotype and viability.

Non-viral vector delivery is not as prominent as viral-based methods. However, non-viral vectors possess several advantages over viral vectors. Many transfection reagents are commercially available and offer an advanced, efficient solution, and the development of delivery systems is a very active area of research. Non-viral vector systems include systems such as lipid nanoparticles, cell-penetrating peptides (CPPs) [168], or more recently DNA 'nanoclews' and gold nanoparticles [169]. Researchers are still investigating additional innovative vector delivery such as inorganic nanoparticles, carbon nanotubes (CNTs) [170], bare mesoporous silica nanoparticles (MSNPs), and dense silica nanoparticles (SiNPs) [171].

9.3.4.2 Check for Anticipated Knockout/Knock-In

Direct Polymerase Chain Reaction (PCR)-mediated assays using primers targeting mutation sites are basically unable to measure tight indel genomic modification. To better evaluate gene editing, efficient solutions such as Surveyor assay or mismatch detection assay (MDA or T7E1 assay) have been developed. The T7 endonuclease 1 (T7E1) MDA is a widely used method for evaluating the activity of site-specific nucleases such as Cas9, but compared with NGS, the T7E1 assay underestimates the activity observed in edited cells [172]. Indeed, enzyme mismatch cleavage (EMC) assays such as MDA and T7E1 are not able to provide accurate identification of a unique insertion and deletion that are likely observed and are the most common type of modification in gene editing following DSB generation and NHEJ-mediated repair. Therefore these assays should be used with caution.

To precisely determine indel modifications, Sanger sequencing is also performed on PCR products amplified from the genomic region flanking the gRNA target site. To better decode the specific mutations on all alleles, the PCR products must be cloned and sequenced. However, Sanger sequencing is costly, time and labour intensive, and poorly suited for high-throughput screening. Editing efficiencies can also be predicted by Sanger-based techniques such as the Tracking of Indels by Decomposition (TIDE) assay or Indel Detection by Amplicon Analysis (IDAA) that are reported to enable more precise and reliable identification but are still time and labour intensive and, in some instances, show puzzling results in edited clones [172].

New sequencing technologies such as NGS allow high-throughput generation of sequencing data and greatly contribute to better detect and characterize indel formation induced by CRISPR. This technology is useful to study large sample numbers due to its tremendous progress in terms of speed, throughput, and cost. Indeed, NGS has been increasingly used for the analysis of CRISPR/Cas9 gene editing experiments. Many public tools for gene editing assessment are available for analysing the CRISPR NGS data such as CRISPR-GA [173], CRISPResso [174], BATCH-GE [175], and Cas-Analyzer [176]. Massive parallelized NGS analysis opens the way to wide genome editing-based studies for drug discovery. This massive evolution in DNA sequencing technology is also mandatory to increase feasibility, accuracy, and specificity of the deconvolution step in CRISPR screens thanks to direct gRNA deep sequencing [177]. However, all of these techniques are not able to directly detect translocations and other major structural changes that could happen in genome editing investigations. Recent NGS pipeline experimental adaptation shows promising results to tackle these issues. For example, CRISPR-DAV can analyse a large number of samples in parallel or serial [178].

9.4 Further Developments of the CRISPR/Cas Technology Facilitates Additional Modes of Genetic Perturbation

9.4.1 CRISPRi

Besides generating functional knockouts, the CRISPR/Cas technology has undergone further development that enables additional modes of genetic perturbation. In particular, mutation of Cas9 catalytic domains has opened up new possibilities. A catalytically dead dCas9 will still engage a DNA target locus when an appropriate gRNA is present; but no DNA cleavage will occur. The presence of dCas9 on target genes can cause a roadblock for transcriptional elongation, RNA polymerase binding, or transcription factor binding. This principle is used by the CRISPRi technology and facilitates knocking down gene expression [179]. CRISPRi may be preferred over a functional knockout in cases such as the study of essential genes, where a complete loss of function would be lethal. In an attempt to further enhance CRISPRi gene repression, Gilbert et al. fused dCas9 to transcriptional repressor domains such as Krüppel-associated box (KRAB) and achieved robust as well as highly specific silencing, and they argued that CRISPRi may be complementary or even advantageous over RNAi [180]. An important consideration for the setup of a CRISPRi experiment is again the design of the gRNA that should be in the promoter region of a gene of interest to efficiently interfere with transcription.

9.4.2 CRISPRa

As in the case of CRISPRi and transcriptional repression, the principle of using dCas9 as a targetable DNA-binding entity that can be fused to effector domains with distinct regulatory functions can also be harnessed to achieve gene activation. Coupling of a potent transcriptional activator domain such as VP16 (virus protein 16 from *herpes simplex* virus-1) to ZFNs or TALENs [181] has been successfully used for transcriptional activation of various endogenous genes and is also feasible with dCas9. The complex facilitates the assembly of the pre-initiation complex at the promoter region of targeted genes, and expression of the dCas9-activator domain fusion in combination with gRNAs in human cells induces specific expression of endogenous targeted genes [180]. Thus, in addition to CRISPRi, dCas9 is also central to CRISPR/Cas-mediated gene activation (CRISPRa) suggesting that the catalytically inactive dCas9 protein can serve as a general platform for RNA-guided DNA targeting [180]. The CRISPRa technology was subjected to further improvement by Tanenbaum et al. who attached a peptide array (SunTag) to dCas9 [182]. By co-expressing dCas9-SunTag with a fusion protein consisting of VP16 and a SunTag-binding domain, they created a potent synthetic transcription factor that recruits multiple copies of a transcriptional activation domain.

9.4.3 Base Editing

Yet another recently developed mode of genetic manipulation by the CRISPR/Cas technology is base editing. In particular, combining dCas9 or nickase Cas9 with a cytidine deaminase domain (e.g. from the APOlipoprotein B mRNA Editing Catalytic polypeptide-like family; APOBEC) offers the possibility of mutating single bases at a target site without DSBs [161]. The cytidine deaminase domain modifies cytidine to uridine within a small window of bases in the vicinity of the PAM site, thereby creating a DNA lesion that can be subjected to several repair mechanisms [183]. Further technology developments increased the efficiency of repair mechanisms that result in a C > T substitution, e.g. by addition of the uracil glycosylase inhibitor that blocks base-excision repair. Thus, base editing provides a useful strategy for precise genetic manipulation that is orthogonal to template-mediated gene editing involving DNA cleavage and thus may offer improvements in efficiency while limiting damage.

9.5 The CRISPR/Cas Technology in Target Discovery and Validation

9.5.1 CRISPR/Cas Technology for Early Target Validation

In light of the continuing issue of failing pharmaceutical programs, increased efforts have to be put into strengthening the scientific basis for new programs. A critical step in this process is the early validation of a molecular target to warrant that the target is of key importance in a disease and that target engagement has the potential to result in a desired therapeutic benefit. Early target validation can be performed by different and complementary techniques as described in other chapters throughout this book and includes the manipulation of functional gene expression of a predicted target and subsequent analysis of downstream signalling pathways and phenotypes in relevant cellular models (see Chapter 11 for more details). RNAi technologies have been the main tool for gene expression manipulation in the past [10] but have suffered from insufficient target depletion and confounding off-target effects. On the other hand, ZFNs as well as TALENs often involve substantial time investment for reagent design and identification of rare cells with desired manipulations. In this regard, the CRISPR/Cas technology offers the advantage of a quick and precise model generation for early target validation. The technology is compatible with classical rescue experiments where a catalytically dead version of a target is re-expressed after knockout to better represent a therapeutic scenario in which a drug interferes with target activity rather than its abundance. Furthermore, as the CRISPR/Cas technology allows template-based genome engineering, precise mutations can also be introduced into the endogenous locus. The power of this approach is exemplified by the case of rocaglates that display antineoplastic activity by preferentially inhibiting the translation of key oncogenic mRNAs and for which several targets had been proposed [184]. By CRISPR/Cas-mediated introduction of a drug resistance-conferring mutation into the endogenous eukaryotic initiation factor

4F gene, Chu et al. were able to validate eIF4A1 as the primary molecular target of rocaglates. The use of the CRISPR/Cas technology for target validation in a slightly different context also expands on the follow-up of large-scale functional genetic screens for target discovery efforts, and several examples will be discussed below. It is also noteworthy that the CRISPR/Cas technology has been quickly embraced by the mouse modelling community to perform genetic manipulations in mouse zygotes for mouse model generation and *in vivo* target validation [185]. CRISPR-modified animal models now allow validation of research findings to reach go/no-go decisions in shorter time frames, particularly when complex strains with stacked modifications are involved [186].

9.5.2 CRISPR Screens and Use for Target Discovery

Target discovery, specifically the identification and subsequent validation of novel and potentially druggable biological targets, remains a challenging discipline in biomedical research. In target discovery, genetic manipulation is a common approach to evaluate whether modulation of the respective protein affects a disease-linked phenotype and can be applied in forward genetic screens. Recent advancements in the research community have revealed the great potential of CRISPR/Cas gene editing. As outlined above, the principle of the CRISPR/Cas gene editing technology (refer to Sections 9.2.1 and 9.3.1 for further details) builds on two factors: (i) an effector nuclease, Cas9, which hydrolyses double-stranded DNA and (ii) an RNA molecule, a gRNA, which targets Cas9 to a specific DNA sequence. The characteristics of the CRISPR/Cas technology enable target discovery by functional genetic screening on a large scale. In large-scale screening campaigns, thousands of individual gRNAs guide Cas9 nucleases to achieve a plethora of directed genomic manipulations in a cell population. A target-related assay read-out such as drug-induced alteration of cell proliferation or probe-based detection of signalling molecules by fluorescence-activated cell sorting (FACS) then allows identification of relevant gRNAs and genes. In the past, loss-of-function genetic screening by RNAi, interfering with target gene expression at the transcript level, was the predominant method for functional genetic screening at large scales. Despite some success with this method including the examples highlighted earlier, this method suffers from insufficient protein depletion and confounding off-target effects [187, 188]. To enable functional genetic screening using the DNA-targeting CRISPR/Cas technology, the RNAi functional genetic screening method was adapted [189]. Head-to-head benchmarking of the CRISPR technology with RNAi technology in most cases resulted in greater sensitivity and specificity when using the CRISPR/Cas9 technology, although both technologies may be compensatory in some cases [190–192]. One example for a complementary potential of both technologies has been highlighted by Morgens et al. who compared the ability of shRNA and CRISPR/Cas screens to identify essential genes in human cells and found little correlation albeit similar precision of both technologies in detecting essential genes. They argued that distinct biological processes are identified with each technology and combining the data improved performance [190]. However, encouraged by the results of the first screens published in December 2013

[107, 189], both industry and academia quickly embarked on more complex CRISPR screening activities to identify disease-relevant targets and support drug discovery efforts. Although having been around for only a few years, a high number of screening campaigns have already been conducted to identify targets for a variety of diseases, and the technology continues to hold great promise.

9.5.3 CRISPR Screens: General Principle and Considerations

From a methodological point of view, the setup of a robust CRISPR screen requires several general considerations including the careful choice of mode of genetic perturbation, screening model, and assay (Figure 9.4). While initially the CRISPR/Cas technology only facilitated knockout mode screens, where the knockout is achieved through NHEJ-mediated indel generation at the gRNA target site, further technology development enabled additional modes. Gene silencing via CRISPRi [179], gene activation via CRISPRa [193–195], and synthetic combination modes are only a few examples of the currently available screening modes (refer to Section 9.4 for further details). Since the reagents of the CRISPR/Cas technology can be delivered by multiple techniques, it is applicable to a variety of cellular models ranging from non-mammalian systems to cancer cell lines, primary cells, iPSCs, and even to mice *in vivo*. Depending on the required sensitivity, relatively crude assays such as induced cell death, e.g. to identify genes conferring resistance to a compound, to very sensitive assays involving FACS analysis, e.g. to identify genes modulating the intracellular abundance of a disease target [196], may be incorporated into the screen design. An additional consideration is the format of the CRISPR screen. Most popular is the pooled format where multiple gRNAs encoded on expression vectors are mixed together and delivered as a pool to the target cells. While this format is cost effective, compatible with large-scale screening, and requires little or no automation, it comes at the expense of limited flexibility in terms of assessable phenotypes. Thus, in cases where a specific phenotype is of interest, e.g. where microscopic evaluation of edited cells is required, and where the focus can be restricted to a smaller set of genes, a screen in an arrayed format may be ideal as individual CRISPR reagents are delivered well by well to cells in a microtiter plate.

While having a variety of options when designing a CRISPR screen, the individual screens conducted so far mostly follow a unifying theme. To explain the general principles, a straightforward setup of a knockout mode pooled CRISPR screen is described (Figure 9.4), followed by key technical considerations to highlight optimization opportunities. To illustrate the application breadth of the technology, selected examples of more complex screens that diverge from the straightforward CRISPR screen setup will be outlined.

A focus of the first CRISPR screens has been the identification of essential genes in human cells, and the setup of those screens can be used to describe the general principles of a knockout mode pooled CRISPR screen [197]. In such a screen, a pool of lentiviral Cas9/gRNA expression vectors, constituting a gRNA library, is virally delivered to a population of proliferating human cancer cells. The individual vectors in the library differ in the gRNA component: up to hundreds of thousands of different gRNAs are included, targeting thousands of different genes. To

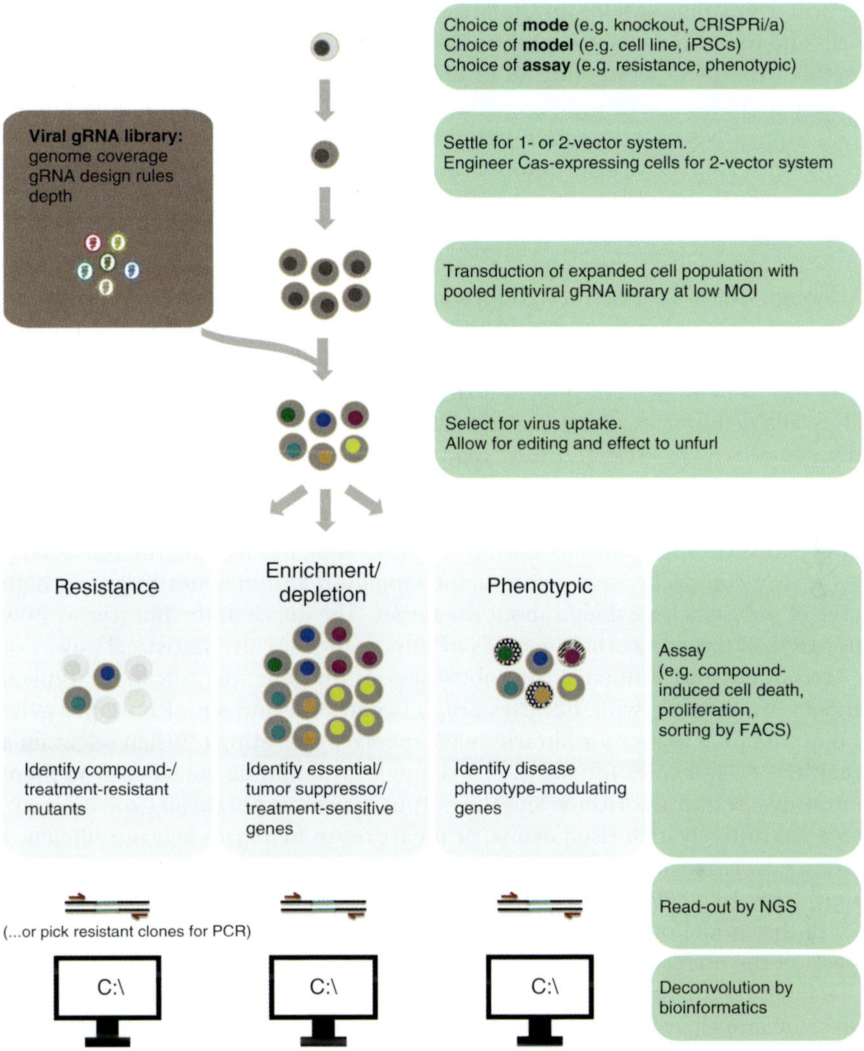

Figure 9.4 CRISPR screens: general principle and considerations. The workflow of a general CRISPR screen is depicted starting with a cellular model at the very top and finishing with the deconvolution of NGS data by bioinformatics for robust hit selection. Key considerations are highlighted in green.

enhance the statistical power in analytical post-processing steps, multiple gRNAs targeting the same gene in different places are often included. A low virus-to-cell ratio multiplicity of infection (MOI) ensures that each cell in the population at maximum receives one viral vector. Following infection, lentiviral expression cassettes integrate into the genome of the host cell, thus making cassette components a heritable trait. Besides the gRNA and the Cas9 nuclease, selectable markers, mostly classical antibiotic resistance genes, are encoded in the lentiviral cassette and allow enrichment of infected cells. Upon expression of Cas9 and gRNAs, those cells that harbour a cassette expressing a gRNA directed against an essential gene will over time cease to proliferate and die, resulting in decreasing numbers of cells and therefore cassettes with respective gRNAs. At a predefined end point, cassettes with gRNAs targeting an essential gene will thus be underrepresented with respect to the starting gRNA pool. Assessment of representation is achieved by counting gRNA cassettes after extraction of genomic DNA from the entire cell population at respective time points and subjection to NGS with cassette-specific primer pairs. The enormous amount of data generated by NGS requires skilled bioinformaticians for deconvolution and to progress from the raw NGS reads to significant gene-level values and biological pathway enrichment analyses.

Although this is a rather straightforward description of a CRISPR screen, several technical considerations should be made by the scientist in order to maximize screening output. Once settled with a particular mode, the choice for a CRISPR library has to be made. For pooled format screens there is a variety of commercially available libraries. These libraries differ in their complexity in terms of how many genes are targeted and how many gRNAs target a single gene. A more focused library may be used when reagents are limited and a narrow biological hypothesis is tested, e.g. a kinase focused library for analysis of a specific signalling pathway in response to a drug. Genome-wide libraries on the other hand allow a very comprehensive genomic interrogation and may not require a high degree of previous knowledge about the target. The depth of the library, i.e. how many gRNAs target a certain gene, is of importance for the statistical power of the screen and will influence the robustness of hit gene identification. Typical numbers for genome-wide libraries are between four and six gRNAs per gene but may be much higher for libraries with special applications. When selecting a library, the design rules for the gRNA sequences should be considered as there are multiple design algorithms and the output may incorporate an exon bias, e.g. for 5′constitutively expressed exons, or measures to increase cleavage efficiency as well as decrease off-target effects (see Section 9.3.3 for more details on gRNA design) [106, 107, 189, 198]. Further important considerations are the delivery of Cas9 to the model of choice and the allelic frequency of the model as both will impact on the effect size. While Cas9 can be delivered together with the gRNA in one large vector, this will limit transfection/infection efficiency as well as Cas9 expression and cleavage efficiency. Alternatively, two vector systems may be used where Cas9 and gRNAs are encoded by different vectors. An advantage of the two vector systems is the possibility of generating and selecting high-performing clonal cell lines, which express Cas9 either constitutively or inducibly for temporal control of expression. Both the one and two vector type of libraries are available. When choosing a model, the specific karyotype may be reviewed as allele frequency could impact on effect size – already from a probabilistic point of view, it is obvious that editing of a diploid genome results in fewer functional alleles with an in-frame mutation than a genome with three or more allele copies.

9.5.4 Selected Examples of Target Discovery Using CRISPR Screens to Illustrate the Breadth of Applications

To date, a high number of complex CRISPR screens have already been performed to identify targets for a range of diseases. Zhang et al. performed a CRISPR/Cas screen to identify host genes that, when edited, result in reduced infection with flaviviruses, which infect hundreds of millions of people annually and against which no antiviral therapy is available [199]. They performed a genome-wide knockout screen with more than 120k gRNAs in human cells and looked for surviving cells upon West Nile virus-induced cell death. gRNAs from individual surviving colonies were amplified by PCR and sequenced. They validated nine human genes required for flavivirus infectivity and identified potential pharmacological targets for inhibiting infection including SPCS1, a protein of the endoplasmic reticulum-associated signal peptidase complex necessary for proper cleavage of flavivirus structural proteins and virus secretion.

Park et al. engineered a physiologically relevant CD4+ T cell line model where productive HIV infection leads to expression of green fluorescent protein (GFP) [200]. After infection with a library comprising more than 180k gRNAs targeting the entire genome as well as infection with HIV, they isolated viable, GFP-negative cells by FACS and used NGS to measure the abundance of all gRNAs from this population. An initial population of cells collected prior to HIV infection and a population of cells propagated without HIV infection served as a reference. They identified five factors that are required for HIV infection yet are dispensible for cellular proliferation and viability, including the HIV co-receptors CD4 and CCR5 as well as proteins in a common pathway to sulfate CCR5 on tyrosine residues, facilitating CCR5 recognition by the HIV envelope. They further validated the results in primary human CD4+ T cells through Cas9-mediated knockout suggesting that biological pathways constituted by these factors can be studied for therapeutic intervention. To further enable research towards HIV treatments, Huang and Nair introduced a platform based on astrocytes, one of the multiple HIV reservoirs in the human body, for identifying candidates for gene editing treatment of HIV latent cells [201].

An interesting example for a CRISPR screen that facilitates future approaches to expand the horizon of anti-parasitic interventions was published by Sidik et al. [202]. They presented the first genome-wide genetic screen in the parasite *Toxoplasma gondii*, which can cause life-threatening disease in immune-compromised individuals or when contracted congenitally, and assessed the contribution of each gene during infection of human fibroblasts. A library containing 10 different gRNAs against ~8k predicted *T. gondii* genes was designed and cloned into an expression vector followed by regular transfection into Cas9-expressing parasites. They defined ~200 previously uncharacterized, fitness-conferring genes from which 16 were further investigated, revealing essential functions during infection of human cells.

A pressing challenge in biomedical research is drug-resistant cancers, and Han et al. [203] presented a CRISPR screening strategy for pairwise genetic interactions to identify synergistic drug combinations. They introduced a CRISPR-based double knockout system that employs effective cloning as well as sequencing of paired gRNA libraries and a statistical scoring method for calculating genetic interactions from CRISPR-deleted gene pairs. Using a library of 490k double gRNAs directed against over 20k pairs of drug targets, they identified synthetic lethal drug target pairs in a leukaemia cell line for which corresponding drugs exhibit synergistic killing, thus providing an effective strategy to screen synergistic drug combinations.

By targeting CRISPR/Cas mutagenesis to exons encoding functional protein domains, Shi et al. overcame limitations of classical CRISPR/Cas approaches that target 5′ exons of candidate genes that often produce in-frame variants that retain functionality [126]. Targeting protein domains generated a higher proportion of null mutations and substantially increased the potency of negative selection, which was exemplified by the targeting of 192 chromatin regulatory domains in murine acute myeloid leukaemia cells, leading to the identification of 6 known drug targets and 19 additional dependencies. The authors suggested that a broader application of this approach may allow comprehensive identification of protein domains that sustain cancer cells and are suitable for drug targeting.

The power of combining multiple CRISPR screening modes is exemplified by the case of rigosertib, a drug in clinical development in high-risk myelodysplastic syndrome for which the molecular target had remained controversial. Jost et al. [204] infected chronic myeloid leukaemia cells either expressing dCas9-KRAB (CRISPRi) [180] or dCas9 fused to the SunTag and a SunTag-binding domain fused to transcriptional activation domains (CRISPRa) with genome-scale CRISPRi and CRISPRa sgRNA libraries targeting roughly 16k genes. After harvesting a subpopulation at the outset of the experiment, they measured the relative abundance of each gRNA in each population by NGS to reveal how each gRNA affects growth in the absence of rigosertib as well as sensitivity to rigosertib. By combining CRISPRi and CRISPRa screening as well as focused, comparative chemical-genetic profiling, they were able to pinpoint microtubules as the target of rigosertib.

Additional examples highlighting the broad range of studies include a screen for functional non-coding elements with paired gRNAs, which identified lncRNAs that have oncogenic or tumour suppressor activities [205] as well as a screen for metastasis driving genes that involved the implantation of CRISPR mutagenized mouse cells into mice *in vivo* and subsequent analysis of distal metastasis for edited genes [206]. Screening in an arrayed format is also feasible as was demonstrated by Kim et al. who employed 4542 arrayed gRNAs and an image-based assay to uncover host genes required for infection by coxsackievirus, human pathogens causing diverse diseases [207].

9.6 Application of CRISPR Genome Editing in Immunology Studies

For a long time, immunologists have lacked straightforward and reliable tools to directly perform gene editing in primary immune cells and had to heavily rely on knock-in or knockout mice for studying the role of genes in immune regulation. While the RNAi technology has been widely used in cancer research, the application of RNAi in immunology is of limited value due to technical challenges with primary immune cells including off-target effects and siRNA/shRNA-associated immunogenicity. The emerging CRISPR/Cas gene editing technology could indeed be a powerful tool for immunologists to dissect disease mechanisms and identify novel therapeutic targets. It is noteworthy that the application of CRISPR/Cas in immunological studies is still limited due to the challenge of manipulating primary immune cells. Herein, we discuss potential technical hurdles and current progress on the application of CRISPR/Cas in immunology studies.

Efficient delivery of the Cas9 protein into primary immune cells has proven difficult with low expression levels achieved by lentivirus-based transduction. To solve this issue, the immune cells isolated from Cas9 knock-in mice were used with stable expression of Cas9. Parnas et al. introduced a lentiviral gRNA library into Cas9 knock-in bone marrow and obtained differentiated dendritic cells. A genome-wide mouse dendritic cell TLR4 pathway screen was successfully performed using this method, and a number of previously unknown lipopolysaccharide/Toll-like receptor (LPS/TLR) pathway regulators (e.g. Tmem258) were identified [208]. This strategy, however, is obviously not applicable for the study of human primary immune cells. To solve this issue, Schumann et al. used electroporation to deliver purified Cas9 protein in complex with a gRNA into primary T cells, and they were able to achieve reasonable knockout efficiencies, resulting in expected cellular phenotypes [209]. For example, electroporation of Cas9 RNP targeting CXCR4 led to about 40% of cells losing high-level expression of CXCR4 on the cell surface. Moreover, the Marson lab developed a new method by combining lentiviral gRNA library infection with Cas9 protein electroporation (termed Single guide RNA (sgRNA) Lentiviral Infection with Cas9 protein Electroporation (SLiCE)) to facilitate genome-wide screening in primary T cells [210]. In this screen, a set of potential regulators of T cell stimulation and immunosuppression were identified. Knockout of new identified immune suppressors could boost T cell activation and *in vitro* cancer cell killing. In addition, Ting et al. developed a guide swap method to increase the efficiency of Cas9 delivery by introducing Cas9 complexed with non-targeting gRNAs, which enabled two genome-scale screens using CD4+ T cells and CD34+ hematopoietic stem and progenitor cells [211].

While significant progress has been made regarding the optimization of Cas9 delivery and expression in primary immune cells, there are still a few other technical caveats. For one, gRNAs or lentiviruses encoding gRNAs may activate the nucleic acid immune sensor(s). This kind of target-independent immune response may change the cell's status and influence the experimental readout. Therefore, it will be helpful to target one gene with multiple gRNAs to get a solid result. Another issue is the difficulty in obtaining sufficient primary cells for genome-wide screens since many immune cell populations do not proliferate and expand *in vitro*. Isolation of desired immune cells from large-size leukopak or buffy coat may partially overcome this issue [212]. Finally, the donor variability may be high in these experiments necessitating multiple donors for reliable data interpretation.

In addition to CRISPR/Cas-based gene knockout, a number of innovative CRISPR/Cas gene editing methods have been developed for immunology studies. Jaitin et al. developed CRISPR-seq, an integrated approach for CRISPR-pooled screens with single-cell transcriptomics [213]. This new method allows profiling of the genetic perturbation at the corresponding transcriptome in the same cell. The authors successfully applied CRISPR-seq in mice to dissect the role of a set of genes following innate immune activation. The *in vivo* gene inactivation-associated transcriptome change could be tracked at single-cell level to determine the specific transcription factor-controlled immune cell differentiation.

In summary, accumulating publications suggest that CRISPR/Cas gene editing is technically feasible in a set of primary immune cells. In the future, CRISPR/Cas will help to dissect the role of genes and genetic pathways and facilitate the discovery of novel drug targets for immune disease.

9.7 Concluding Remarks

As described in this chapter, genetic manipulation technologies have already had a great impact not only on target identification as well as target validation but also on biomedical research in general. Particularly, the CRISPR/Cas technology, despite its youth, is now widely applied and continues to be developed in multiple directions at an astonishing speed. At this point, it should be emphasized that there are certain limitations for the application of the CRISPR/Cas technology. While the issue that targeting options are restricted to the availability of nearby PAM sites can often be tackled by the use of alternative Cas enzymes with different PAM requirements, the delivery of the individual CRISPR components to a model of choice can present the greatest hurdle. Another remaining open issue is the extent of off-target cleavage by the CRISPR/Cas technology. In this regard, a well-designed gRNA is critical and, according to some scientists, may result in the stray mutation frequency falling below the spontaneous background mutation frequency [214]. Furthermore, two recent studies revealed that CRISPR/Cas can induce cell cycle arrest and selection against cells with a functional p53 pathway, something worth paying attention to [122, 215]. Along the same lines, Aguirre et al. [80] observed that gene editing by CRISPR/Cas9 elicits a gene-independent anti-proliferative cell response. They claim that this effect has important practical implications for the interpretation of CRISPR/Cas screening data and confounds the use of this technology for the identification of essential genes in amplified regions. The field is moving rapidly and solutions to tackle major issues may soon be available. Looking ahead, particularly the establishment of catalytically inactive dCas9 protein as a general platform for RNA-guided DNA targeting appears to make the technology fit for the future. New developments such as dCas9/Cas9 fused to an avidin protein open the door for every scientist to build their own flexible tools to recruit biotinylated proteins to genomic target sites and allow action on the genome through numerous mechanisms of action such as epigenetic modification. The Cas9 protein can also be split into two lobes to decrease Cas9 size for efficient delivery, and scientists demonstrated that fusing the two split Cas9 fragments with inteins, which are protein segments excised during protein splicing [216, 217], allowed dimerization and endonuclease reconstitution upon co-expression [218]. New tools derived from CRISPR/Cas9 such as CRISPR-SKIP have been developed for studying specific exon skipping in genes [219] or to investigate epigenetic methylation and acetylation in a pathological context. It is clear that the biomedical terrain accessible with the CRISPR/Cas technology will continue to increase, and ultimately we may be able to comprehensively model an individual patient's biology for the purpose of testing the effectiveness of drug molecules and identifying the right drug for the right patient [220].

References

1 Scherer, S. and Davis, R.W. (1979). Replacement of chromosome segments with altered DNA sequences constructed in vitro. *Proc. Natl. Acad. Sci. U.S.A.* 76: 4951–4955.

2 Smithies, O., Gregg, R.G., Boggs, S.S. et al. (1985). Insertion of DNA sequences into the human chromosomal beta-globin locus by homologous recombination. *Nature* 317: 230–234.

3 Thomas, K.R., Folger, K.R., and Capecchi, M.R. (1986). High frequency targeting of genes to specific sites in the mammalian genome. *Cell* 44: 419–428.

4 Rothstein, R.J. (1983). One-step gene disruption in yeast. *Methods Enzymol.* 101: 202–211.

5 Mansour, S.L., Thomas, K.R., and Capecchi, M.R. (1988). Disruption of the proto-oncogene int-2 in mouse embryo-derived stem cells: a general strategy for targeting mutations to non-selectable genes. *Nature* 336: 348–352.

6 Lu, S. and Zhou, J. (2017). Finding the 'guilty' gene variant of sporadic Parkinson's disease via CRISPR/Cas9. *Neurosci. Bull.* 33: 115–117.

7 Akerman, I., Tu, Z., Beucher, A. et al. (2016). Human pancreatic beta cell lncRNAs control cell-specific regulatory networks. *Cell Metab.* 25: 400–411.

8 Covarrubias, S., Robinson, E.K., Shapleigh, B. et al. (2017). CRISPR/Cas-based screening of long non-coding RNAs (lncRNAs) in macrophages with an NF-kappaB reporter. *J. Biol. Chem.* 292: 20911–20920.

9 Fire, A., Xu, S., Montgomery, M.K. et al. (1998). Potent and specific genetic interference by double-stranded RNA in *Caenorhabditis elegans*. *Nature* 391: 806–811.

10 Dykxhoorn, D.M. and Lieberman, J. (2005). The silent revolution: RNA interference as basic biology, research tool, and therapeutic. *Annu. Rev. Med.* 56: 401–423.

11 Tijsterman, M. and Plasterk, R.H. (2004). Dicers at RISC; the mechanism of RNAi. *Cell* 117: 1–3.

12 Tsherniak, A., Vazquez, F., Montgomery, P.G. et al. (2017). Defining a cancer dependency map. *Cell* 170: 564, e16–576.

13 McDonald, E.R. 3rd,, de Weck, A., Schlabach, M.R. et al. (2017). Project DRIVE: a compendium of cancer dependencies and synthetic lethal relationships uncovered by large-scale, deep RNAi screening. *Cell* 170: 577–592. e10.

14 Marcotte, R., Sayad, A., Brown, K.R. et al. (2016). Functional genomic landscape of human breast cancer drivers, vulnerabilities, and resistance. *Cell* 164: 293–309.

15 Shen, J., Najafi, S., Stable, S. et al. (2018). A kinome-wide RNAi screen identifies ALK as a target to sensitize neuroblastoma cells for HDAC8-inhibitor treatment. *Cell Death Differ.* 25: 2053–2070.
16 Wuestefeld, T., Pesic, M., Rudalska, R. et al. (2013). A Direct in vivo RNAi screen identifies MKK4 as a key regulator of liver regeneration. *Cell* 153: 389–401.
17 Grobler, Y., Yun, C.Y., Kahler, D.J. et al. (2018). Whole genome screen reveals a novel relationship between Wolbachia levels and Drosophila host translation. *PLoS Pathog.* 14: e1007445.
18 Rousseaux, M.W.C., Vazquez-Velez, G.E., Al-Ramahi, I. et al. (2018). A druggable genome screen identifies modifiers of alpha-synuclein levels via a tiered cross-species validation approach. *J. Neurosci.* 38: 9286–9301.
19 Segall, J., Matsui, T., and Roeder, R.G. (1980). Multiple factors are required for the accurate transcription of purified genes by RNA polymerase III. *J. Biol. Chem.* 255: 11986–11991.
20 Miller, T.J. and Mertz, J.E. (1982). Template structural requirements for transcription in vivo by RNA polymerase II. *Mol. Cell. Biol.* 2: 1595–1607.
21 Choo, Y. and Klug, A. (1994). Selection of DNA binding sites for zinc fingers using rationally randomized DNA reveals coded interactions. *Proc. Natl. Acad. Sci. U.S.A.* 91: 11168–11172.
22 Liu, P.Q., Tan, S., Mendel, M.C. et al. (2005). Isogenic human cell lines for drug discovery: regulation of target gene expression by engineered zinc-finger protein transcription factors. *J. Biomol. Screening* 10: 304–313.
23 Davis, D. and Stokoe, D. (2010). Zinc finger nucleases as tools to understand and treat human diseases. *BMC Med.* 8: 42.
24 Urnov, F.D., Rebar, E.J., Holmes, M.C. et al. (2010). Genome editing with engineered zinc finger nucleases. *Nat. Rev. Genet.* 11: 636–646.
25 Jacob, H.J., Lazar, J., Dwinell, M.R. et al. (2010). Gene targeting in the rat: advances and opportunities. *Trends Genet.* 26: 510–518.
26 Geurts, A.M. and Moreno, C. (2010). Zinc-finger nucleases: new strategies to target the rat genome. *Clin. Sci. (London)* 119: 303–311.
27 Chen, C.C., Geurts, A.M., Jacob, H.J. et al. (2013). Heterozygous knockout of transforming growth factor-beta1 protects Dahl S rats against high salt-induced renal injury. *Physiol. Genomics* 45: 110–118.
28 Mattson, D.L., Lund, H., Guo, C. et al. (2013). Genetic mutation of recombination activating gene 1 in Dahl salt-sensitive rats attenuates hypertension and renal damage. *Am. J. Physiol. Regul. Integr. Comp. Physiol.* 304: R407–R414.
29 Gopalakrishnan, K., Kumarasamy, S., Abdul-Majeed, S. et al. (2012). Targeted disruption of Adamts16 gene in a rat genetic model of hypertension. *Proc. Natl. Acad. Sci. U.S.A.* 109: 20555–20559.
30 Le Floch, R., Chiche, J., Marchiq, I. et al. (2011). CD147 subunit of lactate/H+ symporters MCT1 and hypoxia-inducible MCT4 is critical for energetics and growth of glycolytic tumors. *Proc. Natl. Acad. Sci. U.S.A.* 108: 16663–16668.

31 Bentley, C., Jurinka, S.S., Kljavin, N.M. et al. (2013). A requirement for wild-type Ras isoforms in mutant KRas-driven signalling and transformation. *Biochem. J.* 452: 313–320.
32 Provasi, E., Genovese, P., Lombardo, A. et al. (2012). Editing T cell specificity towards leukemia by zinc finger nucleases and lentiviral gene transfer. *Nat. Med.* 18: 807–815.
33 Zou, J., Mali, P., Huang, X. et al. (2011). Site-specific gene correction of a point mutation in human iPS cells derived from an adult patient with sickle cell disease. *Blood* 118: 4599–4608.
34 Goldberg, A.D., Banaszynski, L.A., Noh, K.M. et al. (2010). Distinct factors control histone variant H3.3 localization at specific genomic regions. *Cell* 140: 678–691.
35 Gutschner, T. and Diederichs, S. (2012). The hallmarks of cancer: a long non-coding RNA point of view. *RNA Biol.* 9: 703–719.
36 Chen, W.T., Alpert, A., Leiter, C. et al. (2013). Systematic identification of functional residues in mammalian histone H2AX. *Mol. Cell. Biol.* 33: 111–126.
37 Bonas, U., Stall, R.E., and Staskawicz, B. (1989). Genetic and structural characterization of the avirulence gene avrBs3 from *Xanthomonas campestris* pv. vesicatoria. *Mol. Gen. Genet.* 218: 127–136.
38 Mukherjee, K. and Burglin, T.R. (2007). Comprehensive analysis of animal TALE homeobox genes: new conserved motifs and cases of accelerated evolution. *J. Mol. Evol.* 65: 137–153.
39 Garg, A., Lohmueller, J.J., Silver, P.A., and Armel, T.Z. (2012). Engineering synthetic TAL effectors with orthogonal target sites. *Nucleic Acids Res.* 40: 7584–7595.
40 Gabsalilow, L., Schierling, B., Friedhoff, P. et al. (2013). Site- and strand-specific nicking of DNA by fusion proteins derived from MutH and I-SceI or TALE repeats. *Nucleic Acids Res.* 41: e83.
41 Fontes, A. and Lakshmipathy, U. (2013). Advances in genetic modification of pluripotent stem cells. *Biotechnol. Adv.* 31: 994–1001.
42 Christian, M., Cermak, T., Doyle, E.L. et al. (2010). Targeting DNA double-strand breaks with TAL effector nucleases. *Genetics* 186: 757–761.
43 Cermak, T., Doyle, E.L., Christian, M. et al. (2011). Efficient design and assembly of custom TALEN and other TAL effector-based constructs for DNA targeting. *Nucleic Acids Res.* 39: e82.
44 Hockemeyer, D., Wang, H., Kiani, S. et al. (2011). Genetic engineering of human pluripotent cells using TALE nucleases. *Nat. Biotechnol.* 29: 731–734.
45 Sander, J.D., Cade, L., Khayter, C. et al. (2011). Targeted gene disruption in somatic zebrafish cells using engineered TALENs. *Nat. Biotechnol.* 29: 697–698.
46 Huang, P., Xiao, A., Zhou, M. et al. (2011). Heritable gene targeting in zebrafish using customized TALENs. *Nat. Biotechnol.* 29: 699–700.
47 Clark, K.J., Balciunas, D., Pogoda, H.M. et al. (2011). In vivo protein trapping produces a functional expression codex of the vertebrate proteome. *Nat. Methods* 8: 506–515.

48 Lei, Y., Guo, X., Liu, Y. et al. (2012). Efficient targeted gene disruption in Xenopus embryos using engineered transcription activator-like effector nucleases (TALENs). *Proc. Natl. Acad. Sci. U.S.A.* 109: 17484–17489.

49 Tesson, L., Usal, C., Menoret, S. et al. (2011). Knockout rats generated by embryo microinjection of TALENs. *Nat. Biotechnol.* 29: 695–696.

50 Carlson, D.F., Tan, W., Lillico, S.G. et al. (2012). Efficient TALEN-mediated gene knockout in livestock. *Proc. Natl. Acad. Sci. U.S.A.* 109: 17382–17387.

51 Shi, B., Li, J., Shi, X. et al. (2017). TALEN-mediated knockout of CCR5 confers protection against infection of human immunodeficiency virus. *J. Acquir. Immune Defic. Syndr.* 74: 229–241.

52 Wang, T., Jiao, J., Zhang, H. et al. (2017). TGF-beta induced PAR-1 expression promotes tumor progression and osteoclast differentiation in giant cell tumor of bone. *Int. J. Cancer* 141: 1630–1642.

53 Xiao, L., Wang, Y., Liang, W. et al. (2018). LRH-1 drives hepatocellular carcinoma partially through induction of c-myc and cyclin E1, and suppression of p21. *Cancer Manag. Res.* 10: 2389–2400.

54 Li, B., Qian, M., Cao, H. et al. (2017). TGF-beta2-induced ANGPTL4 expression promotes tumor progression and osteoclast differentiation in giant cell tumor of bone. *Oncotarget* 8: 54966–54977.

55 Karakikes, I., Termglinchan, V., Cepeda, D.A. et al. (2017). A comprehensive TALEN-based knockout library for generating human-induced pluripotent stem cell-based models for cardiovascular diseases. *Circ. Res.* 120: 1561–1571.

56 Adli, M. (2018). The CRISPR tool kit for genome editing and beyond. *Nat. Commun.* 9: 1911.

57 Jansen, R., Embden, J.D., Gaastra, W., and Schouls, L.M. (2002). Identification of genes that are associated with DNA repeats in prokaryotes. *Mol. Microbiol.* 43: 1565–1575.

58 Mojica, F.J., Diez-Villasenor, C., Garcia-Martinez, J., and Soria, E. (2005). Intervening sequences of regularly spaced prokaryotic repeats derive from foreign genetic elements. *J. Mol. Evol.* 60: 174–182.

59 Bolotin, A., Quinquis, B., Sorokin, A., and Ehrlich, S.D. (2005). Clustered regularly interspaced short palindrome repeats (CRISPRs) have spacers of extrachromosomal origin. *Microbiology* 151: 2551–2561.

60 Pourcel, C., Salvignol, G., and Vergnaud, G. (2005). CRISPR elements in *Yersinia pestis* acquire new repeats by preferential uptake of bacteriophage DNA, and provide additional tools for evolutionary studies. *Microbiology* 151: 653–663.

61 Makarova, K.S., Grishin, N.V., Shabalina, S.A. et al. (2006). A putative RNA-interference-based immune system in prokaryotes: computational analysis of the predicted enzymatic machinery, functional analogies with eukaryotic RNAi, and hypothetical mechanisms of action. *Biol. Direct* 1: 7.

62 Barrangou, R., Fremaux, C., Deveau, H. et al. (2007). CRISPR provides acquired resistance against viruses in prokaryotes. *Science* 315: 1709–1712.

63 Brouns, S.J., Jore, M.M., Lundgren, M. et al. (2008). Small CRISPR RNAs guide antiviral defense in prokaryotes. *Science* 321: 960–964.

64 Garneau, J.E., Dupuis, M.E., Villion, M. et al. (2010). The CRISPR/Cas bacterial immune system cleaves bacteriophage and plasmid DNA. *Nature* 468: 67–71.

65 Jinek, M., Chylinski, K., Fonfara, I. et al. (2012). A programmable dual-RNA-guided DNA endonuclease in adaptive bacterial immunity. *Science* 337: 816–821.

66 Gasiunas, G., Barrangou, R., Horvath, P., and Siksnys, V. (2012). Cas9-crRNA ribonucleoprotein complex mediates specific DNA cleavage for adaptive immunity in bacteria. *Proc. Natl. Acad. Sci. U.S.A.* 109: E2579–E2586.

67 Jinek, M., East, A., Cheng, A. et al. (2013). RNA-programmed genome editing in human cells. *eLife* 2: e00471.

68 Cong, L., Ran, F.A., Cox, D. et al. (2013). Multiplex genome engineering using CRISPR/Cas systems. *Science* 339: 819–823.

69 Mali, P., Yang, L., Esvelt, K.M. et al. (2013). RNA-guided human genome engineering via Cas9. *Science* 339: 823–826.

70 Ran, F.A., Hsu, P.D., Wright, J. et al. (2013). Genome engineering using the CRISPR-Cas9 system. *Nat. Protoc.* 8: 2281–2308.

71 Makarova, K.S., Haft, D.H., Barrangou, R. et al. (2011). Evolution and classification of the CRISPR-Cas systems. *Nat. Rev. Microbiol.* 9: 467–477.

72 Chu, H.W., Rios, C., Huang, C. et al. (2015). CRISPR-Cas9-mediated gene knockout in primary human airway epithelial cells reveals a proinflammatory role for MUC18. *Gene Ther.* 22: 822–829.

73 Dekkers, J.F., Wiegerinck, C.L., de Jonge, H.R. et al. (2013). A functional CFTR assay using primary cystic fibrosis intestinal organoids. *Nat. Med.* 19: 939–945.

74 Landry, J.J., Pyl, P.T., Rausch, T. et al. (2013). The genomic and transcriptomic landscape of a HeLa cell line. *G3 (Bethesda Md.)* 3: 1213–1224.

75 Boettcher, M. and McManus, M.T. (2015). Choosing the right tool for the job: RNAi, TALEN, or CRISPR. *Mol. Cell* 58: 575–585.

76 Horii, T. and Hatada, I. (2015). Genome editing using mammalian haploid cells. *Int. J. Mol. Sci.* 16: 23604–23614.

77 Sudmant, P.H., Rausch, T., Gardner, E.J. et al. (2015). An integrated map of structural variation in 2,504 human genomes. *Nature* 526: 75–81.

78 Greene, S.B., Dago, A.E., Leitz, L.J. et al. (2016). Chromosomal instability estimation based on next generation sequencing and single cell genome wide copy number variation analysis. *PLoS One* 11: e0165089.

79 Hart, L. and O'Driscoll, M. (2013). Causes and consequences of structural genomic alterations in the human genome. In: *eLS* (ed. American Cancer Society). Wiley.

80 Aguirre, A.J., Meyers, R.M., Weir, B.A. et al. (2016). Genomic copy number dictates a gene-independent cell response to CRISPR/Cas9 targeting. *Cancer Discovery* 6: 914–929.

81 Piergiorge, R.M., de Miranda, A.B., Guimaraes, A.C., and Catanho, M. (2017). Functional analogy in human metabolism: enzymes with different biological roles or functional redundancy? *Gen. Biol. Evol.* 9: 1624–1636.

82 Karousis, E.D. and Muhlemann, O. (2018). Nonsense-mediated mRNA decay begins where translation ends. *Cold Spring Harbor Perspect. Biol.* 11: a032862.
83 Najm, F.J., Strand, C., Donovan, K.F. et al. (2018). Orthologous CRISPR-Cas9 enzymes for combinatorial genetic screens. *Nat. Biotechnol.* 36: 179–189.
84 Zerbino, D.R., Achuthan, P., Akanni, W. et al. (2018). Ensembl 2018. *Nucleic Acids Res.* 46: D754–D761.
85 O'Leary, N.A., Wright, M.W., Brister, J.R. et al. (2016). Reference sequence (RefSeq) database at NCBI: Current status, taxonomic expansion, and functional annotation. *Nucleic Acids Res.* 44: D733–D745.
86 Lizio, M., Abugessaisa, I., Noguchi, S. et al. (2019). Update of the FANTOM web resource: expansion to provide additional transcriptome atlases. *Nucleic Acids Res.* 47: D752–d758.
87 Doench, J.G. (2018). Am I ready for CRISPR? A user's guide to genetic screens. *Nat. Rev. Genet.* 19: 67–80.
88 Jeziorowska, D., Korniat, A., Salem, J.E. et al. (2015). Generating patient-specific induced pluripotent stem cells-derived cardiomyocytes for the treatment of cardiac diseases. *Expert Opin. Biol. Ther.* 15: 1399–1409.
89 Pan, Q., Shai, O., Lee, L.J. et al. (2008). Deep surveying of alternative splicing complexity in the human transcriptome by high-throughput sequencing. *Nat. Genet.* 40: 1413–1415.
90 Guyot, M. and Pages, G. (2015). VEGF splicing and the role of VEGF splice variants: from physiological-pathological conditions to specific pre-mRNA splicing. *Methods Mol. Biol.* 1332: 3–23.
91 Kikuchi, R., Stevens, M., Harada, K. et al. (2019). Anti-angiogenic isoform of vascular endothelial growth factor-A in cardiovascular and renal disease. *Adv. Clin. Chem.* 88: 1–33.
92 Alnemri, E.S., Fernandes-Alnemri, T., and Litwack, G. (1995). Cloning and expression of four novel isoforms of human interleukin-1 beta converting enzyme with different apoptotic activities. *J. Biol. Chem.* 270: 4312–4317.
93 Sotillo, E., Barrett, D.M., Black, K.L. et al. (2015). Convergence of acquired mutations and alternative splicing of CD19 enables resistance to CART-19 immunotherapy. *Cancer Discovery* 5: 1282–1295.
94 Tabaglio, T., Low, D.H., Teo, W.K.L. et al. (2018). MBNL1 alternative splicing isoforms play opposing roles in cancer. *Life Sci. Alliance* 1: e201800157.
95 Charton, K., Suel, L., Henriques, S.F. et al. (2016). Exploiting the CRISPR/Cas9 system to study alternative splicing in vivo: application to titin. *Hum. Mol. Genet.* 25: 4518–4532.
96 Yue, M. and Ogawa, Y. (2018). CRISPR/Cas9-mediated modulation of splicing efficiency reveals short splicing isoform of Xist RNA is sufficient to induce X-chromosome inactivation. *Nucleic Acids Res.* 46: e26.
97 Simeonov, D.R., Gowen, B.G., Boontanrart, M. et al. (2017). Discovery of stimulation-responsive immune enhancers with CRISPR activation. *Nature* 549: 111–115.
98 Bester, A.C., Lee, J.D., Chavez, A. et al. (2018). An integrated genome-wide CRISPRa approach to functionalize lncRNAs in drug resistance. *Cell* 173: 649–664.e20.

99 Liu, S.J. and Lim, D.A. (2018). Modulating the expression of long non-coding RNAs for functional studies. *EMBO Rep.* 19: e46955.
100 Ho, T.T., Zhou, N., Huang, J. et al. (2015). Targeting non-coding RNAs with the CRISPR/Cas9 system in human cell lines. *Nucleic Acids Res.* 43: e17.
101 Popp, M.W. and Maquat, L.E. (2016). Leveraging rules of nonsense-mediated mRNA decay for genome engineering and personalized medicine. *Cell* 165: 1319–1322.
102 Lindeboom, R.G.H., Supek, F., and Lehner, B. (2016). The rules and impact of nonsense-mediated mRNA decay in human cancers. *Nat. Genet.* 48: 1112–1118.
103 Barretina, J., Caponigro, G., Stransky, N. et al. (2012). The Cancer Cell Line Encyclopedia enables predictive modelling of anticancer drug sensitivity. *Nature* 483: 603–607.
104 Forbes, S.A., Beare, D., Boutselakis, H. et al. (2017). COSMIC: Somatic cancer genetics at high-resolution. *Nucleic Acids Res.* 45: D777–D783.
105 Doench, J.G., Hartenian, E., Graham, D.B. et al. (2014). Rational design of highly active sgRNAs for CRISPR-Cas9-mediated gene inactivation. *Nat. Biotechnol.* 32: 1262–1267.
106 Doench, J.G., Fusi, N., Sullender, M. et al. (2016). Optimized sgRNA design to maximize activity and minimize off-target effects of CRISPR-Cas9. *Nat. Biotechnol.* 34: 184–191.
107 Wang, T., Wei, J.J., Sabatini, D.M., and Lander, E.S. (2014). Genetic screens in human cells using the CRISPR-Cas9 system. *Science* 343: 80–84.
108 Kapahnke, M., Banning, A., and Tikkanen, R. (2016). Random splicing of several exons caused by a single base change in the target exon of CRISPR/cas9 mediated gene knockout. *Cells* 5: E45.
109 Lalonde, S., Stone, O.A., Lessard, S. et al. (2017). Frameshift indels introduced by genome editing can lead to in-frame exon skipping. *PLoS One* 12: e0178700.
110 Mou, H., Smith, J.L., Peng, L. et al. (2017). CRISPR/Cas9-mediated genome editing induces exon skipping by alternative splicing or exon deletion. *Genome Biol.* 18: 108.
111 Prykhozhij, S.V., Steele, S.L., Razaghi, B., and Berman, J.N. (2017). A rapid and effective method for screening, sequencing and reporter verification of engineered frameshift mutations in zebrafish. *Dis. Model. Mech.* 10: 811–822.
112 Sui, T., Song, Y., Liu, Z. et al. (2018). CRISPR-induced exon skipping is dependent on premature termination codon mutations. *Genome Biol.* 19: 164.
113 Kosicki, M., Tomberg, K., and Bradley, A. (2018). Repair of CRISPR–Cas9-induced double-stranded breaks leads to large deletions and complex rearrangements. *Nat. Biotechnol.* 36: 765–771.
114 Hinnebusch, A.G. (2011). Molecular mechanism of scanning and start codon selection in eukaryotes. *Microbiol. Mol. Biol. Rev.* 75: 434–467. first page of table of contents.

115 Kozak, M. (1986). Point mutations define a sequence flanking the AUG initiator codon that modulates translation by eukaryotic ribosomes. *Cell* 44: 283–292.
116 Bazykin, G.A. and Kochetov, A.V. (2011). Alternative translation start sites are conserved in eukaryotic genomes. *Nucleic Acids Res.* 39: 567–577.
117 Gunišová, S., Hronová, V., Mohammad, M.P. et al. (2018). Please do not recycle! Translation reinitiation in microbes and higher eukaryotes. *FEMS Microbiol. Rev.* 42: 165–192.
118 Calvo, S.E., Pagliarini, D.J., and Mootha, V.K. (2009). Upstream open reading frames cause widespread reduction of protein expression and are polymorphic among humans. *Proc. Natl. Acad. Sci. U.S.A.* 106: 7507–7512.
119 Kochetov, A.V., Ahmad, S., Ivanisenko, V. et al. (2008). uORFs, reinitiation and alternative translation start sites in human mRNAs. *FEBS Lett.* 582: 1293–1297.
120 Kozak, M. (2001). Constraints on reinitiation of translation in mammals. *Nucleic Acids Res.* 29: 5226–5232.
121 Tsai, S.Q., Zheng, Z., Nguyen, N.T. et al. (2015). GUIDE-seq enables genome-wide profiling of off-target cleavage by CRISPR-Cas nucleases. *Nat. Biotechnol.* 33: 187–198.
122 Haapaniemi, E., Botla, S., Persson, J. et al. (2018). CRISPR–Cas9 genome editing induces a p53-mediated DNA damage response. *Nat. Med.* 24: 927–930.
123 Ihry, R.J., Worringer, K.A., Salick, M.R. et al. (2018). p53 inhibits CRISPR-Cas9 engineering in human pluripotent stem cells. *Nat. Med.* 24: 937–946.
124 Munoz, D.M., Cassiani, P.J., Li, L. et al. (2016). CRISPR screens provide a comprehensive assessment of cancer vulnerabilities but generate false-positive hits for highly amplified genomic regions. *Cancer Discovery* 6: 900–913.
125 Schoonenberg, V.A.C., Cole, M.A., Yao, Q. et al. (2018). CRISPRO: Identification of functional protein coding sequences based on genome editing dense mutagenesis. *Genome Biol.* 19: 1–19.
126 Shi, J., Wang, E., Milazzo, J.P. et al. (2015). Discovery of cancer drug targets by CRISPR-Cas9 screening of protein domains. *Nat. Biotechnol.* 33: 661–667.
127 Chari, R., Mali, P., Moosburner, M., and Church, G.M. (2015). Unraveling CRISPR-Cas9 genome engineering parameters via a library-on-library approach. *Nat. Methods* 12: 823–826.
128 Gagnon, J.A., Valen, E., Thyme, S.B. et al. (2014). Efficient mutagenesis by Cas9 protein-mediated oligonucleotide insertion and large-scale assessment of single-guide RNAs. *PLoS One* 9: e98186.
129 Hsu, P.D., Scott, D.A., Weinstein, J.A. et al. (2013). DNA targeting specificity of RNA-guided Cas9 nucleases. *Nat. Biotechnol.* 31: 827–832.
130 Liu, X., Homma, A., Say, J. et al. (2016). Sequence features associated with the cleavage efficiency of CRISPR/Cas9 system. *Sci. Rep.* 6: 19675.
131 Moreno-Mateos, M.A., Vejnar, C.E., Beaudoin, J.D. et al. (2015). CRISPRscan: designing highly efficient sgRNAs for CRISPR-Cas9 targeting in vivo. *Nat. Methods* 12: 982–988.

132 Xu, H., Xiao, T., Chen, C.H. et al. (2015). Sequence determinants of improved CRISPR sgRNA design. *Genome Res.* 25: 1147–1157.

133 Thyme, S.B., Akhmetova, L., Montague, T.G. et al. (2016). Internal guide RNA interactions interfere with Cas9-mediated cleavage. *Nat. Commun.* 7: 11750.

134 Wu, X., Scott, D.A., Kriz, A.J. et al. (2014). Genome-wide binding of the CRISPR endonuclease Cas9 in mammalian cells. *Nat. Biotechnol.* 32: 670–676.

135 McVey, M. and Lee, S.E. (2008). MMEJ repair of double-strand breaks (director's cut): deleted sequences and alternative endings. *Trends Genet.* 24: 529–538.

136 Bae, S., Kweon, J., Kim, H.S., and Kim, J.S. (2014). Microhomology-based choice of Cas9 nuclease target sites. *Nat. Methods* 11: 705–706.

137 van Overbeek, M., Capurso, D., Carter, M.M. et al. (2016). DNA repair profiling reveals nonrandom outcomes at Cas9-mediated breaks. *Mol. Cell* 63: 633–646.

138 Horlbeck, M.A., Witkowsky, L.B., Guglielmi, B. et al. (2016). Nucleosomes impede cas9 access to DNA in vivo and in vitro. *eLife* 5: e12677.

139 Chen, X., Rinsma, M., Janssen, J.M. et al. (2016). Probing the impact of chromatin conformation on genome editing tools. *Nucleic Acids Res.* 44: 6482–6492.

140 Daer, R.M., Cutts, J.P., Brafman, D.A., and Haynes, K.A. (2017). The impact of chromatin dynamics on Cas9-mediated genome editing in human cells. *ACS Synth. Biol.* 6: 428–438.

141 Clarke, R., Heler, R., MacDougall, M.S. et al. (2018). Enhanced bacterial immunity and mammalian genome editing via RNA-polymerase-mediated dislodging of Cas9 from double-strand DNA breaks. *Mol. Cell* 71: 42–55.

142 Fu, Y., Foden, J.A., Khayter, C. et al. (2013). High-frequency off-target mutagenesis induced by CRISPR-Cas nucleases in human cells. *Nat. Biotechnol.* 31: 822–826.

143 Fu, B.X.H., Hansen, L.L., Artiles, K.L. et al. (2014). Landscape of target: guide homology effects on Cas9-mediated cleavage. *Nucleic Acids Res.* 42: 13778–13787.

144 Lin, Y., Cradick, T.J., Brown, M.T. et al. (2014). CRISPR/Cas9 systems have off-target activity with insertions or deletions between target DNA and guide RNA sequences. *Nucleic Acids Res.* 42: 7473–7485.

145 Kuscu, C., Arslan, S., Singh, R. et al. (2014). Genome-wide analysis reveals characteristics of off-target sites bound by the Cas9 endonuclease. *Nat. Biotechnol.* 32: 677–683.

146 Duan, J., Lu, G., Xie, Z. et al. (2014). Genome-wide identification of CRISPR/Cas9 off-targets in human genome. *Cell Res.* 24: 1009–1012.

147 Frock, R.L., Hu, J., Meyers, R.M. et al. (2015). Genome-wide detection of DNA double-stranded breaks induced by engineered nucleases. *Nat. Biotechnol.* 33: 179–188.

148 Liang, X., Potter, J., Kumar, S. et al. (2015). Rapid and highly efficient mammalian cell engineering via Cas9 protein transfection. *J. Biotechnol.* 208: 44–53.

149 Cao, J., Wu, L., Zhang, S.M. et al. (2016). An easy and efficient inducible CRISPR/Cas9 platform with improved specificity for multiple gene targeting. *Nucleic Acids Res.* 44: 1–10.

150 Kleinstiver, B.P., Pattanayak, V., Prew, M.S. et al. (2016). High-fidelity CRISPR-Cas9 nucleases with no detectable genome-wide off-target effects. *Nature* 529: 490–495.

151 Slaymaker, I.M., Gao, L., Zetsche, B. et al. (2016). Rationally engineered Cas9 nucleases with improved specificity. *Science* 351: 84–88.

152 Vakulskas, C.A., Dever, D.P., Rettig, G.R. et al. (2018). A high-fidelity Cas9 mutant delivered as a ribonucleoprotein complex enables efficient gene editing in human hematopoietic stem and progenitor cells. *Nat. Med.* 24: 1216–1224.

153 Kulcsár, P.I., Tálas, A., Huszár, K. et al. (2017). Crossing enhanced and high fidelity SpCas9 nucleases to optimize specificity and cleavage. *Genome Biol.* 18: 1–17.

154 Chuai, G.-h., Wang, Q.-L., and Liu, Q. (2017). In silico meets in vivo: towards computational CRISPR-based sgRNA design. *Trends Biotechnol.* 35: 12–21.

155 Liu, H., Wei, Z., Dominguez, A. et al. (2015). CRISPR-ERA: a comprehensive design tool for CRISPR-mediated gene editing, repression and activation. *Bioinformatics* 31: 3676–3678.

156 Labun, K., Montague, T.G., Gagnon, J.A. et al. (2016). CHOPCHOP v2: a web tool for the next generation of CRISPR genome engineering. *Nucleic Acids Res.* 44: W272–W276.

157 Haeussler, M., Schönig, K., Eckert, H. et al. (2016). Evaluation of off-target and on-target scoring algorithms and integration into the guide RNA selection tool CRISPOR. *Genome Biol.* 17: 148.

158 Listgarten, J., Weinstein, M., Kleinstiver, B.P. et al. (2018). Prediction of off-target activities for the end-to-end design of CRISPR guide RNAs. *Nat. Biomed. Eng.* 2: 38–47.

159 Concordet, J.P. and Haeussler, M. (2018). CRISPOR: Intuitive guide selection for CRISPR/Cas9 genome editing experiments and screens. *Nucleic Acids Res.* 46: W242–W245.

160 Chakrabarti, A.M., Henser-Brownhill, T., Monserrat, J. et al. (2018). Target-specific precision of CRISPR-mediated genome editing. *Mol. Cell* 73: 699–713.e6.

161 Schuster, A., Erasimus, H., Fritah, S. et al. (2019). RNAi/CRISPR screens: from a pool to a valid hit. *Trends Biotechnol.* 37: 38–55.

162 Braun, S.M.G., Kirkland, J.G., Chory, E.J. et al. (2017). Rapid and reversible epigenome editing by endogenous chromatin regulators. *Nat. Commun.* 8: 560.

163 Nihongaki, Y., Kawano, F., Nakajima, T., and Sato, M. (2015). Photoactivatable CRISPR-Cas9 for optogenetic genome editing. *Nat. Biotechnol.* 33: 755–760.

164 Nihongaki, Y., Yamamoto, S., Kawano, F. et al. (2015). CRISPR-Cas9-based photoactivatable transcription system. *Chem. Biol.* 22: 169–174.

165 Lee, K., Yu, P., Lingampalli, N. et al. (2015). Peptide-enhanced mRNA transfection in cultured mouse cardiac fibroblasts and direct reprogramming towards cardiomyocyte-like cells. *Int. J. Nanomed.* 10: 1841–1854.

166 Li, L., He, Z.Y., Wei, X.W. et al. (2015). Challenges in CRISPR/CAS9 delivery: potential roles of nonviral vectors. *Hum. Gene Ther.* 26: 452–462.

167 Glass, Z., Lee, M., Li, Y., and Xu, Q. (2018). Engineering the delivery system for CRISPR-based genome editing. *Trends Biotechnol.* 36: 173–185.

168 Radis-Baptista, G., Campelo, I.S., Morlighem, J.R.L. et al. (2017). Cell-penetrating peptides (CPPs): from delivery of nucleic acids and antigens to transduction of engineered nucleases for application in transgenesis. *J. Biotechnol.* 252: 15–26.

169 Sun, W., Ji, W., Hall, J.M. et al. (2015). Self-assembled DNA nanoclews for the efficient delivery of CRISPR-Cas9 for genome editing. *Angew. Chem. Int. Ed.* 54: 12029–12033.

170 Yue, H., Zhou, X., Cheng, M., and Xing, D. (2018). Graphene oxide-mediated Cas9/sgRNA delivery for efficient genome editing. *Nanoscale* 10: 1063–1071.

171 Glass, Z., Li, Y., and Xu, Q. (2017). Nanoparticles for CRISPR-Cas9 delivery. *Nat. Biomed. Eng.* 1: 854–855.

172 Sentmanat, M.F., Peters, S.T., Florian, C.P. et al. (2018). A survey of validation strategies for CRISPR-Cas9 editing. *Sci. Rep.* 8: 888.

173 Guell, M., Yang, L., and Church, G.M. (2014). Genome editing assessment using CRISPR genome analyzer (CRISPR-GA). *Bioinformatics* 30: 2968–2970.

174 Pinello, L., Canver, M.C., Hoban, M.D. et al. (2016). Analyzing CRISPR genome-editing experiments with CRISPResso. *Nat. Biotechnol.* 34: 695–697.

175 Boel, A., Steyaert, W., De Rocker, N. et al. (2016). BATCH-GE: batch analysis of next-generation sequencing data for genome editing assessment. *Sci. Rep.* 6: 30330.

176 Park, J., Lim, K., Kim, J.S., and Bae, S. (2017). Cas-analyzer: an online tool for assessing genome editing results using NGS data. *Bioinformatics* 33: 286–288.

177 Yau, E.H. and Rana, T.M. (2018). Next-generation sequencing of genome-wide CRISPR Screens. *Methods Mol. Biol.* 1712: 203–216.

178 Wang, X., Tilford, C., Neuhaus, I. et al. (2017). CRISPR-DAV: CRISPR NGS data analysis and visualization pipeline. *Bioinformatics* 33: 3811–3812.

179 Qi, L.S., Larson, M.H., Gilbert, L.A. et al. (2013). Repurposing CRISPR as an RNA-guided platform for sequence-specific control of gene expression. *Cell* 152: 1173–1183.

180 Gilbert, L.A., Larson, M.H., Morsut, L. et al. (2013). CRISPR-mediated modular RNA-guided regulation of transcription in eukaryotes. *Cell* 154: 442–451.

181 Zhang, F., Cong, L., Lodato, S. et al. (2011). Efficient construction of sequence-specific TAL effectors for modulating mammalian transcription. *Nat. Biotechnol.* 29: 149–153.

182 Tanenbaum, M.E., Gilbert, L.A., Qi, L.S. et al. (2014). A protein-tagging system for signal amplification in gene expression and fluorescence imaging. *Cell* 159: 635–646.

183 Hess, G.T., Tycko, J., Yao, D., and Bassik, M.C. (2017). Methods and applications of CRISPR-mediated base editing in eukaryotic genomes. *Mol. Cell* 68: 26–43.

184 Chu, J., Galicia-Vazquez, G., Cencic, R. et al. (2016). CRISPR-mediated drug-target validation reveals selective pharmacological inhibition of the RNA helicase, eIF4A. *Cell Rep.* 15: 2340–2347.

185 Dow, L.E. (2015). Modeling disease in vivo with CRISPR/Cas9. *Trends Mol. Med.* 21: 609–621.

186 Smalley, E. (2016). CRISPR mouse model boom, rat model renaissance. *Nat. Biotechnol.* 34: 893–894.

187 Jackson, A.L., Burchard, J., Schelter, J. et al. (2006). Widespread siRNA "off-target" transcript silencing mediated by seed region sequence complementarity. *RNA* 12: 1179–1187.

188 Echeverri, C.J., Beachy, P.A., Baum, B. et al. (2006). Minimizing the risk of reporting false positives in large-scale RNAi screens. *Nat. Methods* 3: 777–779.

189 Shalem, O., Sanjana, N.E., Hartenian, E. et al. (2014). Genome-scale CRISPR-Cas9 knockout screening in human cells. *Science* 343: 84–87.

190 Morgens, D.W., Deans, R.M., Li, A., and Bassik, M.C. (2016). Systematic comparison of CRISPR/Cas9 and RNAi screens for essential genes. *Nat. Biotechnol.* 34: 634–636.

191 DeJesus, R., Moretti, F., McAllister, G. et al. (2016). Functional CRISPR screening identifies the ufmylation pathway as a regulator of SQSTM1/p62. *eLife* 5: e17290.

192 Evers, B., Jastrzebski, K., Heijmans, J.P. et al. (2016). CRISPR knockout screening outperforms shRNA and CRISPRi in identifying essential genes. *Nat. Biotechnol.* 34: 631–633.

193 Perez-Pinera, P., Kocak, D.D., Vockley, C.M. et al. (2013). RNA-guided gene activation by CRISPR-Cas9-based transcription factors. *Nat. Methods* 10: 973–976.

194 Maeder, M.L., Linder, S.J., Cascio, V.M. et al. (2013). CRISPR RNA-guided activation of endogenous human genes. *Nat. Methods* 10: 977–979.

195 Gilbert, L.A., Horlbeck, M.A., Adamson, B. et al. (2014). Genome-scale CRISPR-mediated control of gene repression and activation. *Cell* 159: 647–661.

196 Potting, C., Crochemore, C., Moretti, F. et al. (2018). Genome-wide CRISPR screen for PARKIN regulators reveals transcriptional repression as a determinant of mitophagy. *Proc. Natl. Acad. Sci. U.S.A.* 115: E180–E189.

197 Wang, T., Birsoy, K., Hughes, N.W. et al. (2015). Identification and characterization of essential genes in the human genome. *Science* 350: 1096–1101.

198 Hart, T., Chandrashekhar, M., Aregger, M. et al. (2015). High-resolution CRISPR screens reveal fitness genes and genotype-specific cancer liabilities. *Cell* 163: 1515–1526.

199 Zhang, R., Miner, J.J., Gorman, M.J. et al. (2016). A CRISPR screen defines a signal peptide processing pathway required by flaviviruses. *Nature* 535: 164–168.

200 Park, R.J., Wang, T., Koundakjian, D. et al. (2017). A genome-wide CRISPR screen identifies a restricted set of HIV host dependency factors. *Nat. Genet.* 49: 193–203.

201 Huang, Z. and Nair, M. (2017). A CRISPR/Cas9 guidance RNA screen platform for HIV provirus disruption and HIV/AIDS gene therapy in astrocytes. *Sci. Rep.* 7: 5955.

202 Sidik, S.M., Huet, D., Ganesan, S.M. et al. (2016). A genome-wide CRISPR screen in toxoplasma identifies essential Apicomplexan genes. *Cell* 166: 1423–1435 e12.

203 Han, K., Jeng, E.E., Hess, G.T. et al. (2017). Synergistic drug combinations for cancer identified in a CRISPR screen for pairwise genetic interactions. *Nat. Biotechnol.* 35: 463–474.

204 Jost, M., Chen, Y., Gilbert, L.A. et al. (2017). Combined CRISPRi/a-based chemical genetic screens reveal that rigosertib is a microtubule-destabilizing agent. *Mol. Cell* 68: 210–223 e6.

205 Zhu, S., Li, W., Liu, J. et al. (2016). Genome-scale deletion screening of human long non-coding RNAs using a paired-guide RNA CRISPR-Cas9 library. *Nat. Biotechnol.* 34: 1279–1286.

206 Chen, S., Sanjana, N.E., Zheng, K. et al. (2015). Genome-wide CRISPR screen in a mouse model of tumor growth and metastasis. *Cell* 160: 1246–1260.

207 Kim, H.S., Lee, K., Kim, S.J. et al. (2018). Arrayed CRISPR screen with image-based assay reliably uncovers host genes required for coxsackievirus infection. *Genome Res.* 28: 859–868.

208 Parnas, O., Jovanovic, M., Eisenhaure, T.M. et al. (2015). A genome-wide CRISPR screen in primary immune cells to dissect regulatory networks. *Cell* 162: 675–686.

209 Schumann, K., Lin, S., Boyer, E. et al. (2015). Generation of knock-in primary human T cells using Cas9 ribonucleoproteins. *Proc. Natl. Acad. Sci. U.S.A.* 112: 10437–10442.

210 Shifrut, E., Carnevale, J., Tobin, V. et al. (2018). Genome-wide CRISPR screens in primary human T cells reveal key regulators of immune function. *Cell* 175: 1958–1971.

211 Ting, P.Y., Parker, A.E., Lee, J.S. et al. (2018). Guide swap enables genome-scale pooled CRISPR-Cas9 screening in human primary cells. *Nat. Methods* 15: 941–946.

212 Biotec. (2018) M. MACS Online Handbook. https://www.miltenyibiotec.com/US-en/resources/macs-handbook/human-cells-and-organs/human-cell-sources/blood-human.html (accessed 20 December 2018).

213 Jaitin, D.A., Weiner, A., Yofe, I. et al. (2016). Dissecting immune circuits by linking CRISPR-pooled screens with single-cell RNA-seq. *Cell* 167: 1883–1896 e15.

214 (2018). Keep off-target effects in focus. *Nat. Med.* 24: 1081.

215 Ihry, R.J., Worringer, K.A., Salick, M.R. et al. (2018). p53 inhibits CRISPR-Cas9 engineering in human pluripotent stem cells. *Nat. Med.* 24: 939–946.

216 Shao, Y., Xu, M.Q., and Paulus, H. (1995). Protein splicing: characterization of the aminosuccinimide residue at the carboxyl terminus of the excised intervening sequence. *Biochemistry* 34: 10844–10850.

217 Xu, M.Q. and Perler, F.B. (1996). The mechanism of protein splicing and its modulation by mutation. *EMBO J.* 15: 5146–5153.

218 Truong, D.J., Kuhner, K., Kuhn, R. et al. (2015). Development of an intein-mediated split-Cas9 system for gene therapy. *Nucleic Acids Res.* 43: 6450–6458.

219 Gapinske, M., Luu, A., Winter, J. et al. (2018). CRISPR-SKIP: programmable gene splicing with single base editors. *Genome Biol.* 19: 107.

220 Lino, C. A., Harper, J. C., Carney, J. P., and Timlin, J. A. (2018). Delivering CRISPR: a review of the challenges and approaches. *Drug Delivery,* 25(1), 1234–1257. doi:10.1080/10717544.2018.1474964.

10

Computational Approaches for Target Inference

Gerhard Hessler, Christoph Grebner, and Hans Matter

Integrated Drug Discovery, Sanofi-Aventis Deutschland GmbH, Industriepark Höchst, D-65926, Frankfurt-am-Main, Germany

10.1 Introduction

In recent decades, drug discovery often followed the 'one target–one disease' hypothesis, which resulted in many target-based discovery programs [1]. In a recent analysis of compounds entering clinical trials in 2016 and 2017, most examples originated from those target-based projects [2]. However, the mechanism of action for pharmaceuticals is often linked to interactions with multiple target proteins. Not all interactions may cause a desirable pharmacological effect, but also undesirable ones, thus leading to 'off-target' side effects. Therefore, early *in vitro* profiling plays a critical role, which allows deriving target hypotheses about the desirable pharmacology, as well as off-target liabilities. Moreover, evidence from network and systems biology analyses suggests that most diseases are regulated by robust and highly interconnected pathways and thus may be better modulated using molecules across a range of modalities that bind to multiple disease-relevant proteins [3, 4].

Phenotypic screening is a lead finding approach to handle this complexity. Here, the informed analysis of the read-out from a complex but biologically relevant assay system might lead to the identification of biologically active compounds showing the desired phenotype. Therefore, phenotypic screening has regained a steadily increasing interest during recent years [5, 6]. Phenotypic assays are focused on a physiologically relevant read-out, but are agnostic with respect to molecular target(s). Hence, they offer the opportunity to discover novel disease pathways, which can result in first-in-class therapies [7, 8]. Although compound optimization can be guided on phenotypic read-outs, the identification of the molecular target is often beneficial. Knowledge of molecular targets ensures that a novel mechanism of action was identified. It further allows for the exploitation of a detailed structure–activity relationship (SAR) from target-directed biological assays, which guides compound optimization. Accordingly, many experimental methods are established for target deconvolution and are reviewed elsewhere and described in other chapters in this book [9–11].

Target Discovery and Validation: Methods and Strategies for Drug Discovery,
First Edition. Edited by Alleyn T. Plowright.

Computational approaches are well established for prediction of target–ligand interactions and are thus widely used in lead identification by virtual screening, in the optimization of biological activity, and for prediction of side affinities [12–17]. For target deconvolution of phenotypic screening hits, the problem is reversed. Biologically active compounds have been identified in phenotypic assays, and a reasonable target hypothesis must be derived. Nevertheless, both problems are only two sides of the same coin, namely, the prediction of protein–ligand interactions. Therefore, similar computational technologies are applied in lead finding and optimization and off-target prediction as well as in drug repurposing and target deconvolution. Multiple reviews address the development of *in silico* tools for linking ligands with target and off-target proteins towards prediction of polypharmacology and drug repurposing [12–18]. Thus, *in silico* methods provide highly relevant tools for analysis of phenotypic screening outcomes to generate target hypotheses, which link the observed effect in the complex assay system to protein targets, and also for analysis of target-based screens to develop hypotheses of off-targets. These hypotheses have to be evaluated using pharmacological knowledge about pathways and by an experimental validation to identify a potentially underlying mechanism. In this chapter, we will summarize novel trends for *in silico* target identification. In addition to highlighting their interesting theoretical basis, we will provide prospective applications for some of these tools and discuss practical considerations for applying them in drug discovery projects.

10.2 Data Annotation for Target Identification

The amount of public bioactivity data has increased significantly over the past decade in both scope and precision [19]. PubChem [20] currently is the largest source of bioactivity data, while other databases such as DrugBank [21, 22], Liceptor [23], ChEMBL [24], or WOMBAT [25] also comprise extensive publically available bioactivity data. Other large collections such as GOSTAR [26] or ReaxysMedChem [27] are commercially available. As data sources can be redundant with differing data quality and noise levels, it is important to check input sources carefully for consistency, duplicates, and completeness [28, 29]. Detailed listings of databases and resources are given elsewhere [12, 15, 16, 30, 31].

Data mining employs automated extraction of patterns and associations from large annotated databases. Associations between targets and chemical substructure, features, or descriptor motifs can be automatically extracted across different targets, thus offering large opportunities for phenotypic screening either for the design of phenotypic screening collections or for the annotation of screening hits. This also provides valuable information on potential other targets for those compounds, which originated from target-based approaches.

Well-annotated biological activities can guide the compilation of informative collections for phenotypic screening [32]. Ideally, such screening libraries contain compounds with well-known biological activity. The compounds should be potent against their primary target, selective against other targets, and also exhibit cellular permeability (see Personal foreword for further details). The ideal collection also covers as broad as possible biological space to allow for the identification of many different mechanisms of action [32]. Typically, these goals cannot be fully met due to challenges such as incomplete knowledge about selectivity of many compounds or limited availability of chemical probe molecules for numerous targets. Nevertheless, screening hits from well-annotated libraries can provide important hints for target hypotheses. In the Open PHACTS Discovery Platform [33], numerous workflows have been described, which retrieve biological activity as well as gene ontology (GO) terms [34, 35] and pathway information [36] and thus facilitate the annotation of screening hits with their putative biological function.

In a typical phenotypic screen, historic screening data reveal promiscuity for numerous hits, i.e. those compounds hitting several different targets. In this situation, phenotypically inactive compounds hitting the putative targets can help to discard several false positive target hypotheses. In addition, clusters of similar compounds with activity towards the same target give more credibility to certain target hypotheses. Comparing the number of actives in historic target-based screens with the number of actives in the phenotypic screens can also yield target hypotheses based on the overlap between the two sets. Accordingly, a systematic analysis of assay data from ChemBank [37] has shown that biological assays that share non-promiscuous hits tend to indicate a biological relation between the two assays [38]. Similar observations were reported by Wassermann et al. [39].

Nevertheless, the simple counting scheme can result in artefacts, since a large number of compounds might have been included in the screening set for this particular target. Therefore, enrichment analysis has been established recently for finding statistically sound associations between target-based and phenotypic screening-based hit lists, which can significantly increase the statistical confidence in the suggested target hypothesis [40]. Polyakov et al. could link glycogen synthase kinase 3 (GSK3) to sensitization of tumour cells to TNF-related apoptosis-inducing ligand (TRAIL). In a similar approach, Bornot et al. used combined bioactivity data from in-house sources at AstraZeneca and from external sources such as ChEMBL [24], GOSTAR [26], and Bio-Print [41] to identify inhibitors of tumour necrosis factor-α production in lipopolysaccharide-stimulated THP-1 cells by enrichment analysis [42]. Interestingly, the combined bioactivity data were used to select a reduced screening set of ~10 000 compounds, which should be capable of identifying as many targets as possible as significantly enriched in the phenotypic screen. Later, the target-based enrichment analysis was supplemented with pathway enrichment analysis combining cheminformatics with bioinformatics pathway information to generate hypotheses for which targets and pathways might drive the observed phenotypic effect. Such enrichment analysis-based approaches make use of the full set of available bioactivity data. The value of joining external and internal data for different types of screening analysis has recently been underscored by researchers from Merck with the systematic integration of data into the CHEMGENIE informatics platform [43].

Comparison of hit lists from phenotypic screens with data from target-based screens can provide clear hints for target hypotheses and guide further follow-up work. Compounds active against the putative mechanism of action target can be systematically tested in the phenotypic screen for the observed phenotype to discover chemotypes, which have not been tested in the initial phenotypic screen. Nevertheless, data annotation-based analysis only relies on available data and reflects the amount of available data for given targets. In particular, the discovery of target hypotheses is not possible for targets, for which only few bioactivity data are available. Here, different *in silico*-based technologies allow for additional opportunities, which capitalize on the available bioactivity data by generation of predictive *in silico* models. Nevertheless, data quality, assay harmonization, and compound standardization are essential steps to derive relevant datasets for *in silico* modelling. In particular, for some more advanced assay formats involving cell-based assays, data quality and multiple underlying mechanisms might add significant noise and thus uncertainty for interpretation. This becomes critical when using only public databases due to the inherent difficulty to standardize assay data from multiple laboratories, conditions, or read-outs. The impact of such uncertainties on data modelling has been critically discussed by Kramer et al. [44] and Wenlock and Carlsson [45]. Consequently, data management and integration are essential for building and maintaining *in silico* models, and only reliable training data will produce significant models.

10.3 *In Silico* Methods for Target Identification

Available biological activity data for well-annotated molecules provide a fast and efficient way to derive a target hypothesis for hits in a phenotypic screen as well as information on broader biological activity for hits from a target-based screen. Nevertheless, such data are typically sparse, since most compounds have only been tested against a limited number of targets, and accordingly not all biological activities of compounds are annotated. Therefore, the prediction of activity for a certain target by *in silico* methods provides an important opportunity to uncover additional targets for existing compounds. Computational approaches for *in silico* target identification can be broadly grouped into the following categories:

- Ligand-based approaches such as two-dimensional (2D) and three-dimensional (3D) ligand-based similarity or pharmacophore methods.
- Machine learning and quantitative structure–activity relationship (QSAR) models derived from structure–activity data for ligand–target series.
- Structure-based methods employing 3D structure of proteins including panel docking.
- Protein–protein and ligand–target networks.

For an overview of *in silico* methods used for target identification, see Figure 10.1, while examples of publically available web tools are given in Table 10.1. Furthermore, Table 10.2 gives an overview of selected successful prospective *in silico* target identification studies discussed in the following paragraphs.

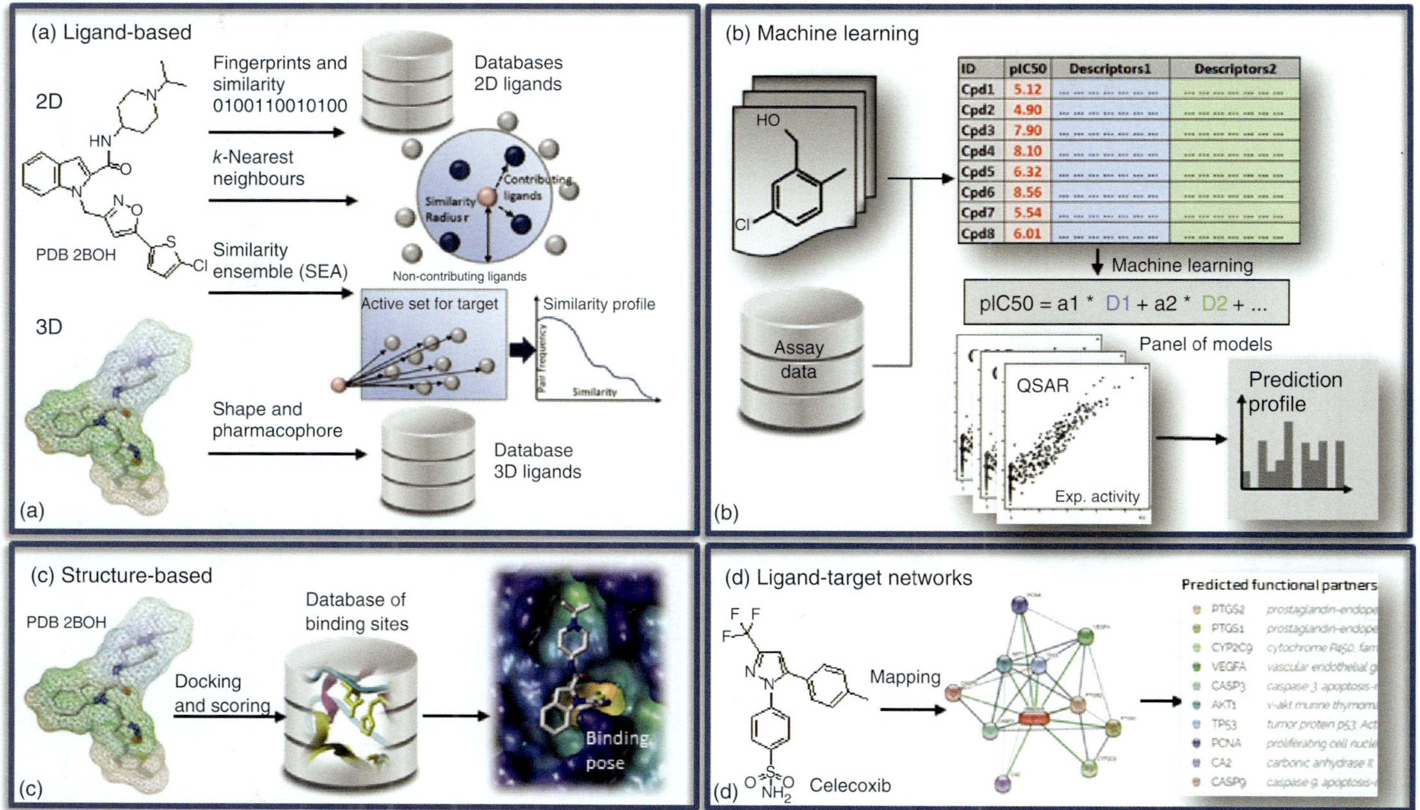

Figure 10.1 Overview of different computational approaches for *in silico* target identification described in this chapter. The ligand and protein structures are taken from a public factor Xa structure in complex with compound 1 (PDB 2BOH, resolution 2.20 Å) [46]. (a) Ligand-based approaches such as 2D or 3D ligand-based similarity, shape, or pharmacophore. (b) Machine learning and QSAR models from structure–activity data for target series. (c) Structure-based approaches including docking into protein binding site databases. (d) Methods based on ligand–target networks. See text for details on individual approaches. Source: Nazaré et al. 2005 [46]. Reproduced with permission of ACS Publications.

Table 10.1 Examples of publically available tools for *in silico* target identification.

Tool	Link	Method	References
SuperPred	http://prediction.charite.de/	Similarity searching	[47, 48]
SEA	http://sea.bkslab.org/	Similarity searching against a ligand ensemble	[49, 50]
ChemProt	http://www.cbs.dtu.dk/services/ChemProt/	Similarity searching	[51]
SwissTarget Prediction	http://swisstargetprediction.ch/	2D and 3D similarity searching in approx. 280 000 compounds from ChEMBL	[52]
TargetHunter	https://www.cbligand.org/TargetHunter/	Similarity searching in ChEMBL ligand set	[53]
PharmMapper	http://lilab-ecust.cn/pharmmapper/index.html	3D pharmacophore-based queries against more than 50 000 pharmacophore models	[54, 55]
FINDSITEcomb2.0	http://pwp.gatech.edu/cssb/FINDSITE-COMB-2	Threading combined with ligand similarity	[56]
HitPick	http://mips.helmholtz-muenchen.de/hitpick/cgi-bin/index.cgi?content=help.html	Similarity search in combination with machine learning based upon ~150 000 interactions extracted from STITCH	[57]
CSNAP	https://services.mbi.ucla.edu/CSNAP/index.html	Chemical similarity network analysis	[58]
Scaffold Hunter	http://scaffoldhunter.sourceforge.net/	Visual analysis of datasets	[59]
PASS	http://www.pharmaexpert.ru/passonline/index.php	Prediction of Activity Spectra for Substances	[60]
GUSAR	http://www.pharmaexpert.ru/GUSAR/antitargets.html	Quantitative structure–activity relationships for chemical compounds	[61]

Table 10.2 Selected successful prospective *in silico* target identification studies cited in this chapter.

Method	Technology	Description	References
SEA	Similarity search	Identification of targets in zebrafish phenotypic assay	[62]
TIGER	Similarity search with SOM	Identification of unknown targets for natural product	[63]
LigandScout	Pharmacophore searching	Identification of targets for natural products	[64]
Fragments (Reker)	Similarity based on fragments	Revealing targets for Archazolid A	[65]
Fragments	Similarity based on fragments	Discover unknown targets for fragment-like natural products	[66]
TIGER and SPiDER	Similarity search with SOM	Discovery of novel inhibitors of the Hedgehog signalling pathway	[63]
Clarity	Similarity search linked to databases	Linking cyclobenzaprine to serotonin syndrome	[67]
Clarity	Similarity search linked to databases	Multi-target activity profile for maslinic acid	[68]
SuperTarget	Similarity search in 2D and 3D	Unveil new functions for known kinase inhibitors	[69]
Scaffold Hunter	Hierarchical scaffold trees	Target annotations for γ-pyrone natural products	[70]
HTS-FP	Experimental fingerprints	Identifying new targets with HTS-FP	[71]

10.3.1 2D Similarity Methods for Target Inference

The similarity principle formulated by Johnson and Maggiora [72] forms the basis for ligand-based 2D and 3D similarity approaches. Its assumption is that similar molecules exhibit similar physico-chemical and biological properties. This assumption is extensively exploited in medicinal chemistry and cheminformatics methods [73] such as similarity searching [74] and QSAR [75]. Similarity searching can be conducted using a multitude of descriptors capturing different molecular features. While classical 2D descriptors and 2D fingerprints are tailored to retrieve close analogues [76], advanced 2D methods or 3D similarity searching can be employed for more distant relationships [77]. This might be beneficial for query molecules without close 2D analogues in an annotated ligand–target set. Instructive exceptions from the similarity principle with surprising activity changes by small modifications were compiled by Kubinyi [78], thus revealing that structure–activity landscapes [79] are extremely complex [80]. Compounds that are similar to an active compound only have a limited chance to be active on the same target [81, 82].

The similarity principle is explored in many *in silico* profiling tools. One of these is SuperPred by Nickel et al. combining similarity searching with target protein information [47, 48]. 665 000 experimental ligand–target interactions are compiled involving 341 000 ligands and 1800 targets. This dataset was derived from the public databases SuperTarget [83], ChEMBL [24], and BindingDB [84], broadly covering publically known target interactions. The authors reported that extended-connectivity fingerprints (ECFP) [85] performed best for similarity searching in retrospective tests. Retrospective predictions of drug classes in the form of the Anatomical Therapeutic Chemical (ATC) classification provided by the WHO were used for validation, resulting in 75% correct classification.

The similarity ensemble approach (SEA) is another similarity approach to identify target hypotheses (Figure 10.2) [49, 50]. SEA uses similarity-based queries, in which molecules are compared with ensembles of actives for distinct targets.

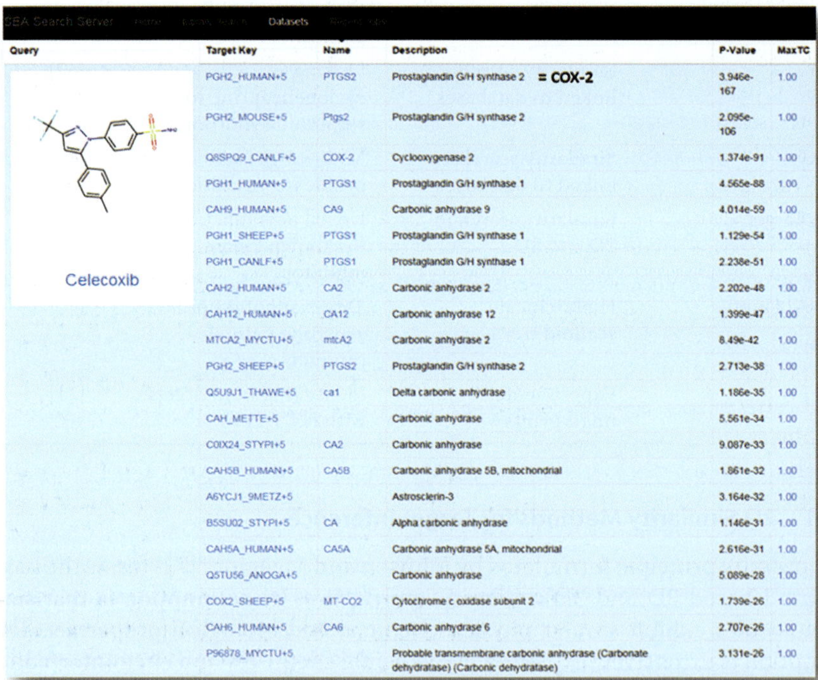

Figure 10.2 Result of a search with the similarity ensemble approach (SEA) search server using the non-steroidal anti-inflammatory drug (NSAID) celecoxib as a query. The listing displays targets, names, P-values from SEA to illustrate the significance of a prediction, and similarity coefficients (T_c) to the nearest analogue in the target ensemble set. The pharmacological target for celecoxib is COX-2 (i.e. PTGS2 = prostaglandin G/H synthase 2).

The resulting distribution of similarity coefficients is compared with a random distribution to explore its significance. The methodology has been used successfully to identify novel targets for a number of molecules, which then could be confirmed experimentally [86]. Keiser et al. profiled a collection of 3665 approved and investigational pharmaceuticals against a panel of 1400 targets using SEA. Out of 3832 predicted non-trivial ligand–targets associations, 30 were subjected to testing, resulting in 5 potent and 14 moderate to low potent hits against 23 previously unknown targets. This validation was extended by Lounkine et al. to a set of 656 drugs with 73 side effect targets [87]. From 1042 off-target interactions predicted by SEA, 48% could be validated using literature or experimental testing. Furthermore, the relevance of some interactions for *in vivo* effects could be demonstrated. While hit rates are promising, activity is only predicted based on classification without discriminating potent from less potent hits.

In another example, the SEA approach identified target hypotheses for active molecules from a zebrafish phenotypic screen [62]. 20 compounds, predicted with a high score for different targets, were experimentally tested for the proposed target hypothesis. Eleven of those molecules were active on 22 of the predicted 31 targets with potencies ranging from nanomolar to micromolar activity. In another example, a target hypothesis for feeding behaviour could be derived for hits from a *C. elegans*-based phenotypic screen, in which the *in silico*-derived hypotheses were credentialized by genetic knockdowns for four targets [88]. Recently, the SEA approach has been combined with Tanimoto similarity-based queries into an approach called SEA+TC [89]. While SEA evaluates similarity against an ensemble of ligands for each target, the Tanimoto based similarity complements this approach by a single-nearest neighbour view. Cross-validation studies indicate that the combined approach is more often correct compared with the classical SEA approach. SEA+TC was used to predict biological activities for 2629 targets against commercially available compounds from the ZINC database [90]. For about 40% of the commercially available compounds, target predictions were possible and are available for download [91], while for 60% of the compounds, no target hypothesis could be derived. It is unclear if these compounds are truly dark chemical matter [92] or if this simply reflects the fact that no similar compounds with biological activity are yet known.

Similarity approaches rely on available ligands to allow predictions for biological activity. Thus, the chemical space for meaningful predictions is constrained to the space defined by available ligands. Target hypotheses cannot be derived for novel chemotypes, which are not represented in the ligand space, thus limiting the possibility to identify novel hypotheses for targets without known ligands.

One strategy to address limitations of similarity approaches is the use of descriptors that capture molecules in a more abstract way, e.g. by pharmacophoric features. Such a strategy is combined with self-organizing maps (SOMs) [93] in the Target Inference Generator (TIGER) approach [94]. TIGER represents query molecules by the Chemically Advanced Template Search (CATS) representation [95], a molecular descriptor employing a topological pharmacophore description, to find previously unknown targets of active compounds. The compound representation is projected onto two SOMs of annotated reference compounds with known targets. The clusters with the most similar reference compounds are used to calculate the scores for each annotated target. While similarity between two compounds is in many other approaches measured directly between those query molecules, SOMs offer an extension, since similar compounds are grouped and similarity to novel compounds is computed using the centroid vector of these molecules.

This method was applied to a phenotypic hit, the natural product Marinopyrrole A with an unknown mode of action. Testing the top-scored hypotheses revealed novel targets and supported the current working hypothesis published by Gomez-Bougie et al. [96]. Later, this method was further explored using two examples, where the authors identified new targets for the COX-2 inhibitor celecoxib [97] and analysed functional drug–drug relationships [98]. The conceptually related SPiDER approach [99] also uses SOMs and the topological pharmacophore representation CATS. Therefore, there is a certain overlap between results of both methods.

Kremer et al. [63] combined cell-based bioactive compound screening with cheminformatics target prediction, i.e. SPiDER [99] and TIGER [94] as consensus, to discover the target for a novel inhibitor of the Hedgehog signalling pathway. This pyrazolo-imidazole compound, smoothib, was reported as an inhibitor of hedgehog signalling and as an antagonist of the protein smoothened (SMO) with a novel chemotype. Smoothib targets the heptahelical bundle of SMO and reduces the expression of Hh target genes [63].

The combination of activity databases with similarity searching and *k*-nearest neighbour (kNN) statistics [100] also forms the basis for methods from Mestres et al. kNN statistics refers to a non-parametric method for classification and regression. For a compound to be predicted, property values for all neighbours within a particular similarity radius are averaged. These concepts are integrated in the commercial software Clarity [101] based on a curated training set of 2.6 million compounds from the patent literature, journals, and public databases that broadly cover chemical space. The current version includes public structure–activity databases, such as BindingDB [84], PubChem [20, 102], ChEMBL [24], DrugBank [103], and IUPHARdb [104]. It comprises models for 3600 targets plus 7 preclinical and 520 clinical toxicological end points. An example search with Clarity is illustrated in Figure 10.3.

First, molecular descriptors were developed, such as feature-based topological Shannon entropy descriptors (SHED) [105–107], feature pairs (FPD), and pharmacophore fragments (PHRAG) [108, 109], which describe molecules with different levels of abstraction. The affinity for ligands is subsequently estimated by a similarity-based approach as the weighted average of a predefined number of neighbours within a similarity radius. This gives importance to close neighbours.

The *in silico* profiling in Clarity was first validated on its ability to predict the experimental interaction matrix between 13 antipsychotic drugs and 34 targets [109] and then prospectively predicting the affinity profile and suggesting additional targets for the drug cyclobenzaprine [67]. Furthermore, the multi-target activity profile for maslinic acid, an antimalarial natural product, was predicted by *in silico* profiling. Among the predicted putative new targets, some activities could also be experimentally confirmed [68]. In another application, Antolín

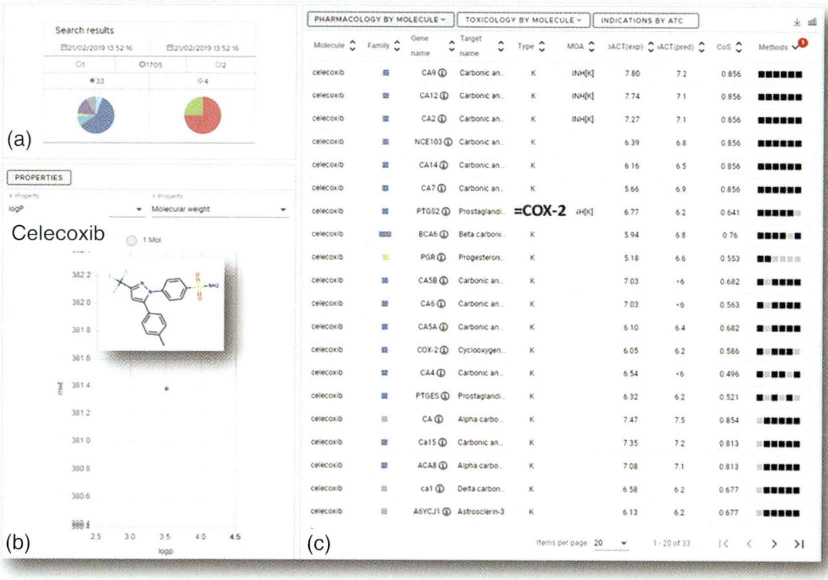

Figure 10.3 Clarity v3.0 summary page with target predictions and experimental knowledge for the non-steroidal anti-inflammatory drug celecoxib. (a) Pie charts summarizing pharmacology interactions by protein target family (left, blue = EC) and by toxicological findings (right, red = cardiotoxicity). (b) Celecoxib and molecular properties. (c) Interactive listing with experimental and predicted targets, interaction constants (predicted: pACT [pred], experimental: pACT [exp]), confidence scores (CoS) for a particular target association, and consensus prediction methods, which indicates how many individual *in silico* prediction methods in Clarity have predicted this particular target (black square). More methods result in higher confidence for a particular interaction.

and Mestres identified ligands interacting with two disease-relevant targets, the PARP1/2 inhibitor UPF1069 and the ROCK1/2 inhibitor hydroxyfasudil [110]. As both compounds were confirmed to be active versus both targets, they could serve to explore the impact of dual inhibitors for PARPs and ROCK kinases in relevant disease models [110].

Recently, the similarity approach in Clarity was augmented by a reduced framework-based algorithm (smallest active subgraphs [SAS]), a comparative assessment of profile similarity (cross-pharmacology index [XPI]), and QSAR models for active subgraphs (SAR) plus an implementation of the similarity ensemble algorithm [49] based on SHED, FPD, and PHRAG descriptors. The SAS is defined for each target as simplest subgraph with pharmacophoric motifs related to activity. This subgraph is then employed to derive 2D-QSAR models for matching compounds, adding predictive models to the similarity-based approach. Integrating these different methods into Clarity now allows for consensus predictions and thus provides additional confidence for any new target hypothesis, once it is found by multiple methods.

Additional value in finding novel ligand–target associations is provided by the concept of cross-pharmacology: closely related target proteins will interact with similar ligands [111, 112]. Such relationships among proteins can possibly be exploited to predict novel target proteins for bioactive molecules and set alerts for side effects. An example is the identification of novel ligand–G-protein-coupled receptor (GPCR) interactions that could be experimentally confirmed [49, 86] and the prediction of potential undesirable profiles for GPCR ligands, as exemplified for nefazodone, fluvoxamine, pergolide, and fluoxetine, which are linked by a panel of different targets involving 5-HT2_A and the sodium-dependent serotonin transporter (SERT) [113]. To capitalize on this concept, Clarity computes XPI for all possible target combinations, defined as the fraction of actives for target A, that also have activity for target B.

As mentioned, each similarity method depends on diversity and coverage of the data sources. Without any analogue, no prediction is possible. Public collections of SAR data are often not sufficient, as SAR data in the pharmaceutical industry only have limited overlap to public databases. Therefore, it is often beneficial to combine public and corporate data which results in a significantly larger coverage of chemical space and more relevant predictions, for example, as described for the prediction of antipsychotics using either public or proprietary modules after integration of Sanofi data [17]. This combined module covers new targets, provides additional data, and allows for more predictions covering a broader target space.

Another interesting application of similarity-based target predictions is the identification of additional targets for molecular probes. Molecular probes are essential to investigate biology, while a clear answer depends on probe selectivity (see Personal foreword for more details). *In silico* target profiling of the full set of chemical probes from the National Institutes of Health (NIH) Molecular Libraries Program (MLP) predicted, and then validated, relevant *in vitro* affinities for proteins distantly related to the primary targets for the chemical probes ML006, ML123, ML141, and ML204 by experimental testing. A better understanding of the polypharmacology behaviour of these MLP probes might provide a better understanding of biological effects in further investigations [114]. Another example for a chemical probe with significant off-target effects is the PARP family inhibitor PJ34, which was predicted and confirmed to exhibit activity for PIM1/2 kinases [115]. This probe molecule is widely used in the literature to explore the role of PARPs. Therefore, *in silico* profiling can contribute to better characterize chemical probe compounds.

Similarity searches are limited to single or sequential ligand analysis, while Chemical Similarity Network Analysis Pulldown (CSNAP) [58, 116] integrates different ligands into a chemical similarity network for chemotype recognition. For biologically active query compounds, similar well-annotated reference compounds are identified and grouped into chemical similarity subnetworks. Network-based scoring was used to guide and quantify putative protein–ligand interactions. CSNAP demonstrated better accuracy in target prediction than SEA for a set of about 200 compounds. Based on the approach, the major mitotic targets for hits from a cell-based screen of cancer cells were found, and novel compounds targeting microtubules were identified.

A prospective application by Gohlke et al. used 2D and 3D similarity to unveil new functions for known kinase inhibitors [69]. More than 10 000 molecules from the SuperTarget database [117] with activity for 12 anticancer targets were compared in a 2D similarity matrix. While VEGFR inhibitors and PARP inhibitors show only low 2D similarity, a 3D analysis suggests higher similarity. In particular PARP off-target activity was shown for the VEGFR inhibitor vatalanib [69].

10.3.2 3D Similarity Methods for Target Inference

2D similarity searching uses molecular descriptors, which capture the absence or presence of chemical groups as well as their topological arrangement. Nevertheless, they do not capture conformational aspects, which are highly relevant for ligand–protein interactions. Shape-based screening methods use the 3D volume of a molecule together with electrostatic or pharmacophoric features to find similar molecules.

One of the fastest and best performing methods is Rapid Overlay of Chemical Structures (ROCS) [118–120]. Molecules are aligned based on maximizing the overlap of volumes between them. The molecular volume is approximated by Gaussian functions and the chemical environment is also included by a so-called colour force field. In contrast to 2D methods, 3D similarity methods require representative conformational ensembles for molecules. ROCS can identify less intuitive analogues with similar shape and electrostatic profiles, i.e. can enable scaffold hopping. While ROCS is mainly used for virtual screening, it can also be applied for target identification by linking hits from phenotypic screens to compounds with similar bioactivity annotations.

AbdulHameed et al. developed a ligand-based target fishing algorithm [121]. The authors first generated a chemogenomic database grouping 245 targets into 13 groups and correlated activities of 1150 approved drugs with the used targets, resulting in an 1150×245 sized matrix. Thus, each target in the dataset is presented by a number of active ligands, which are used in similarity searches. The maximum similarity score against any of these target representatives is used to indicate a potential target relation for a query compound. A significant number of hits from diverse target sets could be identified with this approach in a validation study with the DUD set [122], including compounds with low similarity in 2D chemical fingerprint space. This DUD set, often employed for benchmarking docking programs, refers to a database containing putatively inactive compounds for a variety of protein targets. In the second step, a drug–drug matrix was generated calculating all ROCS combo similarity scores between all 1150 drugs (1150×1150 matrices). This ROCS combo score provides a sum of scores from shape alignment plus match of chemical functionalities. Both matrices are then used to populate a drug–target matrix, which allows to easily select drug sets for a given target. The authors validated their approach with an external test set of 14 drug molecules with known off-targets.

Another method using 3D shape alignment for structure-based target prediction is called CSNAP3D from Lo et al. [123]. After screening different 3D alignment algorithms (Shape-it [124, 125], Align-it [124, 125], and ROCS [118–120]), the authors used a combination of pharmacophore metrics and shape-similarity metrics. Adding 2D fingerprints further improved the prediction rate.

The authors used this approach to identify several novel Taxol mimetics from a list of antimitotic compounds as hits in a cell-based screening assay.

The main limitation of shape-based approaches such as ROCS for finding novel targets is the size of the ligands. As molecules are aligned based on their volume, it is more likely to retrieve hits of similar size. Very small or very large molecules might produce misguiding similarity scores or incorrect alignments. These problems can be avoided by subROCS, although in this case computational costs increase by a factor of ~20 [126].

Pharmacophore models provide a different view on the spatial arrangement of chemical functionalities in a series and can also be employed as a 3D method to predict protein–ligand interactions. A pharmacophore model describes the ensemble of steric and electronic features, which are necessary for binding of a ligand to a particular protein [127]. Therefore, a pharmacophore model represents a more abstract description, which typically contains features such as hydrogen-bond donors and acceptors and positive or negative charged features as well as different hydrophobic characteristics. A key interest for using pharmacophore models is the chemical scaffold-independent description of molecular features relevant for biological activity, which gives the technology a significant potential for scaffold hopping. 3D pharmacophore models are a well-established concept in medicinal chemistry, described in numerous recent reviews [128–130]. Pharmacophore models can be derived from a set of different biologically active ligands. Different conformations are generated and compared in 3D to identify common pharmacophoric features, which are responsible for the biological activity. On the other hand, pharmacophore models can also be derived from protein–ligand complexes, extracting directly the pharmacophoric features facilitating protein–ligand interactions [131]. For target identification, a panel of pharmacophore models has been generated for different targets, which allows for *in silico* screening for novel ligands [132, 133]. This methodology with model panels was successfully applied to derive target hypotheses. In one example, micromolar activity against three different targets could be confirmed for natural products [64]. Numerous panels of pharmacophore models are available today. Inte:Ligand [134] provides the Pharmacophore ActivityProfiler, which encompasses a database of ~10 000 pharmacophore models (PharmacophoreDB) covering ~300 pharmaceutically relevant targets. The database was derived from protein–ligand 3D complexes as well as from ligand datasets. The Discovery Studio Suite from BIOVIA [135] contains a database of pharmacophore models derived from the scPDB [136, 137], a database of druggable binding sites extracted from the PDB database [138].

10.3.3 Fragment-Based Approaches

Since similarity queries rely on similarity to existing molecules captured in databases, predictions for novel chemical matter or complex molecules are challenging. Modification of the chemical descriptor to more abstract representations is one popular approach. Another interesting approach was described by Reker et al. to predict targets for natural products [65]. Their method relies on dissecting, i.e. retrosynthetic splitting, of the natural product into fragments and comparing the fragments to synthetic reference drugs. In principle, fragments represent small chemical portions of a compound mimicking pharmacophoric features, which can be experimentally validated, thus extending and building on the pharmacophore concept. As with the earlier described SPiDER method [99], the approach uses SOMs to cluster the reference compounds with annotated target activity. Within the study, the authors also investigate the performance of the method when starting from the parent natural product in comparison with starting from the pool of fragments. While the complete natural product seems to be more selective for target engagement, fragments can help to predict promising alternative targets and by this may help to reveal the mechanism of action of pharmacologically active natural products. This approach was successfully applied for target identification of the complex macrocyclic natural product Archazolid A [65].

Furthermore, Rodrigues et al. used this approach to discover and experimentally validate so far unknown targets for the fragment-like natural products goitrin, isomacroin, and graveolinine (Figure 10.4) [66]. Brand et al. used the related SPiDER method [99] combined with proteomic analysis to reveal 5-lipoxygenase (5-LO) as the target of lipoxygenin in the Wnt pathway [139]. Lipoxygenin and the chemically distinct 5-LO inhibitor CJ-13610 also promote cardiac differentiation of human induced pluripotent stem cells and inhibit Hedgehog, TGF-β, BMP, and Activin A pathway signalling, thus clearly suggesting a yet unknown role of 5-LO in these pathways [139]. Rodrigues et al. unveiled (−)-englerin as a modulator of L-type calcium channels using SPiDER and a pharmacophoric probe compound [140], while Schneider at al. presented a proof-of-concept study for *in silico* de-orphanization of phenotypic screening hits by suggesting prostanoid E receptor as a target of the cyclodepsipeptide doliculide, a natural anticancer compound [141]. The target hypothesis was subsequently validated by experimental testing.

Schuffenhauer et al. [142] proposed another approach that uses hierarchical scaffold trees. A scaffold is a chemical representation of a molecule, where all acyclic side chains are removed. As the method focuses on central motifs, it is complementary to 2D similarity methods. A removal of rings in the scaffold itself then leads to higher hierarchy levels. As scaffolds are well-defined entities, classification and searching is intuitive. Scaffold trees plus bioactivity are criteria for tree construction and allow efficient mapping, visualization, and navigation of

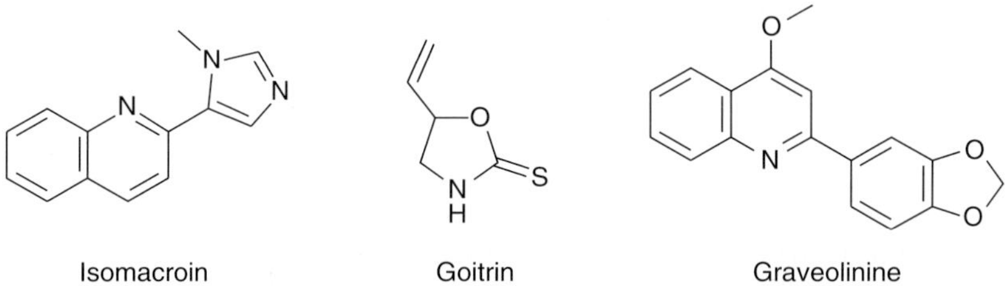

Figure 10.4 The natural products isomacroin, goitrin, and graveolinine used for fragment-based *in silico* target identification by Rodrigues et al. [66].

the chemical space, enabling the correlation of scaffolds to bioactivity. This can guide the design of new molecules, as shown by identification of new scaffolds for 5-LO and estrogen receptor α (ERα) [143].

The interactive exploration of the chemical space with the software Scaffold Hunter for complex SAR was described by Wetzel et al. [144]. Scaffold Hunter is a chemical data organization and analysis tool with an interactive visualization of the hierarchical scaffold tree [59, 145].

Applications of this scaffold organization concept involve the identification of structural features linked to mutagenicity [146] or identification of scaffolds linked to biological promiscuity from collections screened against 100 unrelated proteins or 172 kinases [147]. The method was also applied for dataset enrichment to identify active chemical series in high-throughput screens (HTS) [148, 149]. Furthermore, this approach served to identify prospective target and bioactivity annotations for a series of γ-pyrone natural products [70]. This was inspired by the hypothesis that natural product scaffolds could be linked to scaffolds with known bioactivity to identify potential target proteins [150], which led to the identification of monoamine oxidases, sphingomyelinases, and STATs with a conserved Src homology 2 domain [70].

10.3.4 QSAR Models and Machine Learning

Similarity searching typically considers all parts of a query molecule as equally important. However, medicinal chemistry experience suggests that some parts of the molecule are highly relevant for biological activity, while others are dispensable. This aspect is covered in the concepts of fragments, privileged motifs, and pharmacophores.

Machine learning algorithms take this aspect into account by capturing SAR, since weights are derived for different molecular descriptors, giving more emphasis to features linked to activity. An example workflow for generating QSAR models can be found in Figure 10.5. Machine learning [151] uses bioactivity data to correlate structure-derived descriptors with activity for a target or assay. Such descriptors include representations of atoms and their properties, bonds, substructures, and fragments, aromaticity, general molecule topology, surfaces, physico-chemical properties, and many others. Many linear and non-linear statistical approaches such as partial least squares (PLS) [152, 153], support vector machines (SVM) [154], random forest (RF) [155, 156], and deep neural networks (DNN) [157–159] have been successfully applied for modelling larger datasets to either build QSAR models [75], which predict the strength of protein–ligand interactions, or to derive classification models, which distinguish active molecules from inactive ones. Such *in silico* models provide good tools to predict if compounds are active on certain targets and thus can also be used for target inference or off-target predictions. A recent analysis further revealed that machine learning methods can outperform similarity-based methods for drug repurposing, thus identifying novel targets [160].

Poroikov and coworkers developed Prediction of Activity Spectra for Substances (PASS) to predict activities using 2D descriptors in the early 2000s [60, 161]. PASS classifies molecules for their activity to >3600 end points

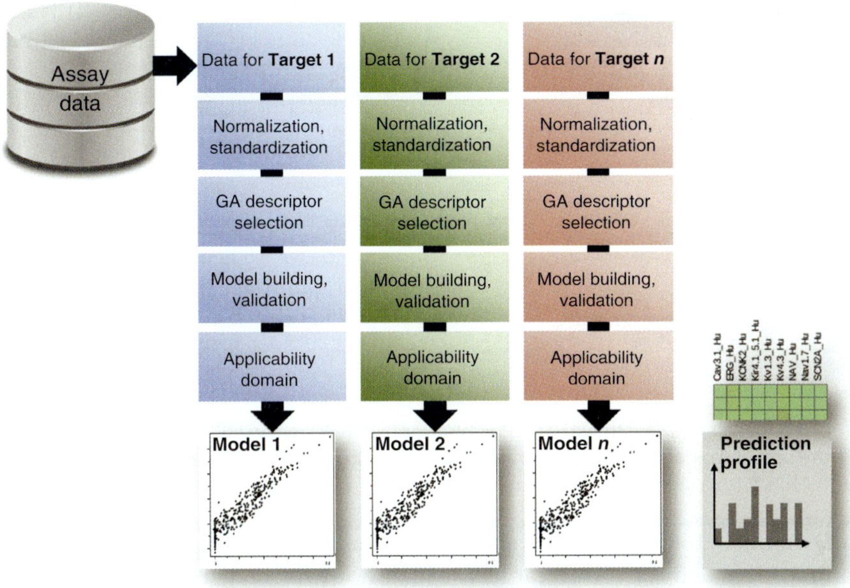

Figure 10.5 *In silico* model building and validation workflow for establishing a panel of QSAR models covering diverse protein targets and off-targets. Those QSAR model panels find applications for *in silico* profiling and off-target predictions.

containing target proteins as well as pharmacological activity. Recently, an *in silico* profiling for 18 important off-targets (13 receptors, 2 enzymes, 3 transporters) on a dataset of 4000 compounds was described [61, 162]. The approach was then extended using a ligand–target dataset from ChEMBL in combination with a Bayesian-like method to derive predictive models for >2500 targets [163]. Linking results of such a method to phenotypic screening read-outs can help to infer related targets.

As an alternative approach, Reymond and coworker proposed the Polypharmacology Browser version 2 (PPB2) [164] as a target prediction tool based on ChEMBL (v22) bioactivity data. Ligand similarities are evaluated using three different fingerprints encoding composition (MQN), shape and pharmacophores (Xfp), or substructures (ECFP4). The combination of nearest neighbour searching with local Naïve Bayesian machine learning models from substructure fingerprints led to best statistical quality. The method successfully predicted off-targets including hERG for CIS22a [165], a TRPV6 inhibitor. Clearly, the results of a PPB2 search can also be used to locate potential targets of a molecule to phenotypic effects. Screenshots of the web server [166] are shown in Figure 10.6.

Naïve Bayesian classification combines the presence of features such as substructures and functional groups in a statistical approach in a training set to obtain a probability for a compound to be active. This approach can also be used to derive both broad target family and focused single-target statistical models, as demonstrated for kinase inhibitor series [167]. Bayesian multi-class models are described as an efficient approach to combine multiple targets within a single

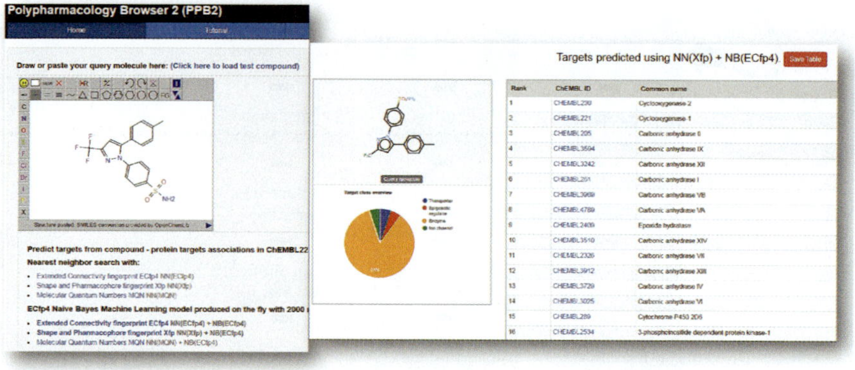

Figure 10.6 Result of a search with the Polypharmacology Browser 2 (PPB2, ppb2.gdb.tools) using the non-steroidal anti-inflammatory drug celecoxib as a query. The result page ranks potential hits with a link to the most similar compound in ChEMBL and the target name.

in silico model [168]. Molecules not classified as 'active' then contribute to the definition of 'inactives' for all targets, which however may not reflect the true activity.

In silico affinity fingerprints derived from such a Naïve Bayesian classification were applied by Bender et al. for off-target profiling [169]. For this approach, Bayes affinity fingerprints encoding information about the ligand bioactivity space are applied. In contrast to conventional similarity searching, where molecules are directly compared on the basis of molecular descriptors, molecules are compared to several sets of molecules from different activity classes. Each chemical structure is described by a set of Bayes scores for a panel of reference ligands comprising about 1000 activity classes from the WOMBAT database. Pairwise structural comparisons using the Pearson correlation coefficient then captures the degree similarity of pairs of Bayes scores, i.e. panel activity classes. The *in silico* panel is named 'Bayes affinity fingerprints'. These fingerprints showed improved retrieval of known actives when used in similarity searches compared with chemical fingerprints. These fingerprints therefore can be viewed as an extension of *in vitro* affinity fingerprints [170] to ligand bioactive chemical space.

Based on Bayesian multi-class models, Martin et al. reported a 2D-QSAR approach named Profile-QSAR [171] for *in silico* profiling of kinases. It is described as a meta-QSAR method, since activity of a molecule for a novel protein kinase is expressed as a linear combination of predicted activities against a panel of 92 reference kinases. Firstly, a set of Bayesian models for the 92 training kinases is derived as a complete prediction matrix. This computed matrix is then used to derive a PLS model for predicting activities for novel kinases. The method was extended to cover a significant subset of kinome target proteins using structure-based chemogenomics [172]. The method was also extended to proteases [173] and applied in drug discovery projects. In Profile-QSAR 2.0, the Naïve Bayesian models were replaced by RF regression due to improved performance [174]. Further improvements in predictivity resulted from using deep learning as a statistical engine for Profile-QSAR 2.0 [175].

Merget et al. [176] reported ligand-based activity prediction models for >280 kinases by machine learning on a large proprietary kinase bioactivity dataset combined with open-source ligand–target data. High-quality and statistically significant RF models were derived for ~200 kinases by combining open data with proprietary data. RF models outperformed other machine learning models like Naive Bayesian classifiers or deep learning models. The derived models with potential application in selectivity profiling and virtual screening are evenly distributed across the kinome tree, allowing reliable profiling for all branches. Interestingly, the authors could enhance the prediction quality by employing experimental bioactivity fingerprints of a small kinase subset.

We have developed an internal *in silico* approach for prediction for diverse targets and off-targets [17, 177] based on the program Cubist [178–180] as the statistical engine, which has been applied to *in silico* profiling and for building off-target models, e.g. for pregnane X receptor (PXR) [181]. Cubist employs a regression tree algorithm, which partitions a dataset by rules into homogeneous SAR groups. Each node defined by this tree has an associated multiple linear regression (MLR) model describing the SAR for molecules in this particular group [182]. Cubist classifies molecules using structural parameters according to rules and evaluates a separate SAR model for each subset, rather than fitting a single model to the entire dataset. This approach provides more accurate predictions than classical decision trees. Using this approach, global models for ~600 off-targets from profiling data in the Sanofi corporate database were built as described earlier [17]. The final model ensemble allows efficient prediction of novel compounds. Quantitative predictions for each target are returned, which are translated into a classification scheme at a threshold of 10 μM for target interaction. The applicability domain for each model is explored by a chemical similarity approach [183], which is defined for a new compound as a threshold of 50% similarity to the training set, as evaluated by UNITY [184]. For a reported case study involving kinase inhibitors, predictions for molecules not in the training set show good correlation to experimental data and confirm a trend for *in vivo* cardiotoxic effects observed for these molecules [17]. An illustration of such a prediction is given in Figure 10.7. In addition to the identification of off-target effects, the model panel is also used to identify target hypotheses for phenotypic screening hits.

An alternative method is Gaussian processes [185], which is widely used in machine learning, but not yet in drug design. Obrezanova et al. proposed the use of Gaussian processes for QSAR and absorption, distribution, metabolism, and excretion (ADME) predictions, discussed its applicability and its capability for automatic model generation and compared it to methods such as artificial neural networks or Bayesian neural networks [186]. Later, Reutlinger et al. applied a Gaussian process model trained on annotated drug targets from the ChEMBL database [24] to predict biological targets for synthesized compounds from a DeanFlow reactor chip. The quick and efficient synthesis in a microreactor chip combined with computational target predictions allows the generation of bioactivity-focused libraries, which can be used to identify novel scaffolds [187]. The authors extended their study to generate target-focused compound libraries

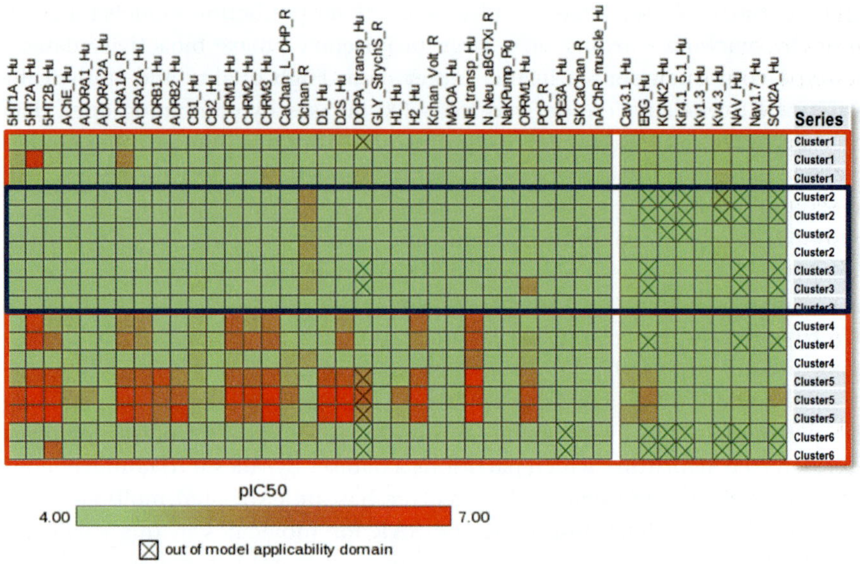

Figure 10.7 *In silico* off-target prediction using the Sanofi internal QSAR model panel for multiple clusters as a heat map. An HTS of the Sanofi collection for positive allosteric modulators of the GLP1 receptor resulted in interesting chemical clusters. Those were subjected during triaging to *in silico* off-target profiling, which resulted in de-prioritizing clusters based on higher predicted target promiscuity. Green fields in the heat map indicate a low predicted pIC_{50} between targets on the *x*-axis and ligands on the *y*-axis, while red indicates a potential interaction (c.f. colour map). An 'X' indicates an unreliable prediction outside of the model applicability domain.

by combining Gaussian process models with ant colony optimization for automated compound picking [188].

Deep learning is an evolving technique with many successful applications, such as for property prediction [189–191]. The complex training process for DNNs including selection of suitable hyperparameters and the lack of large-scale comparisons led Mayr et al. to extensively compare machine learning methods and feature representations of molecules for target predictions using the ChEMBL database [159]. The authors used the area under the receiver operating characteristic curve (ROC-AUC) as a metric for comparison. Feedforward neural networks outperformed other methods such as SVM, kNN, or RF. Furthermore, feedforward neural networks performed better than other neural networks, such as convolutional neural networks using graphs and recurrent neural networks using SMILES, although differences are small. As no feature selection is required for graphs or SMILES-based predictive approaches, those represent a useful alternative for model building.

Recently, machine learning methods have also been described, which use chemical descriptors in combination with protein descriptions, thus directly linking the ligand to its interacting protein. A few prospective applications using deep learning approaches for drug–target interactions are already disclosed. Bosc et al. developed a chemometrics-based approach to model kinase selectivity integrating protein and ligand descriptions [192]. While kinases are represented by 3D descriptors, ligands are represented using 2D fingerprints. The novel protein descriptor is able to classify kinases based on group membership and their DFG-type conformation. Internal validation showed the potential to discriminate 'active' from 'inactive' protein kinase–ligand interactions, while external validation suggests that the number of inactive pairs might be overestimated.

Öztürk et al. proposed a novel idea to use ligand-based SMILES strings and protein sequences to build a regression model for predicting binding affinity [193]. The overall results are comparable to established baseline models; however, the method performed better with larger datasets. As only protein sequences and SMILES are used, the method might be promising for targeting unexplored proteins. Similarly, Feng et al. proposed PADME [194], which combines graph convolutional networks for representing molecules with protein sequence composition descriptors for describing proteins. By including protein information into the network, both approaches are capable of predicting molecule–target interactions for proteins not included in training. Gao et al. presented an end-to-end neural network model. The protein is encoded by its amino acid and GO annotations, while molecules are represented as chemical graphs. By predicting drug–protein interactions without the need of domain knowledge and feature engineering, the method might also generalize to new proteins [195]. Since the last three interesting approaches were not yet prospectively applied, their performance in prospective applications is unclear.

10.3.5 Experimentally Derived Molecular Descriptors

In many applications, the description of molecules is derived from their chemical structure. A very interesting extension is the use of experimentally derived descriptors. The wealth of information for many existing compounds allows generating descriptors from previous experimental results, as shown with high-throughput screening fingerprints (HTS-FP) [196]. In this approach, the molecule is described by a vector capturing the activity in a panel of different biological assays, biochemical as well as cellular assays. Activity is captured by the Z-score of the compound, namely, the deviation of the measured activity from the mean value normalized by the standard deviation. It could be shown that the performance of similarity searching with HTS-FP descriptors depends on the target class. Nevertheless, good results were found for novel scaffolds identifying numerous compounds that are different to those identified by chemical fingerprints. This complementarity makes HTS-FP an interesting extension for target inference with promising applicability to a broader chemical space. Missing data and experimental noise associated with high-throughput data are potential limitations, which might require further optimization of the assays represented in the fingerprint [197].

HTS-FP have also proven useful for building machine learning models to predict target activity, which showed better enrichments and chemotype diversity than chemical descriptors [198]. In a larger study, target hypotheses for natural products and a set of drugs were experimentally confirmed, illustrating the suitability of HTS-FP for target identification [71]. Target predictions were made for 1400 drugs and 1300 natural products, resulting in prediction of 5281 and 2798 previously unknown targets for the natural products and drug sets, respectively. Interestingly, targets identified for the two sets had only little overlap. Drugs were biased towards membrane receptors, and natural products towards soluble enzymes. 65 drug–target predictions were investigated *in vitro*, resulting in a conformation rate of 74%, including the inhibition of COX-1/2 by the HIV protease inhibitor tipranavir [71].

Recently, HTS-FP were used to generate DNN [199]. Multiple end points were trained in a neural network for multitask learning. The biological fingerprint-derived model identified different compounds compared with a model from chemical descriptors, highlighting the added value of using HTS-FP. Inspired by the SEA methodology, BioSEA uses HTS-FP as descriptors and an ensemble-based similarity calculation [200]. The method could be successfully used to identify tubulin inhibitors with different scaffolds than the natural products used as query compounds. However, the identified compounds reproduce the phenotype in the phenotypic assay and the mechanism of action of the natural products.

Gene expression profiles have also been employed as interesting molecular descriptors (see Chapter 11 for more details) [201]. Briefly, data from the high-throughput L1000 platform [202] were used for 31761 samples in combination with SVM-based models for two targets, namely, HSP90 and NR3C1. Additional compounds from the dataset were predicted to be active on either of those targets, which could be experimentally confirmed for 22 out of 275 proposed molecules, representing a 300-fold enrichment compared with the original screening campaigns.

High-content screening (HCS) measures many different cellular parameters in a screening campaign, such as cellular and nuclear morphology. Such changes are captured in cellular images (see also Chapter 11). In a recent disclosure, HCS-derived images were taken as a basis for building machine learning models to predict biological activity [203]. For this purpose, images from an HTS for the detection of nuclear translocation of the three-channel glucocorticoid receptor were analysed with CellProfiler [204] and converted into image-based fingerprints. These image-based fingerprints were used as training data for different machine learning models and applied to predictions for a large panel of 535 different biochemical and cellular assays. DNNs and a method based on Bayesian Matrix Factorization [205] produced models with good predictivity in cross-validation studies. Two of the models could be successfully applied to select biologically active compounds in an oncology and a central nervous system (CNS) project. The methodology allowed the selection of diverse chemical compounds with sub-micromolar activity.

Experimentally derived descriptors capture the biological response of the molecule in different biological assays. Therefore, they offer a different perspective than chemical descriptors and thus broaden the scope of *in silico* methods for target discovery. The potential of such descriptors has been demonstrated in numerous validation studies and in searching for novel chemical matter on some targets. The first prospective applications in target identification illustrate the potential to identify novel ligand–target associations. In the context of target inference, the requirement of experimental results for any molecule used is not as severely limiting as for designing new molecules.

10.3.6 Structure-Based Screening

Structure-based screening methods can be applied when reliable 3D structural information for target proteins is available. This 3D information can be obtained by experimental methods such as X-ray crystallography, NMR spectroscopy, or cryogenic electron microscopy (cryo-EM). In addition, validated homology models based on experimental structures of related proteins can also be used. The main advantage of structure-based methods is that they provide additional information from analysing protein–ligand interactions beyond correlation of bioactivity data for ligand series (see Figures 10.8 and 10.9). A broad overview of structure-based approaches was recently provided [208, 209]. Although the structural coverage of the human proteome has significantly increased over time [210], certain target classes such as membrane proteins are still under-represented.

Usually, methods in structure-based design are more costly than methods in ligand-based design, especially molecular dynamics simulations, Monte Carlo sampling, free-energy-perturbation theory, or Markov state modelling. While these methods can be used to explore binding processes, estimate binding affinity, and exploit binding to different targets, the number of possible targets and simulations is limited by computational resources.

High-throughput methods are required for target inference, where the most important approach is docking, which is significantly faster than simulations. In docking for target inference, a large database of prepared protein structures is used to cross-dock a ligand against all possible binding sites. Sturm et al. studied the structural effect of ligand–protein complexes on ligand promiscuity, i.e. the ability of ligands to bind to different targets. Focusing on drug-like ligands and druggable targets, they found that ligand promiscuity is caused by either similar binding sites in unrelated targets or specific characteristics of the ligand, such as conformational flexibility [211]. Correlating the docking score can then help to identify promising targets [209, 212]. In this context, optimally prepared databases can greatly benefit such screening, for example, the MacroMolecular Data Service (MMDS) database from OpenEye employing the Iridium database of protein–ligand structures [213]. Similarly, Kufareva et al. created the Pocketome database [214, 215], which collects conformational ensembles of druggable binding sites. An augmented pocketome using computationally predicted pockets was proposed later by Bhagavat et al. [216].

Schomburg et al. developed the inverse Rapid Index-based Screening Engine (iRAISE) method [217]. The method is used for reverse docking, i.e. identifying possible targets for a given ligand. In particular, the authors discuss four main challenges that need to be addressed in reverse docking: preprocessing and handling of many proteins, efficient and consistent handling of structural data, ranking of targets, and significant benchmark data such as datasets containing sufficient information about molecules with target and non-target annotations.

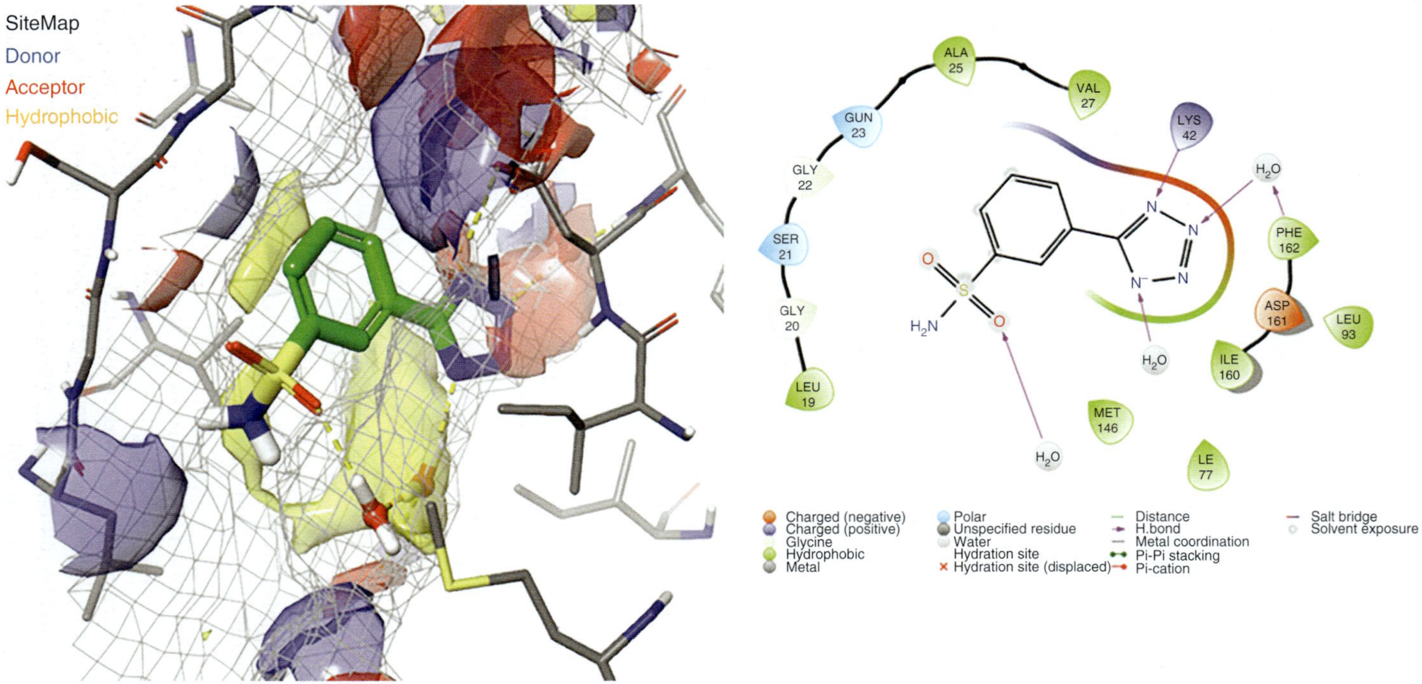

Figure 10.8 X-ray structure of compound 2 in human death-associated protein kinase 3 (DAPK3) (PDB 5A6N, resolution 1.70 Å) [206]. Essential interactions are indicated. Yellow dotted lines indicate hydrogen bonds, and cyan lines indicate aromatic–aromatic interactions. Blue contours indicate protein-derived hydrogen-bond donor regions, red refers to hydrogen-bond acceptor regions, and yellow indicates hydrophobic interactions from a binding site analysis using SiteMap (Schrödinger). Source: Rodrigues et al. 2015 [206]. Reproduced with permission of Wiley.

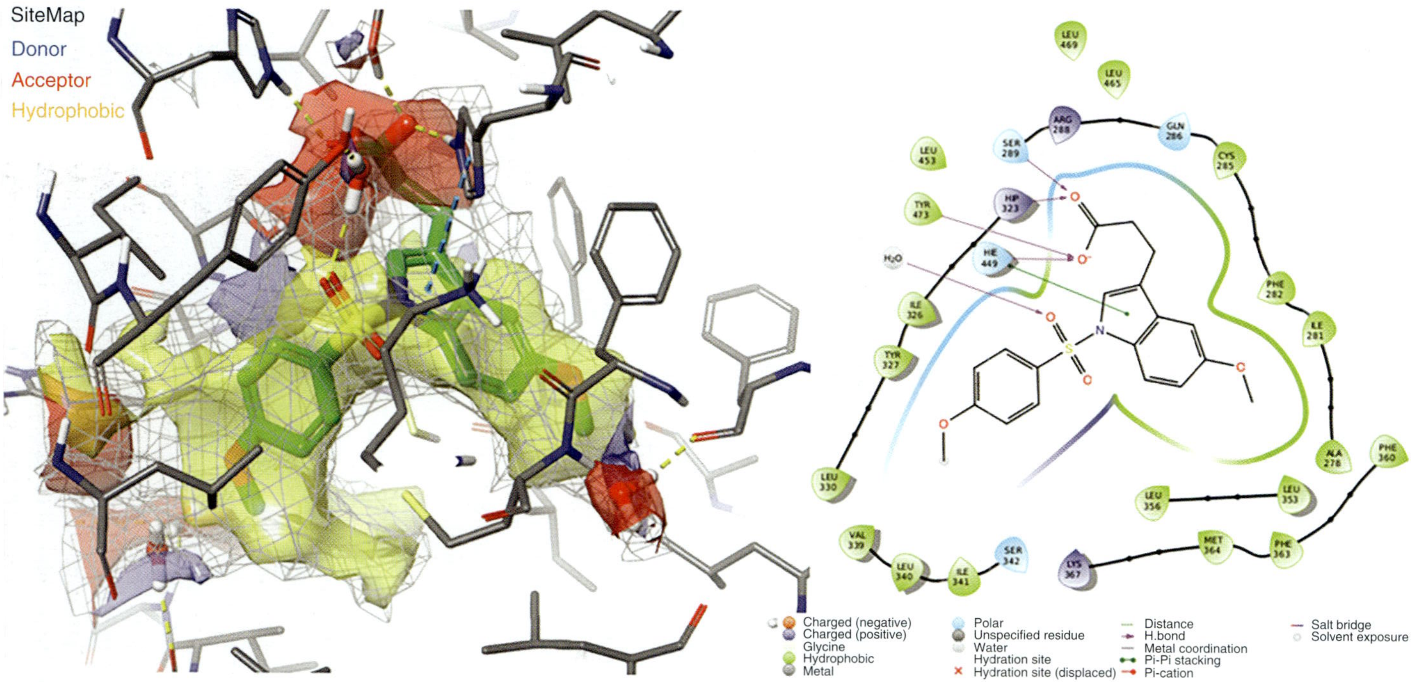

Figure 10.9 X-ray structure of PPARγ with 3-[5-methoxy-1-(4-methoxy-benzenesulfonyl)-1H-indol-3-yl]-propionic acid (PDB 3ET3, resolution 1.95 Å) [207]. See Figure 10.8 for details. Source: Adapted from Artis et al. 2009 [207].

While solutions for the first three challenges are already proposed, the fourth challenge is still a topic of ongoing research.

One approach to overcome one of the major challenges – ranking and scoring hits for different targets – was investigated by Kim et al. [218]. Historically, most scoring functions were developed and parametrized to rank the true positives highest in the list. When results from several targets are mixed, the rate of false positives can increase. Therefore, Kim et al. discuss a combined Z-score using a weighted fraction of ligand and protein Z-scores, which can improve the inverse docking performance. The approach was validated with the Astex, DUD, and DUD-E datasets, where the combined Z-score performed better than the single Z-scores or standard docking scores.

Another common tool is the TarFisDock web server [219], which uses docking into a protein drug target database with ~700 protein structures to predict new targets. Following similar ideas, Málnási-Csizmadia et al. proposed the drug profile matching (DPM) approach [220, 221], which predicts a complete effect profile of a compound, i.e. a vector with activities against distinct targets, using a probability score. When correlating these results to known drug–target activities, several hits were validated. In a follow-up study, novel predicted targets could be validated from a literature search and experiments [222]. This demonstrates the effectiveness of DPM and its usefulness in finding novel targets and repositioning of drugs.

A novel approach is FINDSITEcomb2.0, a hybrid method that combines a threading-based structure prediction method with similarity searches [56]. For a given sequence, threading is used to identify suitable protein structure templates. Based on these templates, protein binding sites are selected with their corresponding ligands from ChEMBL and DrugBank. Finally, the selected ligand set is then compared to the query compound to assess its potential for binding to the given sequence based on the chemical similarity. In validation, the methodology showed good enrichment factors up to ~50. For the predecessor method FINDSITEcomb, numerous predictions were experimentally validated [223]. For eight different proteins, 4–47% of predicted and tested ligands could be experimentally confirmed.

10.3.7 Protein–Protein and Ligand–Target Networks

Complex biological systems involve many protein interactions, which can be represented as networks. Analysis of these networks might provide insights about the mechanism of action for particular molecules [224]. Drug pathway enrichment analysis based on integration of data from various databases was shown to lead to interesting insights for elucidation of the mechanism of action and supported drug repositioning hypotheses [225]. Therefore, these technologies also offer opportunities to generate target hypotheses of phenotypic screening hits.

Some tools [226] were developed for navigating biochemical interaction networks, such as Cytoscape [227, 228], ChEMBLSpace [229], or Search Tool for Interactions of Chemicals (STITCH) (see Figure 10.10) [231, 232]. The latter is an important resource for analysis of ligand–target networks. STITCH integrates information on interactions from diverse sources for 430 000 molecules.

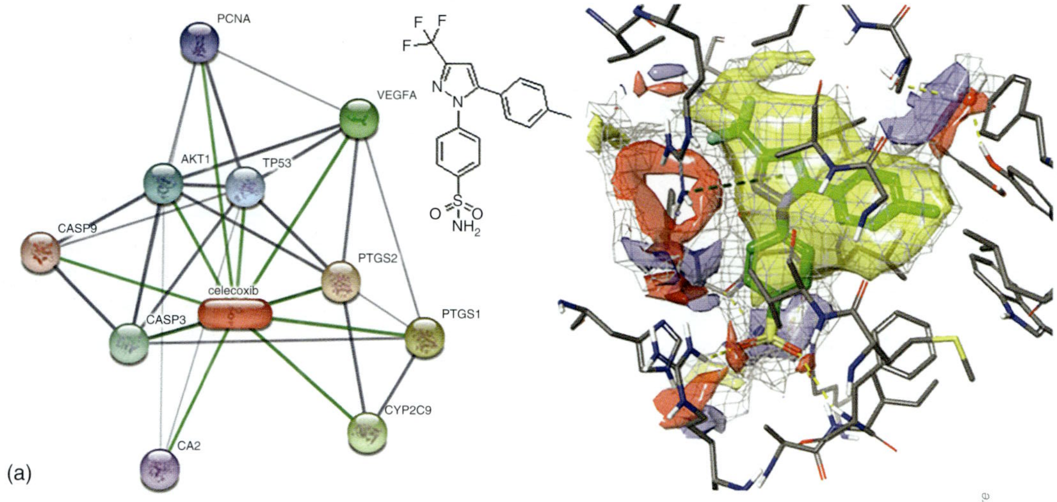

Predicted functional partners:

			Score	
●	PTGS2	prostaglandin-endoperoxide synthase 2 (prostaglandin G/H synthase and cyclooxygenase); Mediates the formation of prostaglandins from arac...	0.999	=COX-2
●	PTGS1	prostaglandin-endoperoxide synthase 1 (prostaglandin G/H synthase and cyclooxygenase); May play an important role in regulating or promotin...	0.998	
●	CYP2C9	cytochrome P450, family 2, subfamily C, polypeptide 9; Cytochromes P450 are a group of heme-thiolate monooxygenases. In liver microsomes, t...	0.990	
●	VEGFA	vascular endothelial growth factor A (412 aa)	0.987	
●	CASP3	caspase 3, apoptosis-related cysteine peptidase; Involved in the activation cascade of caspases responsible for apoptosis execution. At the onse...	0.982	
●	AKT1	v-akt murine thymoma viral oncogene homolog 1; AKT1 is one of 3 closely related serine/threonine- protein kinases (AKT1, AKT2 and AKT3) calle...	0.961	
●	TP53	tumor protein p53; Acts as a tumor suppressor in many tumor types; induces growth arrest or apoptosis depending on the physiological circums...	0.955	
●	PCNA	proliferating cell nuclear antigen; Auxiliary protein of DNA polymerase delta and is involved in the control of eukaryotic DNA replication by increa...	0.929	
●	CA2	carbonic anhydrase II; Essential for bone resorption and osteoclast differentiation (By similarity). Reversible hydration of carbon dioxide. Can hydr...	0.912	
●	CASP9	caspase 9, apoptosis-related cysteine peptidase (416 aa)	0.910	

(b)

Figure 10.10 Target–ligand network constructed using STITCH. The network view (a) is centred at the interaction of the non-steroidal anti-inflammatory drug celecoxib used to treat symptoms of osteoarthritis with its target COX-2 (i.e. PTGS2 = prostaglandin-endoperoxide synthase 2). Network nodes represent proteins; for larger nodes the protein 3D structure is known. Edges represent protein–protein associations (grey). Chemical–protein interactions are shown in green. Stronger associations are represented by thicker lines. The main predicted functional partners and prediction scores are also provided (b). The interaction with its target COX-2 is illustrated using the X-ray structure of the celecoxib/COX-2 complex (PDB 3LN1, resolution 2.40 Å) [230]. Source: Wang et al. 2010 [230]. Reproduced with permission of Elsevier.

Protein–protein interaction networks are well studied and could be potentially explored for drug–target interactions. Proteins that are targeted by drugs with the same mechanism of action are often functionally related. These proteins are then typically closely associated in a protein–protein network, which can be explored for generating drug–protein interaction hypotheses [233, 234]. Hence, a protein related in network space to another one targeted by a drug is likely to also be interacting with this drug. This hypothesis led to the development of drugCIPHER for the prediction of drug–target interactions by integrating drug-therapy information, chemical structures, and protein–protein interaction networks [235]. Other approaches have taken into account network attributes like centrality and degree of characterization of drug targets, assuming that some nodes play a more important role than others in these biological networks. In particular, the interruption of highly interconnected central nodes in a network may cause broad and undesirable pharmacological effects [234].

Ligand–target networks can be represented as models to analyse network topology and identify key features. These approaches were applied, for example, to understand the clinical value of multi-kinase inhibitors in cancer treatment [236]. *In silico* profiling for related patterns in ligand–target networks may provide useful hypotheses for drug repurposing [237]. Although certain pharmaceuticals may target different diseases, they may be linked by structural similarity, share the same interaction of a protein target, or even share side effects. To this end, network profiling led to a hypothesis [238] of the anticancer potential [239] of the antiviral drug nelfinavir due to low-affinity off-target effects on multiple kinases implicated in cell signalling.

Campillos et al. proposed a novel approach to predict drug targets based on drug side effect similarities following the assumption that molecules with related side effects might share common target proteins [240, 241]. Drug associated adverse effects were extracted from the FDA reporting system and stored in the database SIDER [242, 243]. Mining this information led to the discovery of unexpected connections between chemically unrelated drugs for different indications. The integration of chemical structure with side effect profiles significantly improved prediction accuracy and led to novel hypotheses on protein targets. In an application, the authors reported 261 side effect-driven drug–drug relationships by structurally dissimilar molecules. 20 of these unexpected drug–drug relations were experimentally tested, and 13 of those could be validated through binding assays [240].

Despite their values for data analysis, today's network approaches suffer from incomplete ligand–protein interaction data, which are additionally biased towards prominent areas of research, such as kinases and GPCRs, which might limit their applicability.

10.4 Practical Considerations

Rational approaches to target and off-target identification require a tight interplay between *in silico* prediction and experimental validation. This step is a collaborative effort between various departments, namely, medicinal chemistry, molecular modelling, structural biology, molecular biology, and pharmacology.

Knowledge-based approaches capture available information in order to directly apply them for deriving target hypotheses. This provides a huge opportunity for informed decisions for guiding experimental efforts to explore reasonable hypotheses. Example results for celecoxib as the query molecule are shown in Figures 10.2, 10.3, and 10.6 for different approaches. Nevertheless, knowledge-based approaches critically depend on the availability of public and corporate databases containing information from literature and corporate data from HTS, medium-throughput, and profiling campaigns. Mining and navigating this large volume of heterogeneous data also has specific requirements to the underlying database information systems coupled to novel visualization approaches for big data.

Clearly, all these approaches rely heavily on what is previously known. Novel target proteins with only a few exotic ligands cannot usually be exploited. It is also not possible to identify completely novel or undisclosed targets or predict properties for chemical series that have never been associated with a protein family or target. Despite this limitation, it can be expected that this situation will rapidly improve with additional data and enhanced computational approaches to integrate more corporate data into prediction algorithms.

Chemistry-driven lead finding and optimization always intends to identify novel scaffolds, to expand chemical space, and to differentiate and allow patent protection. Patentability here refers to structural novelty, which is complementary to the similarity searching paradigm. Therefore, identification of ligand–target interactions for novel series, using 2D descriptions or knowledge-based methods only, might be challenging in some cases. To improve these limitations, any knowledge-based investigation needs to draw conclusions beyond simple 2D similarity in public databases by use of corporate databases, extending similarity to 3D, docking into proteins, and others as viable complementary approaches for establishing novel ligand–target hypotheses. Therefore, there will be a tremendous impact of novel methods describing relationships in advanced terms beyond simple 2D similarity.

The challenge to capture novel chemical structures can also be addressed using alternative molecular descriptors. A more abstract representation of the chemical structure such as the CATS descriptor, for example, allows the application of similarity-based approaches to more novel chemotypes. Another step in the same direction is the use of experimentally derived fingerprints, for which a good performance for novel scaffolds has been shown in validation studies. The technology capitalizes on large databases within pharmaceutical companies. Nevertheless, even within pharmaceutical companies, such fingerprints are sparsely populated. In addition, they can only be used for compounds that have been tested in many different assays.

3D computational strategies are often applied to overcome this limitation. First, it is possible to apply advanced 3D descriptors involving shape and pharmacophores, which requires an increase in computational costs. A database of prepared protein structures serves for inverse docking of ligands. Moreover, the target protein space could be extended by sequence or 3D similarity of proteins or binding sites. Nevertheless, structural coverage of some protein families by protein structure with sufficient resolution is still relatively sparse, regardless of technical difficulties involving pose and affinity prediction in docking workflows.

Many different machine learning technologies are available to convert sets of active and inactive molecules into knowledge by building predictive models, which can successfully be used to predict target–protein interactions. The majority of tools only consider positive ligand–target interactions, i.e. reported activity of a ligand for a particular target protein. Corporate databases contain even more information about inactive compounds for particular targets from either HTS campaigns or focused optimization programs, which can help to improve predictivity of *in silico* models [244]. However, this also adds some challenge to the computational performance, as typically there are many more inactives than actives for a particular target, at least in corporate databases.

Predictive models have been developed by different technologies such as Bayesian classifiers, RF, or SVM and could be successfully applied for activity prediction and target inference. Recently, deep learning neural networks have been added to the methodological toolbox. While validation studies suggest that this new technology can improve model quality, stringent validation criteria are essential to optimize predictivity, such as the use of external test sets and temporal validation [245].

It is important to keep in mind that the applicability domain of machine learning models is limited and depends on the chemical space represented in the training set and the descriptors used for model building. Useful *in silico* models require a concept for estimating this applicability domain. It is of utmost importance for each prediction to check whether a compound falls within the applicability domain of a method. Otherwise, the risk of false prediction is significantly increased. This helps to provide additional confidence for a computational approach. Other possibilities include the parallel reporting of experimental data for the query molecules, if available, or data for nearest neighbours used for the prediction. Finally, not all computational tools clearly discriminate between different biochemical read-outs, such as binding versus inhibition or activation. Therefore, it has to be checked for individual cases whether the amount of underlying data really justifies biochemical discrimination. Assessment of *in silico* predictions typically comprises a visual inspection step of final results [246] to analyse docking poses and judge the fit to a pharmacophore model. Therefore, more robust and unbiased analysis tools are still required to minimize the necessity for visual inspection, thus allowing the application of these methods to broader panels of proteins and pharmacophore models.

The technical requirements for running *in silico* target inference for a panel of relevant size are relatively demanding. For ligand-based approaches, training data have to be retrieved, and molecules need to be prepared. Input molecules need to be cleaned and checked for consistency. Those with clearly reactive and undesirable chemical substructures and fragments should be flagged and not considered. 2D similarity approaches typically lack information about ligand chirality, and a differentiation between enantiomers and diastereoisomers cannot be expected. In many cases, this information is also not consistently available in large databases. Often, experimental data for less advanced compounds are obtained from stereochemical mixtures (e.g. racemates). While most 3D descriptors are able to discriminate enantiomers, these approaches might not be applied when the underlying data do not justify such discrimination.

10.5 Conclusion

Optimization of protein–ligand interactions is at the heart of drug discovery. Accordingly, many *in silico* methods have been developed to predict interactions, comprising ligand- and structure-based approaches. Different methods ensure systematic exploitation of knowledge either from the protein 3D structure universe or the large volume of ligand bioactivity data. Novel *in silico* approaches also incorporate imaging and phenotypic assay data with the chemical structure to arrive at information systems exploring the 'bioactivity space'. *In silico* target identification can be perceived as reversal of the classical affinity prediction for a target. For selected ligands, the activity against a panel of targets has to be predicted to identify a putative target. Accordingly, all current *in silico* technologies for rapid prediction of protein–ligand interactions are applied for target inference.

Similarity-based approaches are known for their reliability to identify relatively close analogues and thus find wide application in target inference methodology. Numerous successful case studies have been described. Nevertheless, as for all knowledge-based approaches, chemical similarity to known ligands only has a limited reach for prediction of novel targets due to limitations in the number of compounds tested in different assays. Therefore, the advanced description of the chemical moiety is an active area of research. Good improvements in the coverage of chemical space have been achieved by more abstract representations of the chemical compound such as the CATS descriptor in combination with TIGER. Promising results are also reported for experimentally derived descriptors such as HTS-FP. For target discovery, the limitation of such descriptors to compounds that have been broadly tested in many different assays is not as severe as for the design of novel compounds.

Machine learning technologies systematically build models from the available bioactivity data, which can be successfully used for target prediction of diverse chemical compounds. In that area, a number of machine learning technologies such as RF, Bayesian classifier, or SVM have been established as reliable technologies. Recently, the rise of deep learning technologies shows promising results in a number of validation studies, but the number of prospective applications is still limited. For machine learning approaches for a panel of many different targets, a robust workflow has to be established, which includes model validation as well as applicability domain assessments.

Structure-based target predictions use information from the perspective of the protein structure. Systematic docking allows the derivation of target hypotheses, which can be further investigated by bioinformatics. Those approaches can also be combined with ligand-based approaches to obtain further confidence in target predictions for which 3D structure information is available.

In silico methods have proven to be capable of establishing valid target hypotheses and are an established part of target identification efforts. Interestingly, prospective studies are dominated by similarity-based and machine learning approaches. This is certainly partly attributed to the ease of use in particular for similarity-based approaches.

Furthermore, *in silico* methods are well established in classical computer-aided drug design for virtual screening or compound optimization. Therefore, a large body of experience exists for these technologies. In virtual screening, for example, hit rates of 30–40% are certainly at the absolute higher end of what can be achieved. While some of the examples described herein indeed reveal a promising confirmation rate for suggested target hypotheses, those are still far from being optimal. Hence, experimental confirmation remains an essential step, but *in silico* approaches allow the focusing of experimental resources to the most reasonable hypotheses. An obvious step is the analysis if the target hypothesis fits to the observed phenotype. Is the target in a biological pathway in line with the pharmacological effect? Therefore, the combination of cheminformatics with bioinformatics tools is a key element of *in silico* target identification.

Although computational methods will not typically be sufficient to securely identify the target, they are clearly mature enough to guide further experimental efforts for target identification.

References

1 Swinney, D.C. and Anthony, J. (2011). How were new medicines discovered? *Nat. Rev. Drug Discovery* 10 (7): 507–519.

2 Brown, D.G. and Boström, J. (2018). Where do recent small molecule clinical development candidates come from? *J. Med. Chem.* 61 (21): 9442–9468.

3 Hopkins, A.L. (2008). Network pharmacology: the next paradigm in drug discovery. *Nat. Chem. Biol.* 4 (11): 682–690.

4 Antolin, A.A., Workman, P., Mestres, J., and Al-Lazikani, B. (2016). Polypharmacology in precision oncology: current applications and future prospects. *Curr. Pharm. Des.* 22 (46): 6935–6945.

5 Lee, J.A. and Berg, E.L. (2013). Neoclassic drug discovery: the case for lead generation using phenotypic and functional approaches. *J. Biomol. Screen.* 18 (10): 1143–1155.

6 Moffat, J.G., Rudolph, J., and Bailey, D. (2014). Phenotypic screening in cancer drug discovery — past, present and future. *Nat. Rev. Drug Discovery* 13 (8): 588–602.

7 Moffat, J.G., Vincent, F., Lee, J.A. et al. (2017). Opportunities and challenges in phenotypic drug discovery: an industry perspective. *Nat. Rev. Drug Discovery* 16 (8): 531–543.

8 Swinney, D.C. (2013). Phenotypic vs. target-based drug discovery for first-in-class medicines. *Clin. Pharmacol. Ther.* 93 (4): 299–301.

9 Heilker, R., Lessel, U., and Bischoff, D. (2019). The power of combining phenotypic and target-focused drug discovery. *Drug Discovery Today* 24 (2): 526–532.

10 Kubota, K., Funabashi, M., and Ogura, Y. (2019). Target deconvolution from phenotype-based drug discovery by using chemical proteomics approaches. *Biochim. Biophys. Acta, Proteins Proteomics* 1867 (1): 22–27.

11 Schirle, M. and Jenkins, J.L. (2016). Identifying compound efficacy targets in phenotypic drug discovery. *Drug Discovery Today* 21 (1): 82–89.

12 Chen, X., Yan, C.C., Zhang, X. et al. (2015). Drug–target interaction prediction: databases, web servers and computational models. *Briefings Bioinf.* 17 (4): 696–712.

13 Jenkins, J.L., Bender, A., and Davies, J.W. (2006). In silico target fishing: predicting biological targets from chemical structure. *Drug Discovery Today: Technol.* 3 (4): 413–421.

14 Katsila, T., Spyroulias, G.A., Patrinos, G.P., and Matsoukas, M.-T. (2016). Computational approaches in target identification and drug discovery. *Comput. Struct. Biotechnol. J.* 14: 177–184.

15 Koutsoukas, A., Simms, B., Kirchmair, J. et al. (2011). From in silico target prediction to multi-target drug design: current databases, methods and applications. *J. Proteomics* 74 (12): 2554–2574.

16 Lavecchia, A. and Cerchia, C. (2016). In silico methods to address polypharmacology: current status, applications and future perspectives. *Drug Discovery Today* 21 (2): 288–298.

17 Schmidt, F., Matter, H., Hessler, G., and Czich, A. (2014). Predictive in silico off-target profiling in drug discovery. *Future Med. Chem.* 6 (3): 295–317.

18 Chen, R., Liu, X., Jin, S. et al. (2018). Machine learning for drug-target interaction prediction. *Molecules* 23 (9): 2208–2223.

19 James, K. (2012). The evolution of quantitative drug design. In: *Drug Design Strategies: Quantitative Approaches*, Personal foreword (eds. D.J. Livingstone and A.M. Davis), 1–34. The Royal Society of Chemistry.

20 Pubchem project. http://pubchem.ncbi.nlm.nih.gov (last accessed 31 January 2019).

21 DrugBank. www.drugbank.ca (last accessed 02 February 2019).

22 Wishart, D.S., Feunang, Y.D., Guo, A.C. et al. (2017). DrugBank 5.0: a major update to the DrugBank database for 2018. *Nucleic Acids Res.* 46 (D1): D1074–D1082.

23 Evolvus. Liceptor. http://www.evolvus.com/Products/Databases/LiceptorDatabase.html (last accessed 31 January 2019).

24 Gaulton, A., Bellis, L.J., Bento, A.P. et al. (2012). ChEMBL: a large-scale bioactivity database for drug discovery. *Nucleic Acids Res.* 40 (D1): D1100–D1107.

25 Olah, M., Rad, R., Ostopovici, L. et al. (2007). WOMBAT and WOMBAT-PK: bioactive databases for lead and drug discovery. In: *Chemical Biology: From Small Molecules to Systems Biology and Drug Design* (eds. S.L. Schreiber, T.M. Kapoor and G. Wess), 760–786. Wiley-VCH.

26 GOSTAR. https://www.gostardb.com/gostar (last accessed 02 February 2019).

27 ReaxysMedChem. https://www.reaxys.com/#/search/quick (last accessed 02 February 2019).

28 Tiikkainen, P., Bellis, L., Light, Y., and Franke, L. (2013). Estimating error rates in bioactivity databases. *J. Chem. Inf. Model.* 53 (10): 2499–2505.

29 Tiikkainen, P. and Franke, L. (2012). Analysis of commercial and public bioactivity databases. *J. Chem. Inf. Model.* 52 (2): 319–326.

30 Oprea, T.I. and Tropsha, A. (2006). Target, chemical and bioactivity databases – integration is key. *Drug Discovery Today: Technol.* 3 (4): 357–365.

31 Williams, A.J. (2008). Public chemical compound databases. *Curr. Opin. Drug Discovery Dev.* 11 (3): 393–404.

32 Jones, L.H. and Bunnage, M.E. (2017). Applications of chemogenomic library screening in drug discovery. *Nat. Rev. Drug Discovery* 16 (4): 285.

33 Open PHACTS Discovery Platform. www.openphacts.org (last accessed 02 February 2019).

34 Ashburner, M., Ball, C.A., Blake, J.A. et al. (2000). Gene ontology: tool for the unification of biology. The Gene Ontology Consortium. *Nat. Genet.* 25 (1): 25–29.

35 The Gene Ontology Consortium (2019). The Gene Ontology Resource: 20 years and still GOing strong. *Nucleic Acids Res.* 47 (D1): D330–D338.

36 Digles, D., Zdrazil, B., Neefs, J.M. et al. (2016). Open PHACTS computational protocols for in silico target validation of cellular phenotypic screens: knowing the knowns. *MedChemComm* 7 (6): 1237–1244.

37 Seiler, K.P., George, G.A., Happ, M.P. et al. (2007). ChemBank : a small-molecule screening and cheminformatics resource database. *Nucleic Acids Res.* 36 (Suppl. 1): D351–D359.

38 Liu, X. and Campillos, M. (2014). Unveiling new biological relationships using shared hits of chemical screening assay pairs. *Bioinformatics* 30 (17): i579–i586.

39 Wassermann, A.M., Lounkine, E., Davies, J.W. et al. (2015). The opportunities of mining historical and collective data in drug discovery. *Drug Discovery Today* 20 (4): 422–434.

40 Polyakov, V.R., Moorcroft, N.D., and Drawid, A. (2014). Enrichment analysis for discovering biological associations in phenotypic screens. *J. Chem. Inf. Model.* 54 (2): 377–386.

41 Krejsa, C.M., Horvath, D., Rogalski, S.L. et al. (2003). Predicting ADME properties and side effects: the BioPrint approach. *Curr. Opin. Drug Discovery Dev.* 6 (4): 470–480.

42 Bornot, A., Blackett, C., Engkvist, O. et al. (2014). The role of historical bioactivity data in the deconvolution of phenotypic screens. *J. Biomol. Screen.* 19 (5): 696–706.

43 Kutchukian, P.S., Chang, C., Fox, S.J. et al. (2018). CHEMGENIE: integration of chemogenomics data for applications in chemical biology. *Drug Discovery Today* 23 (1): 151–160.

44 Kramer, C., Kalliokoski, T., Gedeck, P., and Vulpetti, A. (2012). The experimental uncertainty of heterogeneous public Ki data. *J. Med. Chem.* 55 (11): 5165–5173.

45 Wenlock, M.C. and Carlsson, L.A. (2015). How experimental errors influence drug metabolism and pharmacokinetic QSAR/QSPR models. *J. Chem. Inf. Model.* 55 (1): 125–134.

46 Nazaré, M., Will, D.W., Matter, H. et al. (2005). Probing the subpockets of factor Xa reveals two binding modes for inhibitors based on a 2-carboxyindole scaffold: a study combining structure-activity relationship and X-ray crystallography. *J. Med. Chem.* 48 (14): 4511–4525.

47 Nickel, J., Gohlke, B.-O., Erehman, J. et al. (2014). SuperPred: update on drug classification and target prediction. *Nucleic Acids Res.* 42 (Web Server issue): W26–W31.

48 SuperPred. http://prediction.charite.de (last accessed 31 January 2019).

49 Keiser, M.J., Roth, B.L., Armbruster, B.N. et al. (2007). Relating protein pharmacology by ligand chemistry. *Nat. Biotechnol.* 25 (2): 197–206.

50 SEA. http://sea.bkslab.org (last accessed 31 January 2019).

51 Bora, A., Edsgärd, D., Roque, F.S. et al. (2010). ChemProt: a disease chemical biology database. *Nucleic Acids Res.* 39 (Suppl. 1): D367–D372.

52 Gfeller, D., Grosdidier, A., Wirth, M. et al. (2014). SwissTargetPrediction: a web server for target prediction of bioactive small molecules. *Nucleic Acids Res.* 42 (Web Server issue): W32–W38.

53 Wang, L., Ma, C., Wipf, P. et al. (2013). TargetHunter: an in silico target identification tool for predicting therapeutic potential of small organic molecules based on chemogenomic database. *AAPS J.* 15 (2): 395–406.

54 Liu, X., Ouyang, S., Yu, B. et al. (2010). PharmMapper server: a web server for potential drug target identification using pharmacophore mapping approach. *Nucleic Acids Res.* 38 (Web Server issue): W609–W614.

55 Wang, X., Shen, Y., Wang, S. et al. (2017). PharmMapper 2017 update: a web server for potential drug target identification with a comprehensive target pharmacophore database. *Nucleic Acids Res.* 45 (W1): W356–W360.

56 Zhou, H., Cao, H., and Skolnick, J. (2018). FINDSITEcomb2.0: a new approach for virtual ligand screening of proteins and virtual target screening of biomolecules. *J. Chem. Inf. Model.* 58 (11): 2343–2354.

57 Liu, X., Vogt, I., Haque, T., and Campillos, M. (2013). HitPick: a web server for hit identification and target prediction of chemical screenings. *Bioinformatics* 29 (15): 1910–1912.

58 CSNAP (Chemical Similarity Network Analysis Pull-down) Web. https://services.mbi.ucla.edu/CSNAP/index.html (last accessed 31 January 2019).

59 Scaffold Hunter. http://scaffoldhunter.sourceforge.net (last accessed 31 February 2019).

60 PASS webserver. http://www.pharmaexpert.ru/passonline/index.php (last accessed 31 January 2019).

61 GUSAR webserver. http://www.pharmaexpert.ru/GUSAR/antitargets.html (last accessed 31 January 2019).

62 Laggner, C., Kokel, D., Setola, V. et al. (2011). Chemical informatics and target identification in a zebrafish phenotypic screen. *Nat. Chem. Biol.* 8 (2): 144–146.

63 Kremer, L., Schultz-Fademrecht, C., Baumann, M. et al. (2017). Discovery of a novel inhibitor of the hedgehog signaling pathway through cell-based compound discovery and target prediction. *Angew. Chem. Int. Ed.* 56 (42): 13021–13025.

64 Rollinger, J.M., Schuster, D., Danzl, B. et al. (2009). In silico target fishing for rationalized ligand discovery exemplified on constituents of Ruta graveolens. *Planta Med.* 75 (3): 195–204.

65 Reker, D., Perna, A.M., Rodrigues, T. et al. (2014). Revealing the macromolecular targets of complex natural products. *Nat. Chem.* 6 (12): 1072–1078.

66 Rodrigues, T., Reker, D., Kunze, J. et al. (2015). Revealing the macromolecular targets of fragment-like natural products. *Angew. Chem. Int. Ed.* 127 (36): 10662–10666.

67 Mestres, J., Seifert, S.A., and Oprea, T.I. (2011). Linking pharmacology to clinical reports: cyclobenzaprine and its possible association with serotonin syndrome. *Clin. Pharmacol. Ther.* 90 (5): 662–665.

68 Moneriz, C., Mestres, J., Bautista, J.M. et al. (2011). Multi-targeted activity of maslinic acid as an antimalarial natural compound. *FEBS J.* 278 (16): 2951–2961.

69 Gohlke, B.-O., Overkamp, T., Richter, A. et al. (2015). 2D and 3D similarity landscape analysis identifies PARP as a novel off-target for the drug Vatalanib. *BMC Bioinf.* 16 (1): 308.

70 Wetzel, S., Wilk, W., Chammaa, S. et al. (2010). A scaffold-tree-merging strategy for prospective bioactivity annotation of γ-pyrones. *Angew. Chem. Int. Ed.* 49 (21): 3666–3670.

71 Wassermann, A.M., Lounkine, E., Urban, L. et al. (2014). A screening pattern recognition method finds new and divergent targets for drugs and natural products. *ACS Chem. Biol.* 9 (7): 1622–1631.

72 Johnson, M.A. and Maggiora, G.M. (1990). *Concepts and Applications of Molecular Similarity*, 99–117. New York: Wiley.

73 Wawer, M., Lounkine, E., Wassermann, A.M., and Bajorath, J. (2010). Data structures and computational tools for the extraction of SAR information from large compound sets. *Drug Discovery Today* 15 (15): 630–639.

74 Willett, P., Barnard, J.M., and Downs, G.M. (1998). Chemical similarity searching. *J. Chem. Inf. Comput. Sci.* 38 (6): 983–996.

75 Hansch, C., Leo, A., and Hoekman, D. (1995). *Exploring QSAR: Fundamentals and Applications in Chemistry and Biology*. Washington, DC: American Chemical Society.

76 Matter, H. (1997). Selecting optimally diverse compounds from structure databases: a validation study of two-dimensional and three-dimensional molecular descriptors. *J. Med. Chem.* 40 (8): 1219–1229.

77 Nettles, J.H., Jenkins, J.L., Bender, A. et al. (2006). Bridging chemical and biological space: "target fishing" using 2D and 3D molecular descriptors. *J. Med. Chem.* 49 (23): 6802–6810.

78 Kubinyi, H. (1998). Similarity and dissimilarity: a medicinal chemist's view. In: *3D QSAR in Drug Design: Ligand-Protein Interactions and Molecular Similarity* (eds. H. Kubinyi, G. Folkers and Y.C. Martin), 225–252. Dordrecht: Springer Netherlands.

79 Bajorath, J., Peltason, L., Wawer, M. et al. (2009). Navigating structure–activity landscapes. *Drug Discovery Today* 14 (13): 698–705.

80 Maggiora, G.M. (2006). On outliers and activity cliffs–why QSAR often disappoints. *J. Chem. Inf. Model.* 46 (4): 1535–1535.

81 Martin, Y.C., Kofron, J.L., and Traphagen, L.M. (2002). Do structurally similar molecules have similar biological activity? *J. Med. Chem.* 45 (19): 4350–4358.

82 Muchmore, S.W., Debe, D.A., Metz, J.T. et al. (2008). Application of belief theory to similarity data fusion for use in analog searching and lead hopping. *J. Chem. Inf. Model.* 48 (5): 941–948.

83 Hecker, N., Ahmed, J., von Eichborn, J. et al. (2012). SuperTarget goes quantitative: update on drug-target interactions. *Nucleic Acids Res.* 40 (Database issue): D1113–D1117.

84 Liu, T., Lin, Y., Wen, X. et al. (2007). BindingDB: a web-accessible database of experimentally determined protein-ligand binding affinities. *Nucleic Acids Res.* 35 (Database issue): D198–D201.

85 Rogers, D. and Hahn, M. (2010). Extended-connectivity fingerprints. *J. Chem. Inf. Model.* 50 (5): 742–754.

86 Keiser, M.J., Setola, V., Irwin, J.J. et al. (2009). Predicting new molecular targets for known drugs. *Nature* 462 (7270): 175–181.

87 Lounkine, E., Keiser, M.J., Whitebread, S. et al. (2012). Large-scale prediction and testing of drug activity on side-effect targets. *Nature* 486 (7403): 361–367.

88 Lemieux, G.A., Keiser, M.J., Sassano, M.F. et al. (2013). In silico molecular comparisons of *C. elegans* and mammalian pharmacology identify distinct targets that regulate feeding. *PLoS Biol.* 11 (11): e1001712.

89 Irwin, J.J., Gaskins, G., Sterling, T. et al. (2018). Predicted biological activity of purchasable chemical space. *J. Chem. Inf. Model.* 58 (1): 148–164.

90 ZINC 15 database. https://zinc15.docking.org (last accessed 02 February 2019).

91 ZINC 15 predictions. https://zinc15.docking.org/predictions/home (last accessed 02 February 2019).

92 Wassermann, A.M., Lounkine, E., Hoepfner, D. et al. (2015). Dark chemical matter as a promising starting point for drug lead discovery. *Nat. Chem. Biol.* 11 (12): 958–966.

93 Kohonen, T. (1982). Self-organized formation of topologically correct feature maps. *Biol. Cybern.* 43 (1): 59–69.

94 Schneider, P. and Schneider, G. (2017). De-orphaning the marine natural product (±)-marinopyrrole A by computational target prediction and biochemical validation. *Chem. Commun.* 53 (14): 2272–2274.

95 Schneider, G., Neidhart, W., Giller, T., and Schmid, G. (1999). "Scaffold-hopping" by topological pharmacophore search: a contribution to virtual screening. *Angew. Chem. Int. Ed.* 38 (19): 2894–2896.

96 Gomez-Bougie, P., Dousset, C., Descamps, G. et al. (2018). The selectivity of Marinopyrrole A to induce apoptosis in $MCL1^{high}$ $BCL2^{low}$ expressing myeloma cells is related to its ability to impair protein translation. *Br. J. Haematol.* 180 (1): 157–159.

97 Schneider, P. and Schneider, G. (2017). A computational method for unveiling the target promiscuity of pharmacologically active compounds. *Angew. Chem. Int. Ed.* 56 (38): 11520–11524.

98 Schneider, P. and Schneider, G. (2018). Polypharmacological drug–target inference for chemogenomics. *Mol. Inf.* 37 (9–10): 1800050.

99 Reker, D., Rodrigues, T., Schneider, P., and Schneider, G. (2014). Identifying the macromolecular targets of de novo-designed chemical entities through self-organizing map consensus. *Proc. Natl. Acad. Sci. U.S.A.* 111 (11): 4067–4072.

100 Zheng, W. and Tropsha, A. (2000). Novel variable selection quantitative structure–property relationship approach based on the k-nearest-neighbor principle. *J. Chem. Inf. Comput. Sci.* 40 (1): 185–194.

101 Chemotargets SL. Clarity v3.0. https://www.chemotargets.com (last accessed 31 January 2019).

102 Wang, Y., Suzek, T., Zhang, J. et al. (2014). PubChem BioAssay: 2014 update. *Nucleic Acids Res.* 42 (Database issue): D1075–D1082.

103 Law, V., Knox, C., Djoumbou, Y. et al. (2014). DrugBank 4.0: shedding new light on drug metabolism. *Nucleic Acids Res.* 42 (Database issue): D1091–D1097.

104 Harmar, A.J., Hills, R.A., Rosser, E.M. et al. (2009). IUPHAR-DB: the IUPHAR database of G protein-coupled receptors and ion channels. *Nucleic Acids Res.* 37 (Database issue): D680–D685.

105 Gregori-Puigjane, E. and Mestres, J. (2008). A ligand-based approach to mining the chemogenomic space of drugs. *Comb. Chem. High Throughput Screen.* 11 (8): 669–676.

106 Gregori-Puigjané, E. and Mestres, J. (2006). SHED: shannon entropy descriptors from topological feature distributions. *J. Chem. Inf. Model.* 46 (4): 1615–1622.

107 Mestres, J., Martín-Couce, L., Gregori-Puigjané, E. et al. (2006). Ligand-based approach to in silico pharmacology: nuclear receptor profiling. *J. Chem. Inf. Model.* 46 (6): 2725–2736.

108 Vidal, D., Garcia-Serna, R., and Mestres, J. (2011). Ligand-based approaches to in silico pharmacology. In: *Chemoinformatics and Computational Chemical Biology* (ed. J. Bajorath), 489–502. Totowa, NJ: Humana Press.

109 Vidal, D. and Mestres, J. (2010). In silico receptorome screening of antipsychotic drugs. *Mol. Inf.* 29 (6–7): 543–551.

110 Antolín, A.A. and Mestres, J. (2018). Dual inhibitors of PARPs and ROCKs. *ACS Omega* 3 (10): 12707–12712.

111 Schuffenhauer, A., Floersheim, P., Acklin, P., and Jacoby, E. (2003). Similarity metrics for ligands reflecting the similarity of the target proteins. *J. Chem. Inf. Comput. Sci.* 43 (2): 391–405.

112 Hert, J., Keiser, M.J., Irwin, J.J. et al. (2008). Quantifying the relationships among drug classes. *J. Chem. Inf. Model.* 48 (4): 755–765.

113 Garcia-Serna, R. and Mestres, J. (2010). Anticipating drug side effects by comparative pharmacology AU - Garcia-Serna, Ricard. *Expert Opin. Drug Metab. Toxicol.* 6 (10): 1253–1263.

114 Antolín, A.A. and Mestres, J. (2015). Distant polypharmacology among MLP chemical probes. *ACS Chem. Biol.* 10 (2): 395–400.

115 Antolín, A.A., Jalencas, X., Yélamos, J., and Mestres, J. (2012). Identification of pim kinases as novel targets for PJ34 with confounding effects in PARP biology. *ACS Chem. Biol.* 7 (12): 1962–1967.

116 Lo, Y.-C., Senese, S., Li, C.-M. et al. (2015). Large-scale chemical similarity networks for target profiling of compounds identified in cell-based chemical screens. *PLoS Comput. Biol.* 11 (3): e1004153.

117 Günther, S., Kuhn, M., Dunkel, M. et al. (2008). SuperTarget and Matador: resources for exploring drug-target relationships. *Nucleic Acids Res.* 36 (Database issue): D919–D922.

118 Grant, J.A., Gallardo, M.A., and Pickup, B.T. (1996). A fast method of molecular shape comparison: a simple application of a Gaussian description of molecular shape. *J. Comput. Chem.* 17 (14): 1653–1666.

119 Grant, J.A. and Pickup, B.T. (1995). A Gaussian description of molecular shape. *J. Phys. Chem.* 99 (11): 3503–3510.

120 Hawkins, P.C.D., Skillman, A.G., and Nicholls, A. (2007). Comparison of shape-matching and docking as virtual screening tools. *J. Med. Chem.* 50 (1): 74–82.

121 AbdulHameed, M.D.M., Chaudhury, S., Singh, N. et al. (2012). Exploring polypharmacology using a ROCS-based target fishing approach. *J. Chem. Inf. Model.* 52 (2): 492–505.

122 Huang, N., Shoichet, B.K., and Irwin, J.J. (2006). Benchmarking sets for molecular docking. *J. Med. Chem.* 49 (23): 6789–6801.

123 Lo, Y.-C., Senese, S., Damoiseaux, R., and Torres, J.Z. (2016). 3D chemical similarity networks for structure-based target prediction and scaffold hopping. *ACS Chem. Biol.* 11 (8): 2244–2253.

124 Silicos IT. http://silicos-it.be.s3-website-eu-west-1.amazonaws.com/index.html (last accessed 19 February 2019).

125 Taminau, J., Thijs, G., and De Winter, H. (2008). Pharao: pharmacophore alignment and optimization. *J. Mol. Graph. Model.* 27 (2): 161–169.

126 OpenEye Scientific (2015). Webinar: subROCS: A Gold Standard in Molecular Alignment. https://www.eyesopen.com/news/webinars/2015/05/subrocs-gold-standard-molecular-alignment (last accessed 12 February 2019).

127 Wermuth, C.G., Ganellin, C.R., Lindberg, P., and Mitscher, L.A. (1998). Glossary of terms used in medicinal chemistry (IUPAC Recommendations 1998). *Pure Appl. Chem.* 70: 1129.

128 Langer, T. (2010). Pharmacophores in drug research. *Mol. Inf.* 29 (6–7): 470–475.

129 Leach, A.R., Gillet, V.J., Lewis, R.A., and Taylor, R. (2010). Three-dimensional pharmacophore methods in drug discovery. *J. Med. Chem.* 53 (2): 539–558.

130 Lu, X., Yang, H., Chen, Y. et al. (2018). The development of pharmacophore modeling: generation and recent applications in drug discovery. *Curr. Pharm. Des.* 24 (29): 3424–3439.

131 Gaurav, A. and Gautam, V. (2014). Structure-based three-dimensional pharmacophores as an alternative to traditional methodologies. *J. Recept. Ligand Channel Res.* 2014 (7): 27–38.
132 Steindl, T.M., Schuster, D., Laggner, C., and Langer, T. (2006). Parallel screening: a novel concept in pharmacophore modeling and virtual screening. *J. Chem. Inf. Model.* 46 (5): 2146–2157.
133 Steindl, T.M., Schuster, D., Wolber, G. et al. (2006). High-throughput structure-based pharmacophore modelling as a basis for successful parallel virtual screening. *J. Comput.-Aided Mol. Des.* 20 (12): 703–715.
134 Inteligand. www.inteligand.com (last access 03 February 2019).
135 Biovia. https://www.3ds.com/products-services/biovia (last accessed 31 January 2019).
136 Desaphy, J., Bret, G., Rognan, D., and Kellenberger, E. (2014). sc-PDB: a 3D-database of ligandable binding sites—10 years on. *Nucleic Acids Res.* 43 (D1): D399–D404.
137 sc-PDB. http://bioinfo-pharma.u-strasbg.fr/scPDB (last accessed 03 February 2019).
138 RCSB PDB database. www.rcsb.org (last accessed 03 February 2019).
139 Brand, S., Roy, S., Schröder, P. et al. (2018). Combined proteomic and in silico target identification reveal a role for 5-lipoxygenase in developmental signaling pathways. *Cell Chem. Biol.* 25 (9): 1095–1106.e23.
140 Rodrigues, T., Sieglitz, F., Somovilla, V.J. et al. (2016). Unveiling (−)-englerin A as a modulator of L-type calcium channels. *Angew. Chem. Int. Ed.* 128 (37): 11243–11247.
141 Schneider, G., Reker, D., Chen, T. et al. (2016). Deorphaning the macromolecular targets of the natural anticancer compound doliculide. *Angew. Chem. Int. Ed.* 128 (40): 12596–12599.
142 Schuffenhauer, A., Ertl, P., Roggo, S. et al. (2007). The scaffold tree – visualization of the scaffold universe by hierarchical scaffold classification. *J. Chem. Inf. Model.* 47 (1): 47–58.
143 Renner, S., van Otterlo, W.A.L., Dominguez Seoane, M. et al. (2009). Bioactivity-guided mapping and navigation of chemical space. *Nat. Chem. Biol.* 5 (8): 585–592.
144 Wetzel, S., Klein, K., Renner, S. et al. (2009). Interactive exploration of chemical space with Scaffold Hunter. *Nat. Chem. Biol.* 5 (8): 581–583.
145 Schäfer, T., Kriege, N., Humbeck, L. et al. (2017). Scaffold Hunter: a comprehensive visual analytics framework for drug discovery. *J. Cheminf.* 9 (1): 28.
146 Hsu, K.-H., Su, B.-H., Tu, Y.-S. et al. (2016). Mutagenicity in a molecule: identification of core structural features of mutagenicity using a scaffold analysis. *PLoS One* 11 (2): e0148900.
147 Yongye, A.B. and Medina-Franco, J.L. (2013). Toward an efficient approach to identify molecular scaffolds possessing selective or promiscuous compounds. *Chem. Biol. Drug Des.* 82 (4): 367–375.
148 Varin, T., Gubler, H., Parker, C.N. et al. (2010). Compound set enrichment: a novel approach to analysis of primary HTS data. *J. Chem. Inf. Model.* 50 (12): 2067–2078.

149 Varin, T., Schuffenhauer, A., Ertl, P., and Renner, S. (2011). Mining for bioactive scaffolds with scaffold networks: improved compound set enrichment from primary screening data. *J. Chem. Inf. Model.* 51 (7): 1528–1538.

150 van Hattum, H. and Waldmann, H. (2014). Biology-oriented synthesis: harnessing the power of evolution. *J. Am. Chem. Soc.* 136 (34): 11853–11859.

151 Lo, Y.-C., Rensi, S.E., Torng, W., and Altman, R.B. (2018). Machine learning in chemoinformatics and drug discovery. *Drug Discovery Today* 23 (8): 1538–1546.

152 Wold, S., Albano, C., Dunn, W.J. et al. (1984). Multivariate data analysis in chemistry. In: *Chemometrics: Mathematics and Statistics in Chemistry* (ed. B.R. Kowalski), 17–95. Dordrecht: Springer Netherlands.

153 Dunn, W.J. III,, Wold, S., Edlund, U. et al. (1984). Multivariate structure-activity relationships between data from a battery of biological tests and an ensemble of structure descriptors: the PLS method. *Quant. Struct.-Act. Relat.* 3 (4): 131–137.

154 Cortes, C. and Vapnik, V. (1995). Support-vector networks. *Mach. Learn.* 20 (3): 273–297.

155 Chen, B., Sheridan, R.P., Hornak, V., and Voigt, J.H. (2012). Comparison of random forest and Pipeline Pilot Naïve Bayes in prospective QSAR predictions. *J. Chem. Inf. Model.* 52 (3): 792–803.

156 Svetnik, V., Liaw, A., Tong, C. et al. (2003). Random forest: a classification and regression tool for compound classification and QSAR modeling. *J. Chem. Inf. Comput. Sci.* 43 (6): 1947–1958.

157 LeCun, Y., Bengio, Y., and Hinton, G. (2015). Deep learning. *Nature* 521 (7553): 436–444.

158 Schmidhuber, J. (2015). Deep learning in neural networks: an overview. *Neural Netw.* 61: 85–117.

159 Mayr, A., Klambauer, G., Unterthiner, T. et al. (2018). Large-scale comparison of machine learning methods for drug target prediction on ChEMBL. *Chem. Sci.* 9 (24): 5441–5451.

160 Murtazalieva, K.A., Druzhilovskiy, D.S., Goel, R.K. et al. (2017). How good are publicly available web services that predict bioactivity profiles for drug repurposing? *SAR QSAR Environ. Res.* 28 (10): 843–862.

161 Lagunin, A., Stepanchikova, A., Filimonov, D., and Poroikov, V. (2000). PASS: Prediction of activity spectra for biologically active substances. *Bioinformatics* 16 (8): 747–748.

162 Zakharov, A.V., Lagunin, A.A., Filimonov, D.A., and Poroikov, V.V. (2012). Quantitative prediction of antitarget interaction profiles for chemical compounds. *Chem. Res. Toxicol.* 25 (11): 2378–2385.

163 Pogodin, P.V., Lagunin, A.A., Filimonov, D.A., and Poroikov, V.V. (2015). PASS targets: ligand-based multi-target computational system based on a public data and naïve Bayes approach. *SAR QSAR Environ. Res.* 26 (10): 783–793.

164 Awale, M. and Reymond, J.-L. (2019). Polypharmacology browser PPB2: target prediction combining nearest neighbors with machine learning. *J. Chem. Inf. Model.* 59 (1): 10–17.

165 Simonin, C., Awale, M., Brand, M. et al. (2015). Optimization of TRPV6 calcium channel inhibitors using a 3D ligand-based virtual screening method. *Angew. Chem. Int. Ed.* 54 (49): 14748–14752.
166 PPB2. ppb2.gdb.tools (last accessed 11 February 2019).
167 Xia, X., Maliski, E.G., Gallant, P., and Rogers, D. (2004). Classification of kinase inhibitors using a Bayesian model. *J. Med. Chem.* 47 (18): 4463–4470.
168 Bender, A. (2011). Bayesian methods in virtual screening and chemical biology. In: *Chemoinformatics and Computational Chemical Biology* (ed. J. Bajorath), 175–196. Totowa, NJ: Humana Press.
169 Bender, A., Jenkins, J.L., Glick, M. et al. (2006). "Bayes affinity fingerprints" improve retrieval rates in virtual screening and define orthogonal bioactivity space: when are multitarget drugs a feasible concept? *J. Chem. Inf. Model.* 46 (6): 2445–2456.
170 Kauvar, L.M., Higgins, D.L., Villar, H.O. et al. (1995). Predicting ligand binding to proteins by affinity fingerprinting. *Chem. Biol.* 2 (2): 107–118.
171 Martin, E., Mukherjee, P., Sullivan, D., and Jansen, J. (2011). Profile-QSAR: a novel meta-QSAR method that combines activities across the kinase family to accurately predict affinity, selectivity, and cellular activity. *J. Chem. Inf. Model.* 51 (8): 1942–1956.
172 Martin, E. and Mukherjee, P. (2012). Kinase-kernel models: accurate in silico screening of 4 million compounds across the entire human kinome. *J. Chem. Inf. Model.* 52 (1): 156–170.
173 Mukherjee, P. and Martin, E. (2012). Profile-QSAR and Surrogate AutoShim protein-family modeling of proteases. *J. Chem. Inf. Model.* 52 (9): 2430–2440.
174 Martin, E.J., Polyakov, V.R., Tian, L., and Perez, R.C. (2017). Profile-QSAR 2.0: kinase virtual screening accuracy comparable to four-concentration IC_{50}s for realistically novel compounds. *J. Chem. Inf. Model.* 57 (8): 2077–2088.
175 Martin, E.J., Polyakov, V., and Tian, L. (2017). Deep learning profile-QSAR 2.0 IC_{50} predictions as accurate as 4-pt IC_{50}s: applications to polypharmacology; Abstracts of Papers of The American Chemical Society, 253
176 Merget, B., Turk, S., Eid, S. et al. (2017). Profiling prediction of kinase inhibitors: toward the virtual assay. *J. Med. Chem.* 60 (1): 474–485.
177 Baringhaus, K.H., Hessler, G., Matter, H., and Schmidt, F. (2013). Development and applications of global ADMET models. In: *Chemoinformatics for Drug Discovery* (ed. J. Bajorath), 245–265. Hoboken, NJ: Wiley.
178 Aha, D.W., Kibler, D., and Albert, M.K. (1991). Instance-based learning algorithms. *Mach. Learn.* 6 (1): 37–66.
179 Quinlan, R. (1998). Learning with continuous classes. Proceedings of Australian Joint Conference on Artificial Intelligence.
180 Data Mining with Cubist. RuleQuest Research Pty Ltd. Computer software: https://www.rulequest.com/cubist-info.html.
181 Matter, H., Anger, L.T., Giegerich, C. et al. (2012). Development of in silico filters to predict activation of the pregnane X receptor (PXR) by structurally diverse drug-like molecules. *Bioorg. Med. Chem.* 20 (18): 5352–5365.
182 Butina, D. and Gola, J.M.R. (2003). Modeling aqueous solubility. *J. Chem. Inf. Comput. Sci.* 43 (3): 837–841.

183 Sheridan, R.P., Feuston, B.P., Maiorov, V.N., and Kearsley, S.K. (2004). Similarity to molecules in the training set is a good discriminator for prediction accuracy in QSAR. *J. Chem. Inf. Comput. Sci.* 44 (6): 1912–1928.

184 Certara (2018). UNITY Chemical Information Software. St. Lous, MO.

185 Rasmussen, C.E. and Williams, C.K.I. (2006). Gaussian processes for machine learning. In: *Adaptive Computation and Machine Learning* (ed. T. Dietterich). Cambridge, MA: MIT Press.

186 Obrezanova, O., Csányi, G., Gola, J.M.R., and Segall, M.D. (2007). Gaussian processes: a method for automatic QSAR modeling of ADME properties. *J. Chem. Inf. Model.* 47 (5): 1847–1857.

187 Reutlinger, M., Rodrigues, T., Schneider, P., and Schneider, G. (2014). Combining on-chip synthesis of a focused combinatorial library with computational target prediction reveals imidazopyridine GPCR ligands. *Angew. Chem. Int. Ed.* 53 (2): 582–585.

188 Bieler, M., Reutlinger, M., Rodrigues, T. et al. (2016). Designing multi-target compound libraries with Gaussian process models. *Mol. Inf.* 35 (5): 192–198.

189 Ma, J., Sheridan, R.P., Liaw, A. et al. (2015). Deep neural nets as a method for quantitative structure–activity relationships. *J. Chem. Inf. Model.* 55 (2): 263–274.

190 Mayr, A., Klambauer, G., Unterthiner, T., and Hochreiter, S. (2016). DeepTox: toxicity prediction using deep learning. *Front. Environ. Sci.* 3: 80.

191 Wenzel, J., Matter, H., and Schmidt, F. (2019). Predictive multitask deep neural network models for ADME-tox properties: learning from large data sets. *J. Chem. Inf. Model.* https://doi.org/10.1021/acs.jcim.8b00785 53 (3): 1253–1268.

192 Bosc, N., Wroblowski, B., Meyer, C., and Bonnet, P. (2017). Prediction of protein kinase–ligand interactions through 2.5D kinochemometrics. *J. Chem. Inf. Model.* 57 (1): 93–101.

193 Öztürk, H., Özgür, A., and Ozkirimli, E. (2018). DeepDTA: deep drug-target binding affinity prediction. *Bioinformatics* 34 (17): i821–i829.

194 Feng, Q., Dueva, E., Cherkasov, A., and Ester, M. (2018). PADME: A Deep Learning-based Framework for Drug-Target Interaction Prediction. *arXiv:1807.09741.*

195 Gao, K.Y., Fokoue, A., Luo, H. et al. (2018). Interpretable drug target prediction using deep neural representation. Proceedings of the 27th International Joint Conference on Artificial Intelligence, p. 3371–3377.

196 Petrone, P.M., Simms, B., Nigsch, F. et al. (2012). Rethinking molecular similarity: comparing compounds on the basis of biological activity. *ACS Chem. Biol.* 7 (8): 1399–1409.

197 Cortes Cabrera, A. and Petrone, P.M. (2018). Optimal HTS fingerprint definitions by using a desirability function and a genetic algorithm. *J. Chem. Inf. Model.* 58 (3): 641–646.

198 Riniker, S., Wang, Y., Jenkins, J.L., and Landrum, G.A. (2014). Using information from historical high-throughput screens to predict active compounds. *J. Chem. Inf. Model.* 54 (7): 1880–1891.

199 Sturm, N., Sun, J., Vandriessche, Y. et al. (2018). Application of bioactivity profile-based fingerprints for building machine learning models. https://doi.org/10.26434/chemrxiv.6969584.v1.

200 Cortes Cabrera, A., Lucena-Agell, D., Redondo-Horcajo, M. et al. (2016). Aggregated compound biological signatures facilitate phenotypic drug discovery and target elucidation. *ACS Chem. Biol.* 11 (11): 3024–3034.

201 De Wolf, H., Cougnaud, L., Van Hoorde, K. et al. (2018). High-throughput gene expression profiles to define drug similarity and predict compound activity. *Assay Drug Dev. Tech.* 16 (3): 162–176.

202 Subramanian, A., Narayan, R., Corsello, S.M. et al. (2017). A next generation connectivity map: L1000 platform and the first 1,000,000 profiles. *Cell* 171 (6): 1437–1452.e17.

203 Simm, J., Klambauer, G., Arany, A. et al. (2018). Repurposing high-throughput image assays enables biological activity prediction for drug discovery. *Cell Chem. Biol.* 25 (5): 611–618.e3.

204 Gustafsdottir, S.M., Ljosa, V., Sokolnicki, K.L. et al. (2013). Multiplex cytological profiling assay to measure diverse cellular states. *PLoS One* 8 (12): e80999.

205 Simm, J., Arany, A., Zakeri, P. et al. (2015). Macau: Scalable Bayesian Multi-Relational Factorization with Side Information using MCMC. https://arxiv.org/abs/1509.04610v2.

206 Rodrigues, T., Reker, D., Welin, M. et al. (2015). De novo fragment design for drug discovery and chemical biology. *Angew. Chem. Int. Ed.* 54 (50): 15079–15083.

207 Artis, D.R., Lin, J.J., Zhang, C. et al. (2009). Scaffold-based discovery of indeglitazar, a PPAR pan-active anti-diabetic agent. *Proc. Natl. Acad. Sci. U.S.A.* 106 (1): 262–267.

208 Byrne, R. and Schneider, G. (2019). In silico target prediction for small molecules. In: *Systems Chemical Biology: Methods and Protocols* (eds. S. Ziegler and H. Waldmann), 273–309. New York: Springer.

209 Huang, H., Zhang, G., Zhou, Y. et al. (2018). Reverse screening methods to search for the protein targets of chemopreventive compounds. *Front. Chem.* 6 (138): 1–28.

210 Somody, J.C., MacKinnon, S.S., and Windemuth, A. (2017). Structural coverage of the proteome for pharmaceutical applications. *Drug Discovery Today* 22 (12): 1792–1799.

211 Sturm, N., Desaphy, J., Quinn, R.J. et al. (2012). Structural insights into the molecular basis of the ligand promiscuity. *J. Chem. Inf. Model.* 52 (9): 2410–2421.

212 Patel, H., Lucas, X., Bendik, I. et al. (2015). Target fishing by cross-docking to explain polypharmacological effects. *ChemMedChem* 10 (7): 1209–1217.

213 Warren, G.L., Do, T.D., Kelley, B.P. et al. (2012). Essential considerations for using protein–ligand structures in drug discovery. *Drug Discovery Today* 17 (23): 1270–1281.

214 Ilatovskiy, A.V., Kufareva, I., and Abagyan, R. (2011). Pocketome: an encyclopedia of small-molecule binding sites in 4D. *Nucleic Acids Res.* 40 (D1): D535–D540.

215 PockeTome. http://ablab.ucsd.edu/POCKETOME (last accessed 12 February 2019).

216 Bhagavat, R., Sankar, S., Srinivasan, N., and Chandra, N. (2018). An augmented pocketome: detection and analysis of small-molecule binding pockets in proteins of known 3D structure. *Structure* 26 (3): 499–512.e2.

217 Schomburg, K.T., Bietz, S., Briem, H. et al. (2014). Facing the challenges of structure-based target prediction by inverse virtual screening. *J. Chem. Inf. Model.* 54 (6): 1676–1686.

218 Kim, S.S., Aprahamian, M.L., and Lindert, S. (2019). Improving inverse docking target identification with Z-score selection. *Chem. Biol. Drug Des.* 0 (0): 1–12.

219 Zhang, H., Li, H., Jiang, H. et al. (2006). TarFisDock: a web server for identifying drug targets with docking approach. *Nucleic Acids Res.* 34 (Suppl. 2): W219–W224.

220 Peragovics, Á., Simon, Z., Brandhuber, I. et al. (2012). Contribution of 2D and 3D structural features of drug molecules in the prediction of drug profile matching. *J. Chem. Inf. Model.* 52 (7): 1733–1744.

221 Simon, Z., Peragovics, Á., Vigh-Smeller, M. et al. (2012). Drug effect prediction by polypharmacology-based interaction profiling. *J. Chem. Inf. Model.* 52 (1): 134–145.

222 Végner, L., Peragovics, Á., Tombor, L. et al. (2013). Experimental confirmation of new drug–target interactions predicted by drug profile matching. *J. Med. Chem.* 56 (21): 8377–8388.

223 Srinivasan, B., Zhou, H., Kubanek, J., and Skolnick, J. (2014). Experimental validation of FINDSITE(comb) virtual ligand screening results for eight proteins yields novel nanomolar and micromolar binders. *J. Cheminf.* 6: 16.

224 Dai, Y.-F. and Zhao, X.-M. (2015). A survey on the computational approaches to identify drug targets in the postgenomic era. *BioMed Res. Int.* 2015: 1–9.

225 Pan, Y., Cheng, T., Wang, Y., and Bryant, S.H. (2014). Pathway analysis for drug repositioning based on public database mining. *J. Chem. Inf. Model.* 54 (2): 407–418.

226 Gehlenborg, N., O'Donoghue, S.I., Baliga, N.S. et al. (2010). Visualization of omics data for systems biology. *Nat. Methods* 7 (3s): S56–S68.

227 Smoot, M.E., Ono, K., Ruscheinski, J. et al. (2011). Cytoscape 2.8: new features for data integration and network visualization. *Bioinformatics (Oxford, England)* 27 (3): 431–432.

228 Cytoscape. http://www.cytoscape.org (last accessed 31 January 2019).

229 Fechner, N., Papadatos, G., Evans, D. et al. (2012). ChEMBLSpace—a graphical explorer of the chemogenomic space covered by the ChEMBL database. *Bioinformatics* 29 (4): 523–524.

230 Wang, J.L., Limburg, D., Graneto, M.J. et al. (2010). The novel benzopyran class of selective cyclooxygenase-2 inhibitors. Part 2: The second clinical candidate having a shorter and favorable human half-life. *Bioorg. Med. Chem. Lett.* 20 (23): 7159–7163.

231 Szklarczyk, D., Santos, A., von Mering, C. et al. (2016). STITCH 5: augmenting protein-chemical interaction networks with tissue and affinity data. *Nucleic Acids Res.* 44 (D1): D380–D384.
232 STITCH. http://stitch.embl.de (last accessed 31 January 2019).
233 Yıldırım, M.A., Goh, K.-I., Cusick, M.E. et al. (2007). Drug—target network. *Nat. Biotechnol.* 25: 1119–1126.
234 Yao, L. and Rzhetsky, A. (2008). Quantitative systems-level determinants of human genes targeted by successful drugs. *Genome Res.* 18 (2): 206–213.
235 Zhao, S. and Li, S. (2010). Network-based relating pharmacological and genomic spaces for drug target identification. *PLoS One* 5 (7): e11764.
236 Knight, Z.A., Lin, H., and Shokat, K.M. (2010). Targeting the cancer kinome through polypharmacology. *Nat. Rev. Cancer* 10 (2): 130–137.
237 Achenbach, J., Tiikkainen, P., Franke, L., and Proschak, E. (2011). Computational tools for polypharmacology and repurposing. *Future Med. Chem.* 3 (8): 961–968.
238 Xie, L., Evangelidis, T., Xie, L., and Bourne, P.E. (2011). Drug discovery using chemical systems biology: weak inhibition of multiple kinases may contribute to the anti-cancer effect of nelfinavir. *PLoS Comput. Biol.* 7 (4): e1002037.
239 Azmi, A.S. (2012). Network pharmacology for cancer drug discovery: are we there yet? *Future Med. Chem.* 4 (8): 939–941.
240 Campillos, M., Kuhn, M., Gavin, A.-C. et al. (2008). Drug target identification using side-effect similarity. *Science* 321 (5886): 263–266.
241 Kuhn, M., Campillos, M., González, P. et al. (2008). Large-scale prediction of drug–target relationships. *FEBS Lett.* 582 (8): 1283–1290.
242 Kuhn, M., Campillos, M., Letunic, I. et al. (2010). A side effect resource to capture phenotypic effects of drugs. *Mol. Syst. Biol.* 6: 343–343.
243 Kuhn, M., Letunic, I., Jensen, L.J., and Bork, P. (2015). The SIDER database of drugs and side effects. *Nucleic Acids Res.* 44 (D1): D1075–D1079.
244 Mervin, L.H., Afzal, A.M., Drakakis, G. et al. (2015). Target prediction utilising negative bioactivity data covering large chemical space. *J. Cheminf.* 7: 51–51.
245 Sheridan, R.P. (2013). Time-split cross-validation as a method for estimating the goodness of prospective prediction. *J. Chem. Inf. Model.* 53 (4): 783–790.
246 Ripphausen, P., Stumpfe, D., and Bajorath, J. (2012). Analysis of structure-based virtual screening studies and characterization of identified active compounds. *Future Med. Chem.* 4 (5): 603–613.

11

Bioinformatic Approaches in the Understanding of Mechanism of Action (MoA)

Maria-Anna Trapotsi[1], *Ian Barrett*[2], *Ola Engkvist*[3], *and Andreas Bender*[1]

[1] *University of Cambridge, Centre for Molecular Informatics, Department of Chemistry, Lensfield Road, Cambridge CB2 1EW, UK*
[2] *AstraZeneca, Quantitative Biology, Discovery Sciences, Darwin Building 310, Cambridge Science Park, Milton Road, Cambridge, CB4 0WG, UK*
[3] *AstraZeneca, Hit Discovery, Discovery Sciences, Pepparedsleden 1, Gothenburg, SE-43183 Mölndal, Sweden*

11.1 Bioinformatics: Introduction

Bioinformatics is nowadays an established field in the area of drug discovery and development. It has facilitated and accelerated processes such as drug target identification, drug candidate screening and optimization and has also contributed to the characterization of side effects, adverse effects, and drug resistance [1]. Bioinformatics can be considered as an interdisciplinary or hybrid science because it merges the use of biological data with other sciences such as statistics, mathematics, and computer science. The increasing data deposition of high-throughput data in databases in combination with the advances in machine learning techniques has significantly influenced the field of bioinformatics and the drug discovery process [2].

Different types of high-throughput data are used in the field of bioinformatics including genomics, transcriptomics, proteomics, image-based data and others, which contribute to the drug discovery process. Key contributions of bioinformatics to drug discovery include the understanding of connections between diseases and their genetic background, the identification of drug targets that restore the normal cellular function, and the understanding of mechanism of action (MoA) and/or prediction of compounds that are active towards targets (target prediction). In this chapter, we will focus on the third objective and on three different high-throughput data (transcriptomic, pathway, and image-based data), which are shown in Figure 11.1.

In this section, key concepts will be explained. The first is the concept of mechanism versus mode of action, then the concept of target prediction, and finally the use of multilevel information in MoA and target prediction studies.

11.1.1 Some Definitions: Mechanism Versus Mode of Action

A principal challenge in the drug discovery process is the development of therapeutic compounds and the understanding of the mechanism by which they exert

Target Discovery and Validation: Methods and Strategies for Drug Discovery,
First Edition. Edited by Alleyn T. Plowright.

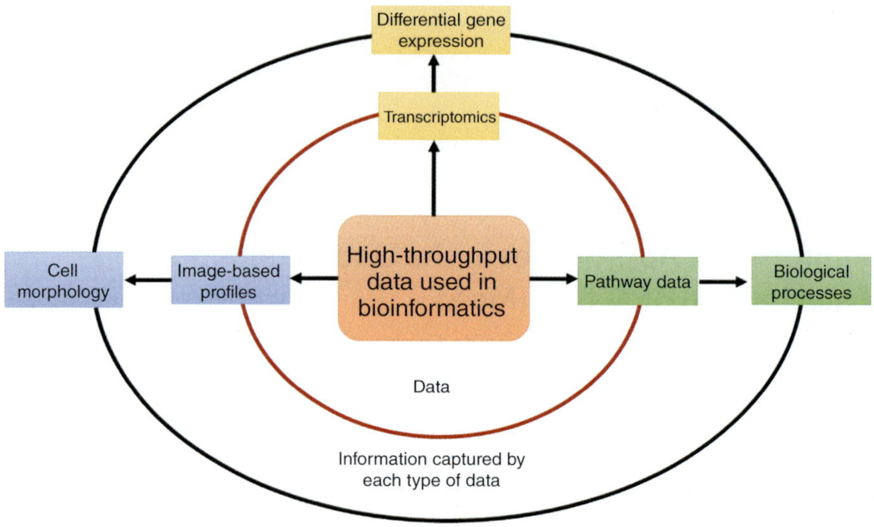

Figure 11.1 The three types of high-throughput data and their biological significance that will be reviewed in this chapter.

their pharmacological effect. When a compound perturbs a biological system, it causes physical, chemical, and functional changes by interacting with different types of biomolecules and biochemical pathways [3, 4]. These changes aim to restore dysfunctions in the human biological system, which are caused by a disease [5]. To better discern how a dysfunction can be restored, it is very important to firstly understand the effect that a compound/drug has on a biological system and secondly to understand how this effect is caused by the biochemical interactions. These two concepts are known as mode of action and MoA and have a different biological interpretation.

The difference between the MoA and mode of action is that the MoA refers to the biological response upon drug administration due to the interaction of the molecule with a specific protein target or targets and it refers to the functional changes on a molecular level [6]. On the other hand, the term mode of action refers to the changes that are observed on a cellular level upon compound administration. These two terms are usually used interchangeably and typically refer to the way by which a drug interacts and produces an effect.

11.1.2 Importance of MoA and Target Prediction in the Drug Discovery Process

The early phases of the drug discovery process often involve the identification of relevant biologically active compounds by performing either phenotypic-based or molecular target-based screening of a molecular library [7]. In both cases the understanding of MoA of hit compounds is important. Briefly, molecular target-based screening is also referred to as 'reverse chemical genetics' [8], and it starts with a known and validated target of a disease. A high-throughput screening (HTS) campaign of chemical libraries is performed to identify binders of the targets to modulate the target in the appropriate fashion [7, 8]. On the other hand, phenotypic screening is also referred to as 'forward chemical genetics' [8]. Compounds are screened in the phenotypic assay to identify those compounds that elicit a response in organs, model organisms, and/or cells relevant to the disease in question [9] and where the response is expected to be therapeutically beneficial. Both screening methods exhibit advantages and limitations, and usually the choice of screening method depends on the disease investigated [10], and in both cases knowledge of compounds' MoA is important.

A method to better understand compound's MoA is to identify the target or targets that it binds to, and that knowledge can facilitate the drug discovery process. Poor target validation and subsequent molecular target-based screening against that target has been linked with high attrition rates in phase II and phase III clinical trials [11]. The underlying reason is that the efficacy of the compounds and their off-target effects are not fully understood until the later stages of drug discovery [6]. An analysis of the factors that contribute to the failure of drugs in phase II and phase III clinical trials highlighted insufficient drug efficacy as the foremost reason of failure [12]. Hence, knowledge of the MoA of a compound could provide an early warning of the efficacy and potential off-target effects, which might be a problem in clinical trials. Phenotypic screening is another hit identification strategy employed in current drug discovery [9]. It provides an understanding of the effect that the screened compound has on complex biological systems. However, it does not consider the information of the biological target. One significant shortcoming of phenotypic screening is the lack of knowledge of the precise MoA. Drugs can be approved by the FDA without the exact knowledge of the MoA and/or molecular target, as long as they are safe and efficacious [13]. However, the deconvolution and understanding of MoA can benefit the design of improved and next-generation compounds, reduce their side and adverse effects, and allow more targeted and precise patient stratification in clinical trials [7].

Although the identification of the MoA and the molecular target of a compound is a key hurdle in the drug discovery process [14], the *a priori* knowledge of a compound's MoA can facilitate and accelerate drug discovery and inform on potential off-target effects. Hence, it is significant to know the mechanism through which a drug exerts its pharmacological effect as this information can pave the way for the development of a therapeutic drug with well-known on- and off-target effects.

11.1.3 Different Levels of Information in Mechanism of Action and Target Prediction

Target prediction is considered as one method to understand the MoA of a compound, and usually computational methods are used to infer protein targets of compounds. The MoA has been extensively investigated on a protein target level by predicting targets based on bioactivity data [15] with the ultimate goal to elucidate the MoA of drugs and possible off-target effects [16]. The rationale behind these methods relies on the assumption that structurally similar compounds are more likely to exhibit similar properties [17]. However, the premise is not always

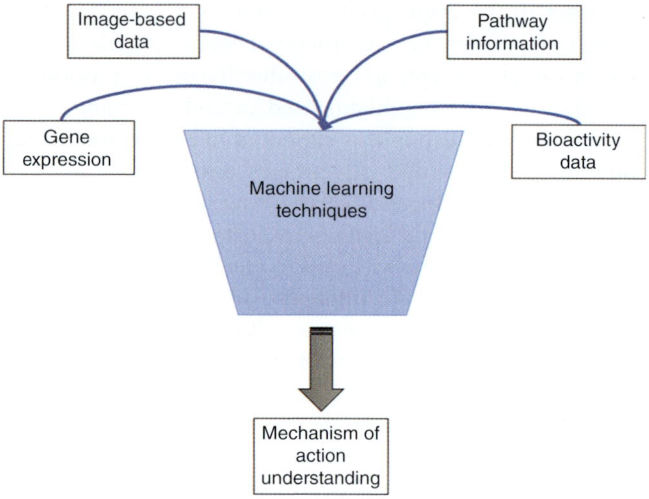

Figure 11.2 Use of different levels of information to better understand compounds' MoA.

valid because of the complex biological processes [18] that occur during a biological dysfunction (i.e. disease) and also because compounds exhibit a broad range of activity that could be beyond the bioactivity effect. The dysfunction can occur in different levels of the biological system such as the expression of genes, biological pathways, and proteins. For example, two structurally similar compounds, the antidiabetic drugs rosiglitazone and troglitazone, exhibit a very different side effect profile due to the different MoA [18].

Human biology is highly complex, and thus it is challenging to develop a safe and efficacious medicine [19]. As such, modern drug discovery has broadened from the classic 'single target-based' approach towards the understanding of the compounds' polypharmacology, gene expression, and activity on biological pathways. Bioinformatic approaches can facilitate the process of MoA understanding by using multilevel information from high-throughput biological assays (e.g. gene expression) with machine learning techniques in order to reveal unexplored connections and interactions of small molecules with the biological system (Figure 11.2). Datasets of gene expression data, biological pathways, and image-based data and methodologies will be discussed further below.

11.2 Transcriptomics Data and Databases

11.2.1 Biological Background of the Transcription Process

The 'central dogma' of molecular biology is based on the principle that genes encode mRNA, which is then translated in the ribosomes to proteins. This can be defined as a biological information flow that links the underlying genetic information with the protein regulation and its clinicopathological effect [20, 21]. Hence, transcriptomics, which refers to the study of transcriptome/mRNA transcripts that are produced by the genome in a specific cell line or under specific circumstances [19], can serve as an intermediate source of information for the understanding of the effect of a compound in a biological system. The information derived from the quantity of mRNA transcripts can reveal information about the effect of perturbations and compounds on protein control at the mRNA level. The differential gene expression profile (the difference between the control and treated samples) of a compound can be considered as an extra indicator of its MoA because it provides a holistic image of the cell upon perturbation or compound treatment. However, there are disadvantages related to gene expression profiles of compounds. Gene expression is one level of information, so it might not be meaningful when considered on its own or a gene expression signature may be noisy, and these two factors should be taken into consideration [22]. Moreover, it is important to mention that different genes can be regulated at different time points. For example, in a study investigating two structurally similar compounds (vincristine and vindesine with Tanimoto coefficient equal to 0.91), these two compounds were tested on the same cell line (A549) and dose (10 μM) but different perturbation times (6 and 24 hours). The two compounds had similar gene expression profiles when the perturbation time was 24 hours but different profiles when the perturbation time was 6 hours [18]. The reason is that genes are regulated at different time points and, as an example in this specific case, the compounds' target topoisomerase 2 alpha (TOP2A) was downregulated for both drugs when the cell is treated for 24 hours, whereas the target is not affected after 6 hours.

The genome-wide expression profiling of transcriptional responses upon compound perturbation has gained increased interest in the exploration of the MoA of bioactive compounds [5]. The reason is that compounds with comparative biological properties could share a commonality in their MoA, and thus compounds with similar gene expression profiles can have a similar MoA [21, 23]. Hence, in recent years compound-induced gene expression repositories have been created and evolved, and gene expression data have become available in public databases for comparison. There are two databases that contain transcriptomic profiles of cultivated cell lines treated with thousands of chemicals and are widely used as reference datasets. These two databases are the Connectivity Map (CMap) and the Library of Integrated Network-Based Cellular Signatures (LINCS), and these will be described in the following sections.

11.2.2 Connectivity Map: CMap

CMap was developed by Lamb et al. in 2006 as a web-based tool to resolve the need to relate diseases, physiological processes, and the action of small molecule therapeutics [24]. The aim of CMap is to help provide solutions to problems by describing biological states (physiological state, disease state, or state induced by a chemical) in terms of transcriptomic signatures. The goal is to identify disease or drug associated signatures that correlate with perturbations on the transcriptomic level [25].

The CMap was developed in two phases: Build 1 and Build 2. The experiments to generate the data were conducted in various cell lines and with a number of perturbations at various doses and perturbation time points. Build 1 included

455 treatment control pairs derived from 165 drugs, 5 cell lines, 42 doses, and 2 perturbation times. Build 2 was a scale-up of the first phase and included 6100 treatment control pairs derived from 1309 compounds, 156 doses, and the same number of cell lines and perturbation times as in Build 1.

11.2.2.1 Applications of CMap in MoA Deconvolution

Data and results from CMap have been extensively used in the elucidation of compounds' MoA, and these methodologies are summarized below.

Methodology 1: Connections with Compound's Gene Expression The first methodology is to submit a compound's gene expression profile into CMap and identify compounds with a similar gene expression profile and thus gain a hypothesis of a compound with similar MoA. This idea relies on the hypothesis that compounds with similar gene expression profiles can share similar MoA, even if they act on different cellular targets [23, 26]. Compounds with similar patterns of performance in biological assays should share a similar MoA [8]. By comparing the gene expression similarity of query compounds with the compounds in CMap, new interactions of existing drugs or new drugs can be identified. This hypothesis can then be validated experimentally either *in vitro* or *in vivo*. Examples from the literature of the use of this approach are shown in Table 11.1.

CMap proved to be efficient in identifying and generating testable hypotheses about MoA of poorly characterized compounds such as celastrol and gedunin. These compounds were found to be able to suppress the gene expression of androgen receptor (AR) activation in prostate cancer cells based on a high-throughput gene expression-based screen for small molecules [24, 34]. Gene expression signatures of these compounds were submitted in CMap and found to have a high connectivity score with three compounds that are known HSP90 inhibitors although they shared a low chemical similarity with these three compounds. Hence, a hypothesis was generated that celastrol and gedunin could potentially act as HSP90 inhibitors. The stability of the AR depends on the HSP90 activity, and thus it was further experimentally validated (*in vitro*) that celastrol and gedunin are able to eliminate AR protein HSP90-interacting proteins in LNCaP and Ba/F3 cell lines.

Another example of better understanding a compound's MoA and repurposing it with CMap is that of a novel compound called F05, which has been identified as an agent able to promote axonal (i.e. neuron) regeneration *in vivo* [35] and could be used for the treatment of the injury of the central nervous system (CNS). Thus, F05 has been submitted in CMap to identify additional neural regeneration promoting compounds [27]. CMap identified compounds that had a similar gene expression profile to the submitted compound although they were not chemically similar. All of the identified compounds were in the same subclass of antipsychotics known as piperazine phenothiazine antipsychotics (PhPAPs). A pharmacological study was also performed and showed that this class of antipsychotics promote regeneration through the antagonism of calmodium signalling. As a result, CMap provided insights and suggestions that PhPAPs could be repurposed for neuron regeneration and antagonism of calmodium signalling can be considered as a new approach to promote neural regeneration.

Table 11.1 Summary of CMap application examples for compounds' understanding of MoA or repurposing.

Chemical	Indication	Mechanism of action	Experimental validation	References
Celastrol and gedunin	Prostate cancer	It was identified to be an HSP90 inhibitor that abrogates androgen receptor (AR) activation in prostate cancer cells	*In vitro*	[24]
Novel compound called F05 and PhPAPs	Neuron regeneration	Antagonism of calmodium signalling	*In vivo*	[27]
N-((8-hydroxy-7-quinolinyl) (4-methylphenyl) methyl)benzamide (HQBA)	Mammary cancer	HQBA has chelating activities that mimics hypoxic response	*In vitro* *In vivo* (rodent)	[28]
VLX 50	Ovarian cancer	VLX 50 identified as an iron chelator with tumour selective activity	*In vitro* *In vivo* (rodent)	[29]
b-AP15	Myeloid leukaemia	Identified as a proteasome inhibitor and showed a deubiquitinating activity in cancer therapy	*In vitro* *In vivo* (rodent)	[30]
Thioridazine	Ovarian cancer	Identified as an inhibitor of P13K/AKT pathway in ovarian cancer cells	*In vitro*	[31]
Epoxy anthraquinone derivative	Neuroblastoma	Identified to be a DNA topoisomerase inhibitor	*In vitro*	[32]
Peptide: Ac2-26	Inflammation	Indicated transcriptional similarity with anti-inflammatory therapeutics	NA	[33]

Compound targets and MoA derived from rationalization of the CMap similarity results.

In another case, CMap was used as an additional independent approach in a setting to better understand the MoA of *N*-((8-hydroxy-7-quinolinyl)(4-methylphenyl)methyl)benzamide (HQBA), which was identified to be active in models of mammary cancers [28]. MCF7 cell lines were treated with HQBA for six hours, and the gene expression signatures were submitted in CMap, which identified four compounds to have high transcriptional similarity (not chemical similarity), and two of these compounds are known iron chelators. It was subsequently hypothesized that HQBA may have chelating activities that mimics the hypoxic response, which was then validated both *in vitro* and *in vivo*. In a similar use of CMap, the compound VLX 50 was identified as an iron chelator with tumour selective activity. In similar research approaches, the antipsychotic drug, thioridazine, was identified as an inhibitor of the phosphatidylinositol-3'-kinase (P13K/AKT) pathway in ovarian cancer cells [31], and some other examples are shown in Table 11.1 [32, 33].

CMap has been benchmarked as a tool that can be used to generate hypotheses of the potential MoA of compounds. The examples in the literature that are discussed above highlight that gene expression similarity can be used as a tool to identify compounds with a similar MoA.

Methodology 2: Small Molecule Target Prediction Based on Drug-Induced Gene Expression Data in a Chemical Structure-Independent Manner In this study, a new method was proposed to predict targets for compounds based on their gene expression profiles extracted from CMap by applying a machine learning classification algorithm [36]. For compounds extracted from CMap, compound-target interactions were obtained from DrugBank and ChEMBL. Initially, compounds' gene expression similarities were examined for their correlation with the similarities of the compounds' chemical structures, and then protein expression similarities were compared with target protein sequence similarities. Results showed that there was no correlation in both cases. As a result, the hypothesis of that work was built on the observation that drug-induced gene expression profiles can provide a different or complementary source of information compared with compound chemical structures and protein amino acid sequences.

Two methods were employed to examine the performance of computational methods for using gene expression data from CMap for compound–target prediction. The first was the direct method, and the second was a classification method for compound–target prediction. The direct method involves the identification of the fold change values of the associated compound–protein pairs in the gene expression matrix because it is hypothesized that the observed gene expression of drug-affected genes is highly variable. A scoring system for compound–protein pairs is then used to identify high scoring compound–protein pairs, where compounds are predicted to be candidate ligands for the proteins. Compound–protein pairs that exhibit a high score are predicted to be candidates for interacting compound–protein pairs. The second method was a supervised classification method, and the pairwise kernel regression algorithm was used, where a similarity function for compounds and a similarity function for proteins are defined. The input of the model was the similarity scores between compound pairs (chemical and transcriptomic similarity) and protein pairs (amino acid sequence similarity), and therefore the performance of the model depends on the similarities of compounds and proteins. Three different approaches were applied: transcriptomic, chemogenomic, and integrative (combination of both).

Different metrics were used to evaluate the models, and results showed that the chemogenomic approach performed poorly when the test compounds were structurally dissimilar to the training set. This was not the case with the transcriptomic similarity approach as its performance was independent of the compound chemical similarity. Moreover, different compound–protein interaction pairs were predicted with a high confidence score depending on the approach used. In more detail, the top predictions from the chemogenomic approach were low substrate-specific proteins such as CYP enzymes, whereas the top predictions from the transcriptomic approach were mostly proteins associated with the mechanism of drug action. It was therefore concluded that the use of transcriptomic information can be useful information in the target prediction of compounds with novel chemical structures.

11.2.3 Library of Integrated Network-Based Cellular Signatures (LINCS)

CMap has proved to be a useful tool in the elucidation of MoA as has been illustrated in the research studies described above. However, there are three limitations associated with the content of CMap. These limitations are the small number of compounds and cell lines, the missing diversity of chemicals [37], and the high cost of commercial gene expression microarrays, which is an obstacle for the genome scale-up of CMap. As a result, Broad Institute has developed a new assay platform called the 'L1000 platform' or 'L1000 methodology', which is considered as a 1000-fold scale-up of CMap [37]. The LINCS program has been developed by the Broad Institute and administrated by the National Institutes of Health (NIH), and it proposes a new method of measuring a compound's gene expression in a high-throughput manner [38].

The L1000 platform is an expansion of CMap, and a comparison of CMap and L1000 is shown in Table 11.2. Firstly, the number of compounds was increased from 1309 to 19 811, including compounds with known MoA. In addition, the L1000 platform contains other biological perturbagens including 18 493 small hairpin RNAs (shRNAs), 3462 cDNAs, and 314 biologics, and in total there are 42 080 perturbagens, thus introducing a significant chemical richness to the LINCS database. Secondly, CMap contains only gene expression data from 3 cancer cell lines, whereas the L1000 platform incorporates 77 cell lines. The breakthrough of the L1000 platform is that it can produce the gene expression profile of compounds at a lower cost compared with CMap and in a high-throughput manner.

The hypothesis behind the L1000 is that it is possible to capture at low cost any cellular state by measuring a reduced representation of the transcriptome [37]. This idea was further validated experimentally. In more detail, 12 031 expression profiles from Gene Expression Omnibus (GEO) were used to identify the optimal number of informative transcripts or as they are called the 'landmark' genes.

Table 11.2 Comparison of CMap and LINCS L1000 (as of January 2018)

	CMap	LINCS L1000
Number of small molecules	1 309	19 811
Cell lines	3	77
Number of gene expression profiles	~7 000	~1 300 000

The number of landmark genes was 978 (~1000), and these genes were sufficient to recover 82% of the information in the transcriptome [37]. In addition, this novel method was compared with the standard gene expression profiling method, RNA-seq. The comparison revealed that there is a strong degree of similarity of the profiles across the L1000 and RNA-seq platforms, and in a further L1000 validation, this new inference methodology was able to infer the gene expression for 83% of transcripts with high precision.

The L1000 datasets are deposited into GEO [39]. There are two available phases in GEO, the LINCS phase I (GSE92742) and LINCS phase II (GSE70138). Phase I represents the earlier phase, and phase II is a newer version, which is updated regularly (every six months) as more L1000 data is produced by the Broad Institute. Broad Institute defined different data levels for the results produced by the assays, which were employed in the L1000 platform. The data is stored in five different levels, and level 4 and level 5 are commonly employed because they represent the gene expression with the Z-score and the moderated Z-score (MOD-Z), respectively [18]. The MOD-Z is considered as a de-noised representation of the gene expression signature.

11.2.3.1 LINCS L1000 Data Exploration

A LINCS L1000 data exploration was conducted to calculate the number of small molecules present per cell line and experimental conditions. When a compound is queried in the L1000 database, it is considered as a vector with three dimensions, which are the cell line, the perturbation time point, and the perturbation dose. These three dimensions are used to query L1000 data, which are stored in a GCTx format. This type of format is an HDF-5-based file format specially designed by the NIH for space efficient storage and rapid access of dense data matrices paired with metadata information [40]. The most populated datasets (more than 2000 small molecules) are shown in the heat map below (Figure 11.3).

The selection of the cell line and experimental conditions (concentration and time point) is very important because the gene expression can vary by altering these three parameters. The reason is that the gene expression changes are highly dependent on the biological conditions. For example, Chen et al. [18] performed an integrative analysis of gene expression data across 11 000 compounds extracted from various cell lines and experimental conditions. Two structurally similar compounds with a Tanimoto coefficient equal to 0.9, testosterone and norethindrone, showed similar transcriptomic profiles in the VCAP cell line and different transcriptomic profiles in A375 cells. For example,

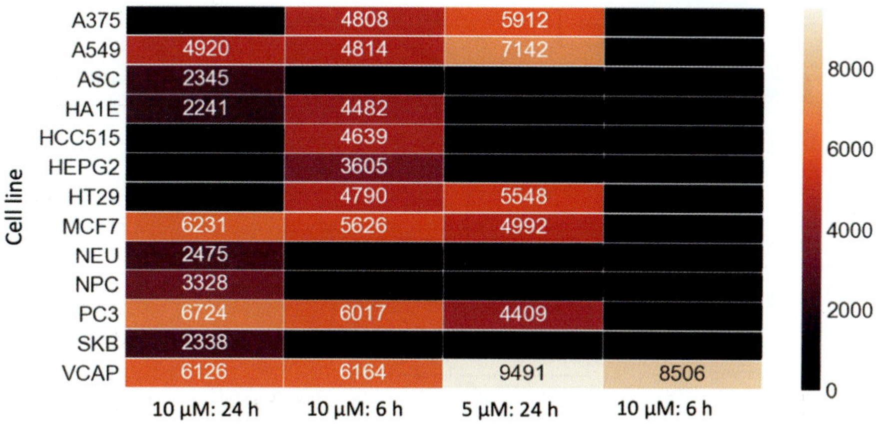

Figure 11.3 Heat map of the most populated datasets (more than 2000 compounds). Values indicate the number of compounds/small molecules present per cell line versus the experimental conditions (perturbation time and perturbation dose). The perturbation dose is measured in micromolar (μM) units and the perturbation time in hours (h). If there are less than 2000 compounds in a combination of cell line and experimental conditions, then no value is displayed in that cell.

four genes were found to be highly differentially expressed in the profiles of the two drugs only in the VCAP cell line and not in the A375 cell line.

In addition to the cell line, the perturbation time is also an important factor. The duration that a compound perturbs a cell can affect the gene expression profiles because if obtained too early the signals might not be robust and if obtained too late the gene expression changes might reflect secondary and tertiary responses [24]. Hence, a good perturbation time for MoA analysis is an early time point of six hours [24]. Moreover, the concentration of the perturbagen is important, and 10 μM is usually selected because high-throughput, cell-based, small molecule screens are often performed at a single relatively high concentration of 10 μM [24].

11.2.3.2 Applications of L1000 Data in MoA Understanding

The aim of LINCS is to systematically determine the cellular effects of compounds on the transcriptomic level or in other words the changes in gene expression that occur when the cells are exposed to perturbing agents [41]. The goal is to provide hypotheses on compounds with shared biological effects for repositioning opportunities and MoA understanding via an extensive catalogue of perturbation response signatures [42]. The great volume of gene expression data in the L1000 platform can give insights into complex and dynamic networks of molecules and biological processes involved in a biological system and/or in a disease state [42, 43].

Methodology 1: Use of Gene Expression Data to Identify Potential Drug Targets LINCS L1000 is a database that a compound can be queried against to identify transcriptional activities that could reveal information about the MoA of a compound and their target gene(s). A target gene is transcribed and then translated into a protein,

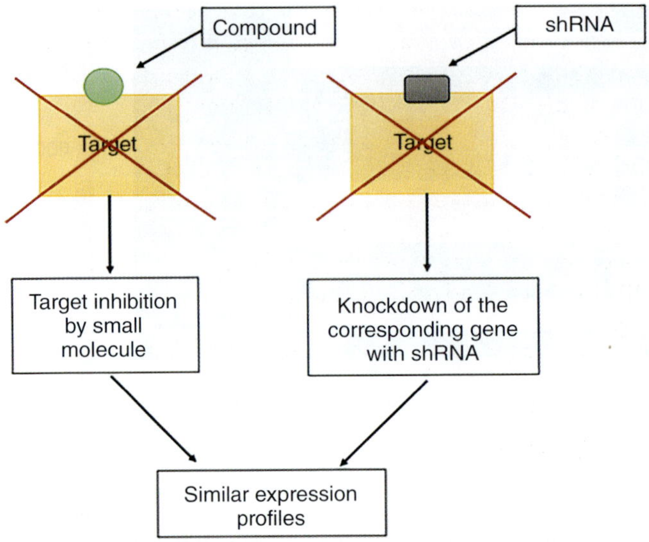

Figure 11.4 The starting hypothesis is that drugs inhibiting their targets should yield similar network level effects to silencing the target gene(s), and thus a drug-induced mRNA signature should correlate with the knockdown signature of the drug's target gene and/or genes on the same pathway(s). Source: Pabon et al. 2018 [22]. Adapted with permission of PLOS.

which the drugs can bind, and therefore a target might refer to either a protein or gene depending on the context [22]. The LINCS database contains both gene expression profiles following treatments in multiple cell lines and also following gene knockdowns (KDs). During KD experiments, the expression of one or more target genes is reduced, and subsequently the amount of target protein(s) in the cell is reduced, and this reduction is the result of treatment with a reagent such as shRNA [44]. Gene expression profiles obtained following KD from LINCS can be used with other types of data to predict drug targets [22]. An example is a method developed by Pabon et al. [22], where they use gene expression profiles following treatments in multiple cell lines and also following KD experiments combined with other genomic data. The hypothesis was that the effect of target inhibition by a compound on gene expression profiles is similar to knocking down the same target with shRNA (Figure 11.4).

For the purpose of this work, a validation set of 29 FDA-approved small molecules was obtained. These compounds were tested on seven cell lines in LINCS, and their known targets were among the 2634 KD genes in the same cell lines. A direct Pearson correlation was measured between the expression profiles from a gene KD and treatment with small molecule expression signatures. Potential targets were ranked based on this direct correlation metric and they were able to predict known targets in the top 100 potential targets for 8/29 validated small molecules. The direct correlation feature was then combined with additional cell-specific protein interaction and gene annotation features, which were used to train a random forest (RF) model to predict targets. Additional features were the cell selection, indirect correlation, and protein–protein interaction (PPI) expression. The cell selection feature was created to reflect the impact that a drug has on a cell line and hence the correlation between the response expression profile of each drug and the control compound for each cell line. A smaller correlation is expected if the drug is active in a cell line, and a higher correlation if the drug is inactive. The indirect correlation and PPI expression features are taking into account PPI information from BioGRID and Human Protein Reference Database (HPRD). The indirect correlation is a feature that measures the correlation of the drug response expression profiles with the KD experiments of each gene's binding partners (identified from a PPI graph). PPI expression or differential expression score is a feature that is also calculated from PPI network information, and for each gene the binding partners are identified and then two scores are computed: the maximum and average absolute value expression level of the interaction partners for each target protein.

The features were used to train a RF model to predict targets, and a leave-one-out cross validation (LOOCV) for each drug was used, and this predicted known targets in the top 100 potential targets for 16/29 drugs (55% accuracy), which is an improvement compared to the direct correlation feature. The set of 29 compounds was tested in seven cell lines, but this method should be applicable also to compounds that have not been tested to all seven cell lines. Therefore, they retrained the model on a set of 152 drugs that were tested on four, five, six, or seven cell lines and compared two different RF methods ('on-the-fly' and '2-level' RF), which can handle missing data. The 'on-the-fly' method learns a drug-specific classifier that is trained on a set of drugs profiled in the same cell lines, whereas the '2-level' RF learns a single classifier trained on profiles from all 152 training drugs. In more detail, during the 'on-the-fly' RF, for a given drug i, they iterate through all the 152 drugs and select the compounds that have been tested in the same cell lines as the drug i. A separate RF is built for each test drug with the 'on-the-fly' method. On the other hand, during the '2-level' RF, an additional step is added during the randomization of features for each tree in the forest. They randomly select four cell lines out of the seven, and they find all drugs that have been tested in those cell lines and use them to train that tree. This process is repeated at least 3500 times in order to ensure that each combination of four cell lines has approximately 100 trees. The '2-level' method performed better with correctly predicting targets for 63 drugs in the top 100 compared with 'on the fly', which predicted targets for 8 drugs in the top 100. Moreover, they further divided the predictions into 'successful' and 'unsuccessful', and they used gene ontology (GO) to test for enrichment. Results showed that intracellular targets were better predicted compared to transmembrane and extracellular targets, and hence this information was encoded into a feature by assigning 1 to the intracellular genes and −1 to transmembrane and extracellular genes.

Finally, they applied this new methodology of predicting targets to 1680 small molecules profiled in LINCS, and 104 compounds were predicted to have carboxy terminus of Hsc70 interacting protein (CHIP) among their top 100 targets. These molecules were further docked to the representative structure of the tetratricopeptide repeat (TPR) domain of CHIP. They visually examined the docking models of top scoring and purchased six compounds for testing. Moreover, they also performed a pharmacophore-based virtual screen of the ZINC database and purchased seven compounds. The ZINC database is a public access database, which is used for virtual screening, ligand discovery, pharmacophore screens, and force field development [45]. Experimental results with these compounds showed that four out of six LINCS compounds reliably reduced substrate binding, whereas three out of seven ZINC compounds did so to a modest degree.

In another study, the expression changes of the landmark genes from L1000 platform experiments were converted into a meaningful barcode of important features by using deep learning techniques [46]. The goal of this study was to increase the sensitivity and specificity of the interpretations and predictions derived from large gene expression datasets from the L1000 platform. Experiments in L1000 are performed in biological replicates, and thus gene expression profiles (Z-scores) can be affected by batch effects. For example, by comparing the similarity of each sample profile to any other in a dataset of 7573 expression profiles from 3699 compounds, there were more than 200 treatment profiles that were more similar to a given treatment than a sample that was treated identically on a different day. Therefore, the first goal of this study was to build a method that distinguishes between replicates and non-replicates and recast the data in a way that maximizes the similarity of replicates in contrast to non-replicates. The machine learning method that was used was not the classic single input sample at a time, which aims to learn on individual samples. In contrast, they used a Siamese neural network method, which allows pairs of compounds as an input and compares them in order to learn a new metric. In total, 7573 landmark gene expression profiles were calculated as Z-scores from 3699 compounds. The input of this model is pairs of 978-dimensional Z-score vectors representing two different gene expression profiles as adjacent vectors. Data is then transformed through two noisy sigmoid layers (400 followed by 100 units). The activation of the second hidden layer is combined in the output layer by calculating a Euclidean distance between the two representations. A margin cost is calculated based on the Euclidean squared distance and the indication of the pair (i.e. replicates or non-replicates). Finally, the cost is used to train the network via backpropagation of the cost gradients. The model was trained on 80% of the data, 10% of the data was used for hyperparameter tuning, and the remaining 10% was used as a test set. The model correctly categorized 97% of the test pairs as replicates or non-replicates.

Therefore, based on the observation that the model is able to distinguish between replicates or non-replicates and the model output is a function of a simple Euclidean distance calculated during the hidden layer activations, the authors hypothesized that this internal representation is capturing the discriminatory power learned by the model. This internal representation was derived from the learned model by using the activation 100-bit second hidden layer of each data point, which was further binarized (values greater or equal to 0.5 were set to 1 and values less than 0.5 were set to 0). The 100-bit binary representation was simply named barcode, which is a reduced representation of gene expression, and the authors further investigated whether biologically interesting aspects are retained in this barcode.

To answer this question, the barcode was compared with gene expression profiles represented as Z-scores and biologically motivated data summaries such as gene set enrichment analysis (GSEA) results. By comparing these three profiles, they concluded that the barcode contains chemical structure and target information and can be used to predict a compound's promiscuity and was found to be more predictive than the initial data measurements, thus revealing underlying features of the expression data that are potentially masked by the noise. Hence, the proposed methodology could be fruitful for other types of data that are high in volume and high-dimensional, and thus there is the possibility to reduce the effects of the noise in the data. In addition, this methodology can be further expanded by combining features from phenotypic information, quantitative structure activity relationships, and pharmacokinetic/pharmacodynamic models.

Methodology 2: MoA Understanding for Bioactive Compounds in a Cell-Specific Manner by Large-Scale Chemically Induced Transcriptomics Another novel approach was developed to better understand the MoA of bioactive compounds by using gene expression signatures from LINCS derived from ~16 000 small molecules and 68 human cell lines [5]. The proposed methodology is able to predict active pathways, target proteins, and therapeutic indications. Firstly, a pathway enrichment analysis is performed and, in more detail, the top and bottom 5% of upregulated and downregulated genes in each compound's expression profiles are mapped onto biological pathway maps, and the statistical significance of the enrichment of the regulated genes per pathway is calculated with a hypergeometric test (Figure 11.5a). As a result, a list of activated and inactivated pathways is produced per compound based on the pathway enrichment analysis of the upregulated and downregulated genes respectively. Moreover, a set of compounds with known target protein is pre-collected, and if a query compound is transcriptionally similar with the pre-collected compounds, then it is predicted

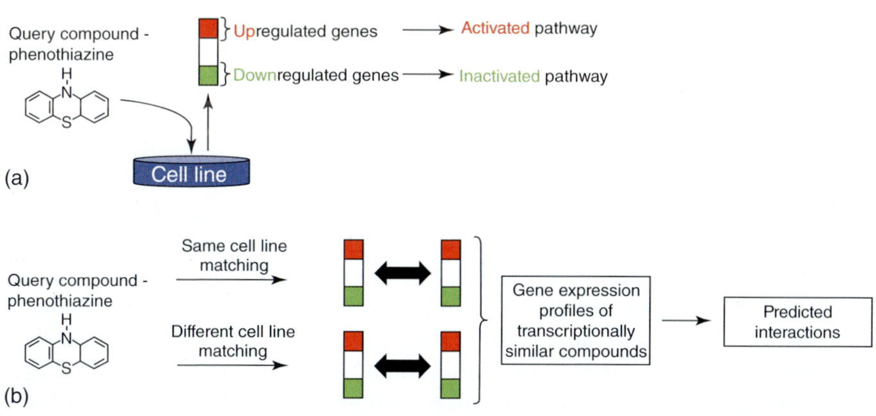

Figure 11.5 Overview of the proposed methodology. Phenothiazine is used as an example of a query compound. (a) The gene expression of a query compound is measured, and then activated and inactivated pathways are obtained based on the compound's differential gene expression. (b) Prediction of potential drug targets.

to bind to the same targets and share the same therapeutic indications as the most transcriptionally similar compound (Figure 11.5b). Two strategies were used for the calculation of transcriptional similarity. The first is the same cell line matching, and the second is the different cell line-matching strategy, where compounds' transcriptional similarity is evaluated on the same or different cell lines respectively.

This study highlighted three important observations. Firstly, they explored the relationships between detected pathways and the drug therapeutic class that the compounds belonged to. Some pathways were highly associated with similarly classified drugs and therefore the pathway enrichment analysis method was able to provide better understanding of the MoA of bioactive compounds at the pathway level. Secondly, the method was evaluated for its ability to predict targets following a fivefold cross validation by using data that overlapped between CMap and LINCS (common data) and also by using all the data available in CMap and LINCS (merged data), following the same cell line matching and different cell line-matching strategy. When the common data was used, the performance of the models was slightly lower or almost the same when the data extracted from LINCS compared with CMap with an area under curve (AUC) equal to 0.82 and 0.83, respectively. This observation suggests that the quality of the gene expression data in LINCS is similar to that present in CMap. However, when the merged data was used, the AUC and area under precision recall (AUPR) scores were much higher than those obtained using CMap, thus highlighting the better data coverage of LINCS. Moreover, this method worked better when they used the same cell line strategy for the similarity searching instead of the different cell line matching, and this suggests that chemically induced gene expression has cell-specific characteristics as well as features common to all cell lines. Finally, they conducted a biological interpretation of the drug–protein–disease network that was obtained based on the compounds' transcriptional similarity and they identified therapeutic indications for 462 diseases based on the target proteins. For example, phenothiazine was predicted to interact with the AR based on its high transcriptional similarity with enzalutamide (these two drugs share a low chemical similarity), which is indicated for prostate cancer. An *in vitro* cellular assay was conducted and experimentally validated the prediction that phenothiazine inhibits AR. In conclusion, this methodology proved to be efficient and could be used in the understanding of MoA and compound repositioning.

Methodology 3: Use of Gene Expression Data to Predict Activatory and Inhibitory Targets
Furthermore, another novel approach was developed to predict activatory and inhibitory targets of drug candidates [47] by integrating chemically induced and genetically perturbed gene expression profiles without dependence on chemical structures of compounds or proteins. The proposed methodology is based on the hypothesis that we are able to predict the inhibition or activation of a target by correlating the inhibition or activation with gene KD of that protein and the overexpression of that protein respectively. Therefore, three signatures were created. The first one was the 'compound profile', which corresponds to the gene expression signature upon compound perturbation. The gene expression profiles of the compounds that inhibit or activate a certain protein can be correlated

with that after gene knockdown of the corresponding protein or with that after overexpression of the protein. Hence, proteins that are inhibited or activated by compounds are represented by gene knockdown signature or by gene expression profiles after overexpression of the protein. A direct correlation method evaluating the correlation coefficients between query compounds and the dataset was then performed, and joint learning predictive models were developed in order to predict the activatory or inhibitory effect of compounds to targets. The ability of the two methods was tested using cross validation and was further compared with the pairwise learning method with AUC and AUPR scores and the joint learning algorithm performed better. The proposed joint learning method was further applied on a drug repositioning setting, and new indications were predicted for 1124 compounds for 365 diseases. For example, it was predicted and further experimentally validated that dienestrol was able to inhibit the retinoic acid receptor α.

11.3 Pathway Data and Databases

11.3.1 What Is a Pathway?

The biological system is a complex network of molecular reactions [48], and therefore the understanding of the complex responses of the human biological system to drug treatments is important in order to identify drug targets and understand MoA. As discussed previously, various levels of high-throughput information can be used to understand the MoA of compounds such as high-throughput gene expression data [2, 49, 50]. However, by using only high-throughput data, it might be possible to fail to provide mechanistic insights into the underlying biology of the data used [51, 52]. To address this limitation of high-throughput data, biological pathway information can be used.

Biological pathways can be considered as a collection of 'nodes', which represent biochemical entities [53]. The nodes are then connected by edges, which represent interactions such as protein–DNA binding and PPI. Hence, a pathway can be considered as an ordered series of molecular events that result in the creation of a new molecular product or the change in a cellular state. Pathways can be categorized in subcategories depending on their role. For example, a pathway can regulate cellular processes such as the cell cycle or can result in the production of a biomolecule (metabolic pathway) or can signal the presence of a hormonal signal (signalling pathway). Therefore, in order to maintain a healthy organism, many pathways are responsible and should all work together. If a pathway becomes dysregulated, then diseases develop, and there is a need of medicines that are able to correct the problematic pathways. Hence many drugs are acting by switching on or inactivating a pathway.

An example of the cell cycle pathway (extracted from Kyoto Encyclopaedia of Genes and Genomes [KEGG] database) is shown in Figure 11.6. This pathway is a representation of the human cell cycle. This pathway is affected, for example, in various diseases such as chronic myeloid leukaemia, which is the result of a reciprocal translocation that forms the Philadelphia (Ph) gene. The result of this

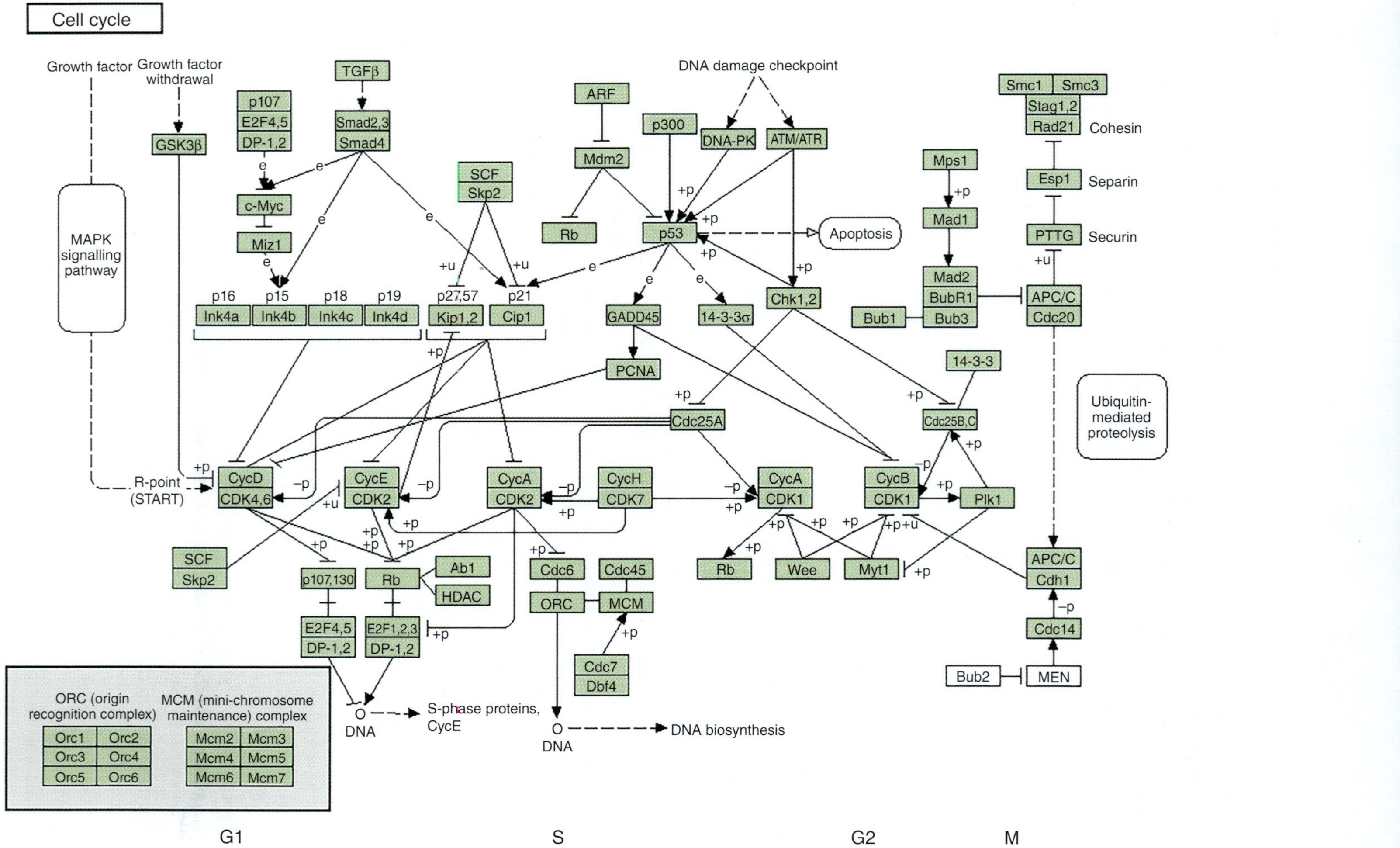

Figure 11.6 Pathway map of the *Homo sapiens* (human) cell cycle pathway downloaded from the KEGG database. Each node in the graph represents an element (e.g. gene), and each edge corresponds to interactions between the nodes. Source: Kanehisa et al. 2016 [54]. Reproduced with permission of Oxford University Press.

translocation is the fusion of ABL gene from chromosome 9, and the BCR gene of chromosome 22 that codes for the BCR-ABL transcript, an oncoprotein that encodes a constitutive kinase activity [55, 56]. Therefore, the ABL gene, which is part of the cell cycle biological pathway (Figure 11.6), is affected and thus to restore the function of the pathway, drugs like imatinib are used. Imatinib is an antineoplastic, which inhibits the BCR-ABL tyrosine kinase, the abnormal kinase created by the Ph chromosome and in more detail, it inhibits proliferation and induces apoptosis in BCR-ABL positive cells. Hence, drugs can target faulty biological pathways to restore the normal function of the cells in various diseases such as cancer, diabetes and others.

11.3.2 Process of Pathway Analysis

The process of pathway analysis is shown in Figure 11.7, but it should be noted that there is no standard or 'consensus' approach to pathway analysis because pathway analysis approaches can be used in various fields of bioinformatics such as the identification of functional roles of genes and proteins in certain phenotypes, prediction of clinical outcome, elucidation of compounds' MoA and others. To begin with, the pathway analysis process starts with either the high-throughput data generation or the data extraction from a database. The majority of methods for pathway analysis were developed with the gene expression in mind as gene expression data is the older, most common, and well-established high-throughput data. Therefore, in this part the gene expression data will be used as an example of data to explain pathway analysis methodologies.

Raw data is then curated appropriately and a pathway database is selected. The choice of the database depends on the types of data and the scope of the research [53]. For example, signalling pathways can be used when the topic of research is cancer, as genetic alterations in cancer cells can be connected with the signalling pathways that control processes associated with tumorigenesis and cancer progression [58]. Moreover, the selection of the pathway database further depends

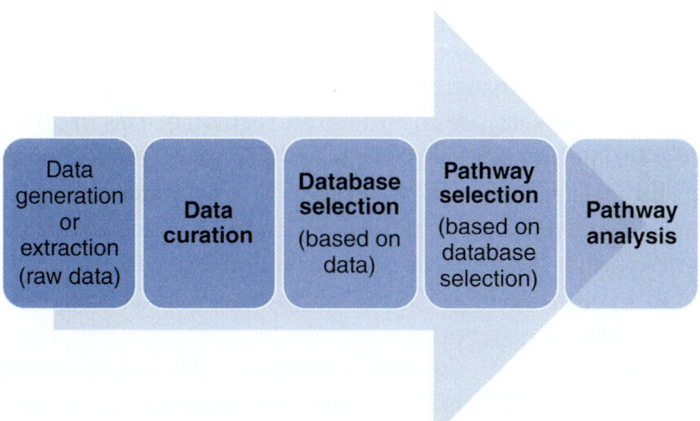

Figure 11.7 Overall process of pathway analysis. Source: Wang et al. 2015 [57]. Reproduced with permission of IGI Global.

on the type of pathways of interest. Several databases have been developed to store metabolic and signalling pathway information and some of them are the Reactome, KEGG, WikiPathways, and BioSystems [59]. A table of some of the most commonly employed databases is shown in Table 11.3. Each database has its own advantages, disadvantages and inaccuracies as all of them might be biased due to the manual curation of the data [51]. In addition, it is very important to use data from different pathway databases as they are often complementary, and thus a better coverage of all the reactions involved in a given pathway can be achieved [59]. For example, BioSystems database incorporates various pathway repositories into the database and allows a comprehensive view of the pathway information available for processes [66]. The existence of these databases and their evolution is a valuable source for the *in silico* model developers for the mathematical interpretation of the emerging properties of the different biological pathways upon their exposure to various perturbations [70].

The annotation of high-throughput data with pathway information offers two advantages. The first is that the grouping of thousands of genes or other types of data by the pathways in which they are involved reduces the complexity and dimensionality of the data [51]. The second is that identifying pathways that differ between a perturbation and a control compound can be more explanatory than a raw list of differentially expressed genes [71]. The two most commonly employed methods to determine the pathways based on high-throughput profiles are the GSEA and the simple hypergeometric test [72]. These two tests will be explained on the basis of annotating differentially expressed gene profiles.

The hypergeometric test is the simplest approach to perform pathway analysis and it quantifies the overlap between a set of differentially expressed genes (or other features) detected in the high-throughput data and a background set of genes [53]. The background can either be the set of genes measured by the microarray/RNA-seq/L1000 experiment or the whole human genome. The null hypothesis of this test is that the genes of a pathway are not enriched in the differentially expressed genes [72]. This method offers the advantage of being simple and computationally inexpensive, but it can be biased from the arbitrary cut-off to define the differentially expressed genes [57].

GSEA on the other hand is a functional class scoring (FCS) method with the underlying hypothesis that the genes that are involved in a similar biological process or pathway (grouped into gene sets) are co-ordinately regulated. This method does not require the differential expressed genes, but on in contrary it uses some comparison metric for all measured genes [72]. Genes are ranked according to a metric (e.g. differential gene expression significance), and then GSEA aims to identify whether the genes from a set/pathway occur in the top or bottom of the ranked gene list. The null hypothesis of GSEA is that no genes in the expression profile are associated with an observation and occur randomly [73]. Then a Kolmogorov–Smirnov test is used to assess the statistical significance of the enrichment. The advantage of the GSEA is that it does not require an arbitrary cut-off to define differentially expressed genes and it provides a more in-depth characterization of pathways representative in the data compared with the hypergeometric test [57].

Table 11.3 Pathway databases.

Database name	Database content	Number of pathways	Peer reviewed	Pathway analysis tool
KEGG	KEGG is an encyclopaedia of genes and genomes, which is used to assign functional meanings to genes and genomes on a molecular and higher level [60]. It consists of 16 main databases and the KEGG PATHWAY is the core of KEGG and consists of a collection of manually drawn maps representing the current knowledge on: metabolism, cellular processes, human diseases etc. [54]	612 685	NA	Yes (KeggArray)
Reactome	Reactome is a free and open-source database of biomolecular pathways that aims to provide visualization, interpretation, and analysis of pathway knowledge to aid systems biology and basic research [48, 61, 62]	2 256 (*Homo sapiens*)	Yes	Yes
WikiPathways	WikiPathways is an open and collaborative platform, which captures and disseminates models of biological pathways [63, 64]	2 761 (over ~25 different species with the human pathway collection being the largest)	Partially yes	Yes (can be performed with a programmatic interface called PathVisioRPC)
BioCyc	BioCyc is a collection of microbial genomes and metabolic pathways (MetaCyc) [65]	14 560	NA	Yes

(*continued*)

Table 11.3 (Continued)

Database name	Database content	Number of pathways	Peer reviewed	Pathway analysis tool
BioSystems	BioSystems database incorporates various pathway repositories like KEGG, BioCyc, Reactome, Pathway Interaction Database, WikiPathways, and Gene Ontology, thus allowing a comprehensive view of the pathway information available for processes [66]	NA	Partially yes	NA
Pathway Commons	Pathway Commons collects and disseminates biological pathways and interaction data. Data is collected from partner databases such as BioGRID, Reactome, PANTHER Pathway, and others [67]	37 600	NA	Yes
Network Data Exchange (NDEx)	NDEx is an open-source software framework that facilitates the sharing of networks of many formats and users are able to manage the sharing and publication of their networks [68]	NA	Yes	NA
OmniPath	OmniPath is a collection of literature-curated human signalling pathways [69]	NA	NA	Yes (pypath – Python module)

11.3.3 Pathways in the Understanding of MoA

11.3.3.1 Methodology 1: MoA Analysis by Annotating Predicted Compounds' Targets with Pathways

Pathway analysis has been used with *in silico* target predictions to elucidate the MoA of compounds and provide further biological insights. In one study, predicted bioactivity profiles (obtained with target prediction) were annotated with pathways and a calculation of enrichment factors revealed targets and pathways that are more likely to be implicated with the studied phenotype, which was the pigmentation phenotype of *Xenopus laevis* tadpoles based on a genetic screen performed on *X. laevis* embryo read-outs [74]. A set of 1364 compounds was extracted from the National Cancer Institute (NCI) diversity set and a target prediction was applied on these compounds with a Laplacian-modified naïve Bayes classifier. Moreover, all predicted targets were annotated with pathways extracted from the KEGG database, and an enrichment calculation against a background distribution was performed to identify enriched targets and pathways. From the total of 1364 compounds, 45 compounds caused the pigmentation phenotype and these compounds were associated with 236 predicted targets. Out of the 236 predicted targets, 33 were found to be enriched. The top 10 enriched targets implicated in pigmentation were confirmed by literature analysis. For example, the top enriched target was the platelet-derived growth factor receptor alpha (PDGFRα), which according to literature findings is important during the *X. laevis* developmental effects such as alterations in the pigmentation.

Similarly, the predicted targets were annotated with KEGG pathways, and 44 out of the total 150 pathways were enriched. Initially, the pathways did not seem to be related to the phenotype, but a literature analysis revealed the link between the pathways and the observed phenotype. For example, one of the top enriched pathways was the mitogen activated protein kinase (MAPK) signalling pathways, whose abnormalities are known to cause malignancies. An additional role of this pathway is that cAMP activation of the MAPK signalling pathway inhibits melanogenesis, hence suggesting a direct association of this cascade with the pigmentation phenotype. Therefore, this study proved that the enrichment calculations for both predicted targets and pathways can reveal a significant correlation with the observed phenotype, thus further revealing underlying biological mechanisms.

The same methodology was utilized in a different concept and was applied to cellular cytotoxic read-outs [6]. In more detail, the pathway annotations improve the MoA information gained from an *in silico* target prediction by providing a better biological interpretation of the results and additionally providing a better mapping of targets onto pathways. In this study two different datasets were used, a cytotoxicity dataset of 1094 compounds and a smaller apoptotic dataset of 10 compounds, and protein targets were also predicted for these compounds. The cytotoxic dataset was extracted from PubChem by selecting 186 bioassays describing molecules that had proved to be cytotoxic to HeLa cells in cell-based assays and the apoptotic dataset was extracted from the Prestwick Chemical Library based on their activity in killing embryonic mouse stem cells detected by a calorimetric assay based on a metabolic activity performed with the Cell Proliferation Kit II. Target predictions for both datasets (cytotoxic and apoptotic) were annotated with pathways, which were extracted from KEGG, GO biological processes, and GO Slim biological processes. The annotated pathways were further subjected to enrichment calculation. Results of the pathway enrichment for the cytotoxic compounds identified pathways important in cancer development and the immune response as well as pathways related to DNA and the cell cycle. For the smaller apoptotic dataset, pathway enrichment revealed only a small number of enriched pathways. A major disadvantage of this methodology and the apoptotic dataset is that on small datasets this methodology needs to be performed differently and an analysis of absolute targets and pathways seems to be more appropriate. Overall, both studies discussed above showed that target prediction with pathway annotations and enrichment calculation can add meaningful biological insights in MoA and target prediction understanding.

11.3.4 Combination of Gene Expression and Pathway Data

11.3.4.1 Methodology 2: Construction of Drug Networks (DNs) with Gene Expression Data and Pathway Annotations

Iorio et al. constructed a 'drug network' (DN) of 1302 drugs (present in CMap database) and 41 047 edges, which indicated the similarity between their gene expression profiles [50, 75]. The drugs in the DN were further partitioned into groups of densely interconnected nodes (i.e. communities). This approach has been implemented into a tool called MANTRA (Mode of Action by NeTwoRk Analysis). The novelty of this tool was that it was using the idea that compounds with high transcriptional similarity can have a similar MoA and identify compounds with similar MoA, but additionally they determined the biological pathways perturbed by these compounds. The results revealed that the communities are significantly enriched with drugs with similar MoA or drugs that act in the same pathway. This tool was validated by correctly predicting the MoA of nine anticancer drugs and also discovered that fasudil (a drug approved in Japan for the treatment of cerebral vasospasm and associated cerebral ischemic symptoms [25, 76]) could be repositioned as an enhancer of cellular autophagy, and this feature of fasudil could potentially be applicable to several neurodegenerative disorders.

In addition, the MANTRA pipeline was further improved by refining the drug neighbourhood (or network community) that shows the highest transcriptomic similarity with a query compound [77]. For a query compound, the DN is searched to identify molecules eliciting a similar transcriptional response. The query results in a neighbourhood of compounds connected to the query compound and clustered onto network communities statistically enriched for certain MoAs. However, the drugs in the neighbourhood might share secondary effects (secondary MoA) with the query compound and not the principal MoA. For example, drugs that are Hsp90 inhibitors are densely interconnected with proteasome inhibitors in the DN. Although these two classes of compounds have a different direct target, they both increase the abundance of unfolded proteins. The explanation behind this observation is that the compounds that are Hsp90 inhibitors inhibit a chaperone protein, which is involved in protein degradation, and the compounds that are proteasome inhibitors inhibit an enzyme responsible for the degradation of misfolded/unfolded proteins. Therefore, Hsp90 and proteasome inhibitors both upregulate genes, which are associated with the response to the unfolded protein stress, and thus they show similarity between their gene expression profiles. Therefore, it is important to be able to distinguish between primary and secondary MoA within a community in the DN. The authors proposed an improved methodology, where the drug neighbourhood of the query compound is refined by taking into account *a priori* known characterization of the drugs in the neighbourhood. This is a supervised approach, and the drug and drug communities that were connected to the query compound are explored for enriched MoA in order to discard effects on drug similarity due to commonalities in secondary MoA. The authors used this proposed methodology to disentangle the indirect mitotic arrest and general microtubule disruption from its primary MoA, which is the microtubule stabilization effect, and further used this method to identify novel microtubule stabilizing compounds such as glizipine and splitomicin.

Moreover, in another study, the MANTRA tool was used together with the group factor analysis (GFA) method as two complementary computational tools in a case study to identify novel and mechanistic insights for the natural compound pinosylvin [23]. GFA decomposes gene expression datasets into 'components'/factors [78]. Each of the components is characterized by a set of drugs that regulate the expression of genes in a similar way, thus creating hypotheses on their common MoA. By using MANTRA the natural polyphenol pinosylvin was predicted to have a G-protein coupled receptor (GPCR)-related mechanism and to be a calmodulin (CaM) inhibitor. In addition, by using GFA, pinosylvin was predicted to increase cAMP levels and to have steroid-like activity. By using the information from both MANTRA and GFA, the authors predicted the potential G-protein-coupled-oestrogen receptor (GPER)-mediated role of the compound in prostate cancer. This case study illustrated that the elucidation of MoA with gene expression data can be challenging, and that often requires multiple computational approaches.

11.3.4.2 Methodology 3: Link Drug Target and Pathway Activation to Understand MoA

Pathway RespOnsive GENes (PROGENy) is a data-driven dimension reduction method that combines both pathway and gene expression data with the aim to infer the activity of cancer relevant signalling pathways by using gene expression data. PROGENy leverages a large compendium of publicly available perturbation experiments that yield a common core of PROGENy to a specified set of stimuli [79]. Comparing PROGENy with other conventional methods of pathway analysis (e.g. GSEA) that uses the genes of the pathway members, PROGENy calculates pathway activity for 11 pathways based on the consensus gene expression signatures derived from perturbation experiments. PROGENy is a simple but at the same time effective linear regression model, which is trained with data from perturbation experiments extracted from ArrayExpress database/GEO. The input of the model is the perturbed pathways and the response variable is the gene expression values as Z-score. PROGENy has been identified as a tool to infer upstream pathway activity in the context of drug responses in cell lines. A Bioconductor package for PROGENy has been developed as well as a web application for the calculation of PROGENy scores from gene expression data.

This tool was further used to explore interactions between drug targets and signalling pathways that can provide new insights on compounds' MoA and drug repositioning and can provide insights about the underlying treatment efficacy in cancer [80]. The aim of this study was to understand how pathway activities modulate response to drugs targeting specific proteins, and the main goal was to get insights of type: 'Activation of pathway Y will confer sensitivity to any drug targeting protein X'. The proposed methodology was applied on the Genomics of Drug Sensitivity in Cancer (GDSC) cell line panel with drug response (IC_{50}) of 265 drugs on 990 cell lines. Firstly, they performed a drug response prediction of the drugs in different cell lines, and secondly, they assessed the interactions between drug targets and signalling pathways. The Macau algorithm has been used to train a multitask learning model to predict drug response taking into account the response in multiple cell lines. The advantage of the multitask learning is that it can bring all the targets and their responses in cell lines into one single model, which can find common patterns reflecting the underlying mechanism. Moreover, by using Macau, side information for both drugs and cell lines can be supplied to the model. Protein targets were used as side information for the compounds and activity scores for 11 signalling pathways derived from the PROGENy tool were used as a side information for the cell lines. The interaction between the features of the compounds and the cell lines was then calculated by computing an interaction matrix. Results of this method indicated that this methodology can guide a tissue-specific combination treatment strategy and suggested modulation of which pathway to maximize the drug response for a given tissue and ultimately help MoA understanding and drug repurposing. For example, brain tissue cells with active epidermal growth factor receptor (EGFR) signalling were found to be resistant to compounds that are PLK1 inhibitors. This result revealed that hypothetically blocking the EGFR pathway while targeting PLK1 could result in a synergistic effect. Overall, the exploration of interactions between drug targets and signalling pathways can shed light in cellular mechanisms and compounds' MoA.

11.4 Image-Based Data

11.4.1 Image Data and Where to Extract Them From

Image-based data or cell morphological phenotypes are an additional source of biological information. Images capture the morphology of the cell and its organelles upon compound administration and can potentially yield biological insights [81] and better understanding of MoA [82]. High-throughput imaging has benefited from advancing technology such as robotic sample preparation and appropriate microscopy equipment and additionally the recent availability

Table 11.4 Databases and image-based datasets reported in public repositories and their potential use in drug discovery

Database	Interesting datasets	Potential uses
Broad Bioimage Benchmark Collection (BBBC)	1600 compound – dataset	• Target identification • Cluster compounds based on image profile similarity to derive potential MoA • Lookup table to identify morphological phenotypes • Assessment of toxicity • Lead hopping
Cell Image Library, Image Data Resource (IDR), and GigaScience DB	~30 000 compound – dataset	

of large libraries of genetic and chemical perturbants (see Chapter 7 for more details) [83]. Hence, the availability of image-based data has resulted in an increasing interest for this type of data. Image-based data is a tool in pharmacological screening to depict cell morphological characteristics or study the phenotype of the cell [83]. Pharmaceutical companies are using high-throughput imaging data to triage compounds to be used in drug discovery projects [81], and additionally there are public databases, where imaging data are stored. The table below summarizes a few imaging datasets that can be used in MoA studies (Table 11.4).

Imaging data can be extracted from publicly available databases such as the Broad Bioimage Benchmark Collection (BBBC) developed by the Broad Institute [84], the 'Cell Image Library' and the Image Data Resource (IDR) [86]. For example, there is a dataset in the BBBC database, which has been obtained by a multiplex cytological profiling assay that measures diverse cellular states upon compound perturbation [85]. In this study, 1600 commercially available bioactive compounds spanning a range of MoA were tested on Human Bone Osteosarcoma Epithelial Cells (U2OS). This dataset was developed using a multiplex assay or in other words, the 'cell painting assay', which uses well-characterized fluorescent morphological labels to broadly stain seven cell components [85]. The seven components are the following: nucleus, endoplasmic reticulum, nucleoli, Golgi apparatus, plasma membrane, F-actin, and mitochondria. Following the multiplex assay, 824 morphological features were extracted from the images with the open-source CellProfiler software. This set of compounds was further validated for its potential use in MoA studies, which is discussed further below.

Following the same cell painting assay, another dataset of image data was created. This is a dataset of 30,616 compounds, which consists of a variety of perturbations including 10 080 compounds from the Molecular Libraries Small Molecule Repository (MLSMR); 2260 compounds, which are part of the Broad Institute known bioactive compound collection (drugs, natural products, small probe molecules); and 18 051 compounds, which are novel compounds from diversity-oriented synthesis approaches [83]. A similar protocol was used for this assay as in the previous dataset with one difference. In this case, fluorescent markers were used to broadly stain eight cellular components, which are the following: nucleus, endoplasmic reticulum, F-actin cytoskeleton, Golgi apparatus, plasma membrane, mitochondria, and the nucleoli and cytoplasmic RNA, which was not fluorescently marked in the previous dataset (Table 11.5). Moreover the raw images were further processed in a quantitative analysis to extract features, and the processed data can be extracted from the GigaDB and in GigaScience GitHub repository [83].

The general workflow that was used to develop the two datasets is summarized in Figure 11.8. Profiles of cells upon various perturbations are obtained in a high-throughput manner [82]. The subcellular structures (i.e. cell components) are stained with fluorescent markers in order to 'paint' cell components and visualize them [83, 85]. Images then have to be analysed to extract meaningful features. It is impossible to extract features by looking at the resulting images by eye and therefore computer vision technology is used. CellProfiler is a software developed for scientists to enable this analysis. It was first published in 2006 and has been cited more than 6000 times since then and currently at a rate of more than 1000 per year [87]. It provides advanced algorithms for image analysis and a series of modules, which can be organized in a sequence/pipeline. This pipeline is applied to identify and measure the morphology of the cells. The derived image-based feature profiles are subsequently used to establish relationships within the datasets, to group compounds based on their profile and identify their MoA, or to suggest drug target pairs or off-target effects.

11.4.2 Application of Image-Based Data in Target Prediction and Better Understanding of MoA

11.4.2.1 Methodology 1: Clustering of Compounds Based on Cell Morphology

One of the first approaches to use image-based data in MoA understanding was to cluster compounds based on their similarity on image-based profiles in order to group molecules with similar activity and MoA. For example, the 1600 compounds in a dataset from BBBC (discussed above) were clustered based on their image-based profile similarity, and it was examined whether the clusters incorporate compounds with similar annotated protein targets or chemical structure [85]. Compounds in the same cluster were identified to have a similar MoA. Furthermore, one of the clusters contained compounds that are modulators of neuronal receptors. The compounds in this cluster showed similar cell profiles with an enhanced Golgi staining and some cells with fused nucleoli. Some examples of drugs that were part of this cluster are the following: metoclopramide and its structural analogue procaine and fluphenazine.

11.4.2.2 Methodology 2: Use of Image-Based Data in the Development of a Cell Morphology Database That Can Facilitate Drug Target Identification

Morphobase is a cellular morphology encyclopaedia/database that consists of cell shape changes induced by various compound perturbations in two cancer

Table 11.5 Example of images obtained with the cell painting assay applied to U2OS cells from the small-molecule Cell Painting experiment. Images in the first row are shown from a DMSO well and columns represent the five channels imaged in the assay. The second and third row display the stained cellular organelle or sub-compartments and the details of dyes respectively [83].

Image example	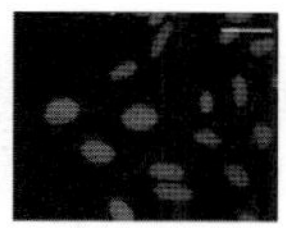	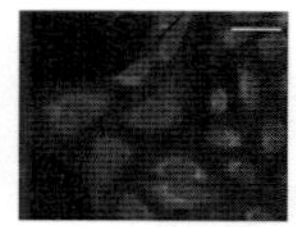	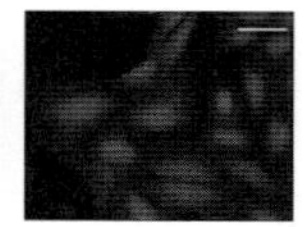	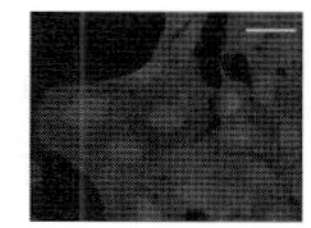	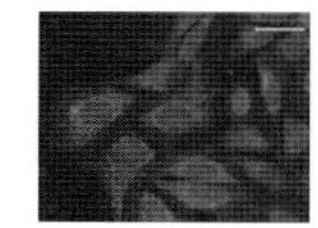
Organelle or cellular component	Nucleus	Endoplasmic reticulum	Nucleoli + cytoplasmic RNA	F-actin cytoskeleton + golgi + plasma membrane	Mitochondria
Fluorescent marker	Hoechst 33 342	Concanavalin A/Alexa Fluor 488 conjugate	Syto 14 green fluorescent nucleic acid stain	Phalloidin/Alexa Fluor 594 conjugate, wheat germ agglutinin (WGA)/Alexa Fluor 594 conjugate	Mito Tracker deep red

The cells were fluorescently labelled for eight cell components shown in the following images (scale bar equal to 50 μm).

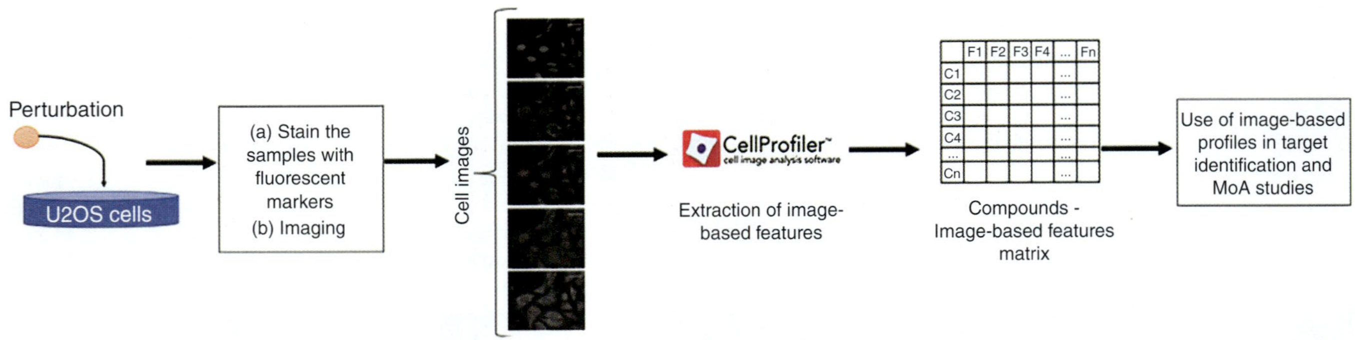

Figure 11.8 Schematic representation of the process to generate images and to extract image features from the images.

cell lines (src^{ts}-NRK [1] and HeLa cells) [88]. In more detail, a high content image analysis was used to examine the effect of 207 compounds on the cell morphology in the two cancer cell lines. Out of the 207 compounds, 54 were drugs with well-characterized MoA, 118 were commonly used experimental drugs, 26 were FDA-approved drugs, 7 were drugs with multiple biological targets and 2 were antibiotics. These compounds were used to perturb two cell lines and then the IN Cell Analyzer was used to calculate descriptors based on the cells' morphology under perturbation.

Following the calculation of the morphological features, a process of multivariate statistical analysis, visualization, and ranking of multiparametric phenotypic datasets was applied in order to evaluate whether the reference dataset of 207 compounds can be used for target identification and MoA understanding. A principal component analysis (PCA) was performed to visualize the multiparametric phenotypic responses. The drugs that had similar activities formed a cluster. For example, a cluster of the compounds were tubulin-targeted compounds. Moreover, the similarities of the morphological changes were calculated with two different statistical metrics: a probability score of being active or inactive and the ranking of query's compound Euclidean distance to the nearest neighbours of the reference compounds.

Three compounds were shown to be able to inhibit the growth of the human promyelocytic leukaemia cell line HL-60, but their exact MoA was unknown. Cell morphological profiles were derived for these three compounds, and the proposed methodology was used to elucidate their MoA. When the three compounds were projected on the principal component (PC) scores, the phenotypic responses of the compounds were similar to each other and in more detail formed a cluster around the tubulin inhibitors. In addition, based on the similarity analysis with Euclidean distance, the molecular target of the compounds was found to be in the microtubule system. The predicted MoA was further experimentally validated with an *in vitro* microtubule assembly assay, and all three of the compounds inhibited the polymerization of tubulin in a dose-dependent manner.

Furthermore, the Morphobase dataset was used in other studies with the aim to identify the MoA of compounds with an unknown mechanism. In one study, a series of indenopyrazoles was synthesized, and one of the compounds was found to show a promising antiproliferative activity against human cancer cells [89]. The Morphobase profiling assay and comparison to the reference compounds within Morphobase suggested that the compound can be classified as a tubulin inhibitor. This observation was further validated *in vitro*, and the compound was shown to inhibit acetylated tubulin accumulation and microtubule formation and the compound-induced G2/M cell cycle arrest in HeLa cells.

11.4.2.3 Methodology 3: Use of Image Data in Drug Repositioning and Biological Activity Prediction

In another study, image data were used to predict assay specific biological activity in two Janssen drug discovery projects [81]. The hypothesis was based on the observation that two chemically very different compounds from any active

1 Rat kidney cells that were infected with ts25, a T class mutant of Rous sarcoma virus Prague strain.

compounds in the training set are unlikely to be predicted as active, and this can be a disadvantage in the bioactivity prediction. Hence, cell image data could be used as additional information as it can reflect compound-induced modulation of diverse targets and biochemical processes independently of the chemical structure of the compounds. The research hypothesis was that imaging data could overcome the limitation of the employed chemical space and that imaging data can be complementary to chemistry-based models for the sparse and poorly annotated chemical space. The workflow of this study is shown on Figure 11.9, and it starts with the image-based feature extraction from cell images with the CellProfiler software. These features were further used in a multitask learning model, which used the Bayesian matrix factorization method Macau to incorporate image-based data as side information. In these two projects, the hit rate was increased by 50- to 250-fold over that of the chemical structure-based models. There were 31 assays with high-quality predictions that were selected and validated with *in vitro* assays. For example, in one of the projects in the field of oncology, a 50-fold increase in the hit rate was observed. By using Macau 60 000 compounds with unknown activity measurements were predicted for their response in a glucocorticoid receptor assay. Out of this compound set 342 with the highest ranking were selected, and 36.3% of these compounds were shown experimentally to have sub-micromolar activity. This compared with the initial hit rate in the high-throughput screen of 0.73%. Hence, the increase to 36.3% with the use of imaging data translates to a 50-fold hit rate enrichment. As a result, image-based data proved to be an important and rich source of information that can be used to predict and even replace biological assays.

11.4.2.4 Methodology 4: Association of Genes with Context-Dependent Morphology Alterations from Cells Exposed to Chemical or Genetic Perturbations for MoA Elucidation

Cell image data is also used to associate changes of cell morphological features with changes in cellular function with the ultimate goal to better understand compounds' MoA. Compounds from the 'cell painting assay' dataset were used with the LINCS gene expression data from the L1000 platform. The overlap between the compounds in the imaging dataset and the LINCS database was equal to 9515 unique compounds. The data from these two sources were used to study the interdependence between transcription and cell morphology in order to create a model, which links transcriptomic changes with corresponding alterations in cell morphology [90]. This model can be applied on a new transcriptomic query to predict associated changes in cellular morphology and get useful insights regarding compounds' MoA.

The methodology proposed consists of five steps. The first step was to identify the compounds that overlapped between the compounds in the imaging dataset and the L1000 platform. As stated above, there were 9515 overlapping compounds, and the gene expression profiles of these compounds were used as a reference dataset. The next step was the query of new gene expression profiles with the reference dataset to identify compounds with similar gene expression changes. The similarity between the gene expression profiles is computed with

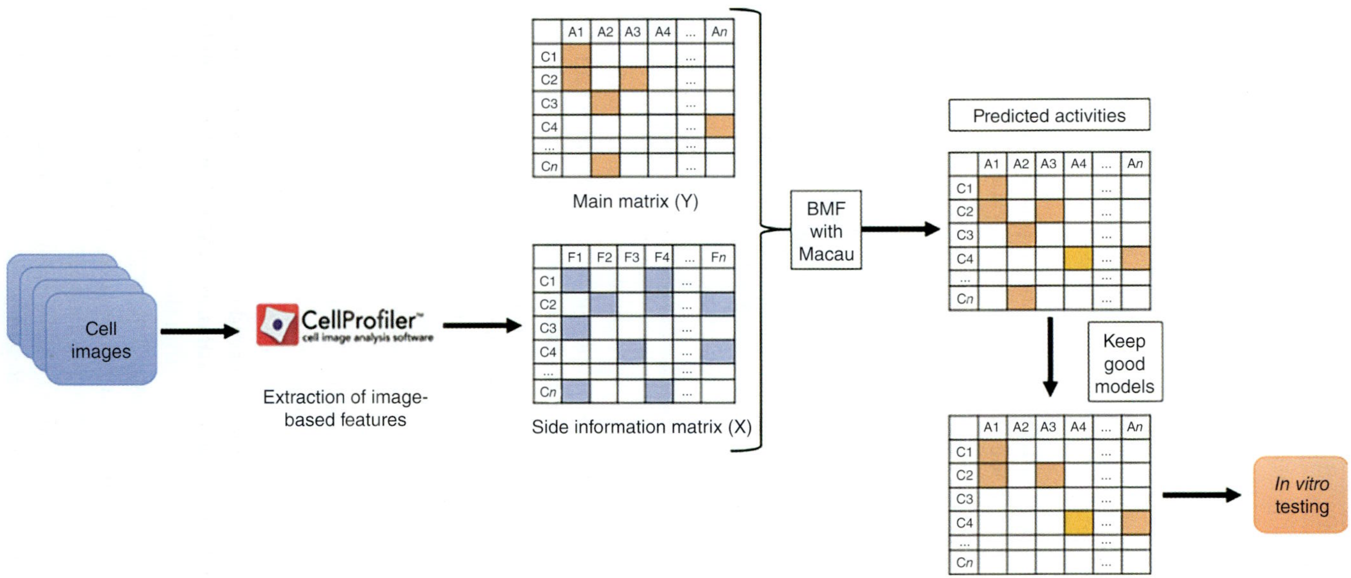

Figure 11.9 Methodology to repurpose image data to efficiently predict biological activity in a range of assays (A1, A2, …, A*n*). Cell morphology features are calculated with the CellProfiler for each compound (C1, C2, …, C*n*), and the features (F1, F2, …, F*n*) are then used as the side information matrix for the main biological activity matrix to perform Bayesian Matrix Factorisation (BMF) Macau. The best performing models are then selected and the results are validated *in vitro*.

the Mathew's correlation coefficient (MCC):

$$MCC = \frac{TP \times TN - FP \times FN}{\sqrt{(TP + FP)(TP + FN)(TN + FP)(TN + FN)}},$$

where TP, TN, FP, and FN are the number of true positives, true negatives, false positives, and false negatives respectively. In this case, the TPs and TNs correspond to the genes that are over- or underexpressed in both the reference and query gene expression profiles. The profiles with MCC greater than 0.1 are selected. The hypothesis is that this set of similar gene expression profiles can reveal shared MoA and phenotypic impact between compounds because compounds with similar gene expression signatures tend to interact with similar protein targets [90, 91].

After the selection of the similar transcriptomic profiles, the next step is the identification of significant associations between alterations in cell morphology and gene expression, and this step is called 'cell morphology enrichment analysis'. A stepwise variable selection approach is used to select landmark genes that are associated with a given image-based feature. Least absolute shrinkage and selection operator (LASSO) was used to assess the association between each image-based feature and the landmark genes, and hence each image feature is modelled as a sparse function of the 978 landmark genes. This method produces a set of genes associated with each image-based feature, and one gene can be assigned to several gene sets if it is associated with more than one image-based feature. Each gene set is representing a set of genes with similar expression patterns and shared phenotypic impact and thus their examination can result in a better understanding of the biological responses to compound perturbations.

The next step is a validation step, where the authors validated the hypothesis that the gene expression changes in response to perturbations can be used to identify associated changes in the image-based features. In more detail, 20 randomly selected genes and the LOOCV were applied to assess how well changes in image-based features can be predicted given the corresponding transcriptomic alterations. For 92% of the queries, the proposed methodology identified associated genes with the image-based features, and a significant positive correlation was observed between the observed and predicted image features.

The proposed methodology was applied on three compounds (nomilin, zardaverine, and hydrocotarnine) to investigate the cell morphological responses. Firstly, a set of compounds with similar gene expression profiles for each compound was identified, and the LASSO-based feature selection produced different gene sets for each compound. The observed and the predicted morphological changes showed a high Spearman correlation, and the largest predicted cell morphology changes were likely to appear within the top 10 experimentally observed image-based features. Moreover, a gene–gene interaction network based on the transcriptomic profiles that are similar to the query compounds was developed. The network edges ($X \geq Y$) are based on the proportion of cell morphological specific gene sets that contain X and also contain Y, and the edge weight shows the strength of the association between two genes. Highly co-expressed gene pairs within the set that are similar to the query gene expression profiles are identified by using the context likelihood of relatedness (CLR) algorithm. The Funrich package was finally used to annotate gene sets with biological pathways. The functional enrichment analysis for the three compounds mentioned above identified genes, which are involved in the regulation of cytoskeletal remodelling and growth activation. For example, changes in the cytoskeleton in addition to its role in determining cell morphology produce changes in gene expression, and therefore this can be an explanation for why we are able to observe associations between gene expression and cell morphology.

11.5 Conclusions

Understanding of the MoA and/or the target that a compound interacts with is of great importance during the drug discovery process. Bioinformatics is a science that can facilitate this understanding by using different levels of information such as gene expression, pathways, and image-based data. In recent years, deposition of high-throughput data in databases in combination with the advances in machine learning techniques has significantly influenced the field of bioinformatics. Various methodologies have been developed to use this information in order to understand compounds' MoA. For example, the similarity of high-throughput profiles can highlight a shared MoA for compounds. Moreover, meaningful features can be extracted from high-throughput data and combined with other features such as PPI information or biological pathway annotations and lead to an improvement in our understanding of a compound's target. Overall, different information can be used alone or in combination to better understand compounds' MoA as shown in the literature examples described above.

Acknowledgement

M.-A.T. would like to thank the BBSRC and AstraZeneca for their funding.

References

1 Xia, X. (2017). Bioinformatics and drug discovery. *Curr. Top. Med. Chem.* 17: 1709–1726.
2 Hassanien, A.E., Al-Shammari, E.T., and Ghali, N.I. (2013). Computational intelligence techniques in bioinformatics. *Comput. Biol. Chem.* 47: 37–47.
3 Rang, H.P., Ritter, J.M., Flower, R.J., and Henderson, G. (2014). *Rang & Dale's Pharmacology: With STUDENT CONSULT Online Access*. Elsevier Churchill Livingstone.
4 Iskar, M., Campillos, M., Kuhn, M. et al. (2010). Drug-induced regulation of target expression. *PLoS Comput. Biol.* 6: e1000925.
5 Iwata, M., Sawada, R., Iwata, H. et al. (2017). Elucidating the modes of action for bioactive compounds in a cell-specific manner by large-scale chemically-induced transcriptomics. *Sci. Rep.* 7 (40164).

6 Liggi, S., Drakakis, G., Koutsoukas, A. et al. (2014). Extending *in silico* mechanism-of-action analysis by annotating targets with pathways: application to cellular cytotoxicity readouts. *Future Med. Chem.* 6: 2029–2056.
7 Zheng, W., Thorne, N., and McKew, J.C. (2013). Phenotypic screens as a renewed approach for drug discovery. *Drug Discovery Today* 18: 1067–1073.
8 Schenone, M., Dančík, V., Wagner, B.K., and Clemons, P.A. (2013). Target identification and mechanism of action in chemical biology and drug discovery. *Nat. Chem. Biol.* 9: 232–240.
9 Koutsoukas, A., Lowe, R., KalantarMotamedi, Y. et al. (2013). In silico target predictions: defining a benchmarking data set and comparison of performance of the multiclass naïve Bayes and Parzen-Rosenblatt window. *J. Chem. Inf. Model.* 53: 1957–1966.
10 Sams-Dodd, F. (2013). Is poor research the cause of the declining productivity of the pharmaceutical industry? An industry in need of a paradigm shift. *Drug Discovery Today* 18: 211–217.
11 Alex, A.A., Harris, C.J., and Smith, D.A. (2015). *Attrition in the Pharmaceutical Industry: Reasons, Implications, and Pathways Forward*. Wiley.
12 Khanna, I. (2012). Drug discovery in pharmaceutical industry: productivity challenges and trends. *Drug Discovery Today* 17: 1088–1102.
13 Gregori-Puigjané, E., Setola, V., Hert, J. et al. (2012). Identifying mechanism-of-action targets for drugs and probes. *Proc. Natl. Acad. Sci. U.S.A.* 109: 11178–11183.
14 Nigsch, F., Hutz, J., Cornett, B. et al. (2012). Determination of minimal transcriptional signatures of compounds for target prediction. *EURASIP J. Bioinf. Syst. Biol.* 2012 (2).
15 Lee, J. and Bogyo, M. (2013). Target deconvolution techniques in modern phenotypic profiling. *Curr. Opin. Chem. Biol.* 17: 118–126.
16 Sleno, L. and Emili, A. (2008). Proteomic methods for drug target discovery. *Curr. Opin. Chem. Biol.* 12: 46–54.
17 Maggiora, G.M. (2006). On outliers and activity cliffs – why QSAR often disappoints. *J. Chem. Inf. Model.* 46: 1535.
18 Chen, B., Greenside, P., Paik, H. et al. (2015). Relating chemical structure to cellular response: an integrative analysis of gene expression, bioactivity, and structural data across 11,000 compounds. *CPT Pharmacometrics Syst. Pharmacol.* 4: 576–584.
19 Berg, E.L. (2014). Systems biology in drug discovery and development. *Drug Discovery Today* 19: 113–125.
20 Lussier, Y.A. and Chen, J.L. (2011). The emergence of genome-based drug repositioning. *Sci. Transl. Med.* 3: 96ps35.
21 Iorio, F., Rittman, T., Ge, H. et al. (2013). Transcriptional data: a new gateway to drug repositioning? *Drug Discovery Today* 18: 350–357.
22 Pabon, N.A., Xia, Y., Estabrooks, S.K. et al. (2018). Predicting protein targets for drug-like compounds using transcriptomics. *PLoS Comput. Biol.* 14: e1006651.
23 Kibble, M., Khan, S.A., Saarinen, N. et al. (2016). Transcriptional response networks for elucidating mechanisms of action of multitargeted agents. *Drug Discovery Today* 21: 1063–1075.

24 Lamb, J., Crawford, E.D., Peck, D. et al. (2006). The connectivity map: using gene-expression signatures to connect small molecules, genes, and disease. *Science* 313: 1929–1935.

25 Musa, A., Ghoraie, L.S., Zhang, S.D. et al. (2017). A review of connectivity map and computational approaches in pharmacogenomics. *Briefings Bioinf.* https://doi.org/10.1093/bib/bbw112.

26 Bezerianos, A., Dragomir, A., and Balomenos, P. (2017). *Computational Methods for Processing and Analysis of Biological Pathways.* Springer International Publishing.

27 Ohnstone, A.L., Reierson, G.W., Smith, R.P. et al. (2012). A chemical genetic approach identifies piperazine antipsychotics as promoters of CNS neurite growth on inhibitory substrates. *Mol. Cell. Neurosci.* 50: 125–135.

28 Coombs, G.S., Schmitt, A.A., Canning, C.A. et al. (2012). Modulation of Wnt/β-catenin signaling and proliferation by a ferrous iron chelator with therapeutic efficacy in genetically engineered mouse models of cancer. *Oncogene* 31: 213–225.

29 Gullbo, J., Fryknäs, M., Rickardson, L. et al. (2011). Phenotype-based drug screening in primary ovarian carcinoma cultures identifies intracellular iron depletion as a promising strategy for cancer treatment. *Biochem. Pharmacol.* 82: 139–147.

30 D'arcy, P., Brnjic, S., Olofsson, M.H. et al. (2011). Inhibition of proteasome deubiquitinating activity as a new cancer therapy. *Nat. Med.* 17: 1636–1640.

31 Rho, S.B., Kim, B.-R., and Kang, S. (2011). A gene signature-based approach identifies thioridazine as an inhibitor of phosphatidylinositol-3′-kinase (PI3K)/AKT pathway in ovarian cancer cells. *Gynecol. Oncol.* 120: 121–127.

32 Gheeya, J., Johansson, P., Chen, Q.R. et al. (2010). Expression profiling identifies epoxy anthraquinone derivative as a DNA topoisomerase inhibitor. *Cancer Lett.* 293: 124–131.

33 Renshaw, D., Montero-Melendez, T., Dalli, J. et al. (2010). Downstream gene activation of the receptor ALX by the agonist annexin A1. *PLoS One* 5: e12771.

34 Hieronymus, H., Lamb, J., Ross, K.N. et al. (2006). Gene expression signature-based chemical genomic prediction identifies a novel class of HSP90 pathway modulators. *Cancer Cell* 10: 321–330.

35 Usher, L.C., Johnstone, A., Ertürk, A. et al. (2010). A chemical screen identifies novel compounds that overcome glial-mediated inhibition of neuronal regeneration. *J. Neurosci.* 30: 4693–4706.

36 Hizukuri, Y., Sawada, R., and Yamanishi, Y. (2015). Predicting target proteins for drug candidate compounds based on drug-induced gene expression data in a chemical structure-independent manner. *BMC Med. Genomics* 8: 82.

37 Subramanian, A., Narayan, R., Corsello, S.M. et al. (2017). A next generation connectivity map: L1000 platform and the first 1,000,000 profiles. *Cell* 171: 1437–1452.e17.

38 Hall, M.L., Calkins, D., and Sherman, W. (2016). Automated protocol for large-scale modeling of gene expression data. *J. Chem. Inf. Model.* 56: 2216–2224.

39 Barrett, T., Wilhite, S.E., Ledoux, P. et al. (2012). NCBI GEO: archive for functional genomics data sets—update. *Nucleic Acids Res.* 41: D991–D995.

40 Enache, O.M., Lahr, D.L., Natoli, T.E. et al. (2017). The GCTx format and cmap{Py, R, M} packages: resources for the optimized storage and integrated traversal of dense matrices of data and annotations. In: *bioRxiv*. https://doi.org/10.1101/227041.

41 Duan, Q., Flynn, C., Niepel, M. et al. (2014). LINCS Canvas Browser: interactive web app to query, browse and interrogate LINCS L1000 gene expression signatures. *Nucleic Acids Res.* 42: W449–W460.

42 Koleti, A., Terryn, R., Stathias, V. et al. (2018). Data Portal for the Library of Integrated Network-based Cellular Signatures (LINCS) program: integrated access to diverse large-scale cellular perturbation response data. *Nucleic Acids Res.* 46: D558–D566.

43 Sun, Y.V. and Hu, Y.-J. (2016). Integrative analysis of multi-omics data for discovery and functional studies of complex human diseases. *Adv. Genet.* 93: 147–190.

44 Taxman, D.J., Moore, C.B., Guthrie, E.H., and Huang, M.T.-H. (2010). Short hairpin RNA (shRNA): design, delivery, and assessment of gene knockdown. In: *RNA Therapeutics: Function, Design, and Delivery* (ed. M. Sioud), 139–156. Humana Press.

45 Sterling, T. and Irwin, J.J. (2015). ZINC 15 – ligand discovery for everyone. *J. Chem. Inf. Model.* 55: 2324–2337.

46 Filzen, T.M., Kutchukian, P.S., Hermes, J.D. et al. (2017). Representing high throughput expression profiles via perturbation barcodes reveals compound targets. *PLoS Comput. Biol.* 13: e1005335.

47 Sawada, R., Iwata, M., Tabei, Y. et al. (2018). Predicting inhibitory and activatory drug targets by chemically and genetically perturbed transcriptome signatures. *Sci. Rep.* 8: 156.

48 Fabregat, A., Jupe, S., Matthews, L. et al. (2018). The reactome pathway knowledgebase. *Nucleic Acids Res.* 46: D649–D655.

49 Ravindranath, A.C., Perualila-Tan, N., Kasim, A. et al. (2015). Connecting gene expression data from connectivity map and *in silico* target predictions for small molecule mechanism-of-action analysis. *Mol. Biosyst.* 11: 86–96.

50 Iorio, F., Bosotti, R., Scacheri, E. et al. (2010). Discovery of drug mode of action and drug repositioning from transcriptional responses. *Proc. Natl. Acad. Sci. U.S.A.* 107: 14621–14626.

51 Khatri, P., Sirota, M., and Butte, A.J. (2012). Ten years of pathway analysis: current approaches and outstanding challenges. *PLoS Comput. Biol.* 8: e1002375.

52 García-Campos, M.A., Espinal-Enríquez, J., and Hernández-Lemus, E. (2015). Pathway analysis: state of the art. *Front. Physiol.* 6: 383.

53 Yuryev, A. and Wiley InterScience (Online service) (2008). *Pathway Analysis for Drug Discovery: Computational Infrastructure and Applications*. Wiley.

54 Kanehisa, M., Furumichi, M., Tanabe, M. et al. (2016). KEGG: new perspectives on genomes, pathways, diseases and drugs. *Nucleic Acids Res.* 45: D353–D361.

55 Zhou, H. and Xu, R. (2015). Leukemia stem cells: the root of chronic myeloid leukemia. *Protein Cell* 6: 403–412.

56 Hehlmann, R., Hochhaus, A., and Baccarani, M. (2007). Chronic myeloid leukaemia. *Lancet* 370: 342–350.

57 Wang, B., Li, R., and Perrizo, W. (2015). *Big Data Analytics in Bioinformatics and Healthcare*. IGI Global.

58 Sever, R. and Brugge, J.S. (2015). Signal transduction in cancer. *Cold Spring Harbor Perspect. Med.* 5: 1–21.

59 Bauer-Mehren, A., Furlong, L.I., and Sanz, F. (2009). Pathway databases and tools for their exploitation: benefits, current limitations and challenges. *Mol. Syst. Biol.* 5: 290.

60 Kanehisa, M., Sato, Y., Kawashima, M. et al. (2015). KEGG as a reference resource for gene and protein annotation. *Nucleic Acids Res.* 44: D457–D462.

61 Croft, D., O'kelly, G., Wu, G. et al. (2010). Reactome: a database of reactions, pathways and biological processes. *Nucleic Acids Res.* 39: D691–D697.

62 Fabregat, A., Sidiropoulos, K., Viteri, G. et al. (2017). Reactome pathway analysis: a high-performance in-memory approach. *BMC Bioinf.* 18: 142.

63 Kutmon, M., Riutta, A., Nunes, N. et al. (2016). WikiPathways: capturing the full diversity of pathway knowledge. *Nucleic Acids Res.* 44: D488–D494.

64 Slenter, D.N., Kutmon, M., Hanspers, K. et al. (2018). WikiPathways: a multifaceted pathway database bridging metabolomics to other omics research. *Nucleic Acids Res.* 46: D661–D667.

65 Karp, P.D., Billington, R., Caspi, R. et al. (2017). The BioCyc collection of microbial genomes and metabolic pathways. *Briefings Bioinf.* https://doi.org/10.1093/bib/bbx085.

66 Geer, L.Y., Marchler-Bauer, A., Geer, R.C. et al. (2010). The NCBI BioSystems database. *Nucleic Acids Res.* 38: D492–D496.

67 Cerami, E.G., Gross, B.E., Demir, E. et al. (2011). Pathway Commons, a web resource for biological pathway data. *Nucleic Acids Res.* 39: D685–D690.

68 Pratt, D., Chen, J., Welker, D. et al. (2015). NDEx, the network data exchange. *Cell Syst.* 1: 302–305.

69 Türei, D., Korcsmáros, T., and Saez-Rodriguez, J. (2016). OmniPath: guidelines and gateway for literature-curated signaling pathway resources. *Nat. Methods* 13: 966–967.

70 Chowdhury, S. and Sarkar, R.R. (2015). Comparison of human cell signaling pathway databases—evolution, drawbacks and challenges. *Database* 2015: 1–25.

71 Glazko, G.V. and Emmert-Streib, F. (2009). Unite and conquer: univariate and multivariate approaches for finding differentially expressed gene sets. *Bioinformatics* 25: 2348–2354.

72 Alexander-Dann, B., Pruteanu, L.L., Oerton, E. et al. (2018). Developments in toxicogenomics: understanding and predicting compound-induced toxicity from gene expression data. *Mol. Omics* 14: 218–236.

73 Maciejewski, H. (2014). Gene set analysis methods: statistical models and methodological differences. *Briefings Bioinf.* 15: 504–518.

74 Liggi, S., Drakakis, G., Hendry, A.E. et al. (2013). Extensions to in silico bioactivity predictions using pathway annotations and differential pharmacology analysis: application to *Xenopus laevis* phenotypic readouts. *Mol. Inf.* 32: 1009–1024.

75 Iorio, F., Saez-Rodriguez, J., and di Bernardo, D. (2013). Network based elucidation of drug response: from modulators to targets. *BMC Syst. Biol.* 7: 139.

76 Ying, H., Biroc, S.L., Li, W.W. et al. (2006). The Rho kinase inhibitor fasudil inhibits tumor progression in human and rat tumor models. *Mol. Cancer Ther.* 5: 2158–2164.

77 Iorio, F., Shrestha, R.L., Levin, N. et al. (2015). A semi-supervised approach for refining transcriptional signatures of drug response and repositioning predictions. *PLoS One* 10: e0139446.

78 Khan, S.A., Faisal, A., Mpindi, J.P. et al. (2012). Comprehensive data-driven analysis of the impact of chemoinformatic structure on the genome-wide biological response profiles of cancer cells to 1159 drugs. *BMC Bioinf.* 13 (112).

79 Schubert, M., Klinger, B., Klünemann, M. et al. (2018). Perturbation-response genes reveal signaling footprints in cancer gene expression. *Nat. Commun.* 9: 20.

80 Yang, M., Simm, J., Lam, C.C. et al. (2018). Linking drug target and pathway activation for effective therapy using multi-task learning. *Sci. Rep.* 8: 8322.

81 Simm, J., Klambauer, G., Arany, A. et al. (2018). Repurposing high-throughput image assays enables biological activity prediction for drug discovery. *Cell Chem. Biol.* 25: 611–618.e3.

82 Scheeder, C., Heigwer, F., and Boutros, M. (2018). Machine learning and image-based profiling in drug discovery. *Curr. Opin. Syst. Biol.* https://doi.org/10.1016/j.coisb.2018.05.004.

83 Bray, M.A., Gustafsdottir, S.M., Rohban, M.H. et al. (2017). A dataset of images and morphological profiles of 30 000 small-molecule treatments using the Cell Painting assay. *Gigascience* 6 (1–5).

84 Ljosa, V., Sokolnicki, K.L., and Carpenter, A.E. (2012). Annotated high-throughput microscopy image sets for validation. *Nat. Methods* 9: 637.

85 Gustafsdottir, S.M., Ljosa, V., Sokolnicki, K.L. et al. (2013). Multiplex cytological profiling assay to measure diverse cellular states. *PLoS One* 8: e80999.

86 Williams, E., Moore, J., Li, S.W. et al. (2017). Image Data Resource: a bioimage data integration and publication platform. *Nat. Methods* 14: 775–781.

87 McQuin, C. et al. (2018). CellProfiler 3.0: next-generation image processing for biology. *PLoS Biol.* 16: e2005970.

88 Futamura, Y., Kawatani, M., Kazami, S. et al. (2012). Morphobase, an encyclopedic cell morphology database, and its use for drug target identification. *Chem. Biol.* 19: 1620–1630.

89 Minegishi, H., Futamura, Y., Fukashiro, S. et al. (2015). Methyl 3-((6-methoxy-1,4-dihydroindeno[1,2-*c*]pyrazol-3-yl)amino)benzoate (GN39482) as a tubulin polymerization inhibitor identified by MorphoBase and ChemProteoBase profiling methods. *J. Med. Chem.* 58: 4230–4241.

90 Nassiri, I. and McCall, M.N. (2018). Systematic exploration of cell morphological phenotypes associated with a transcriptomic query. *Nucleic Acids Res.* 46: –e116.

91 Campillos, M., Kuhn, M., Gavin, A.-C. et al. (2008). Drug target identification using side-effect similarity. *Science* 321: 263–266.

Index

Target Discovery and Validation: Methods and Strategies for Drug Discovery,
First Edition. Edited by Alleyn T. Plowright.